Series Editor
John M. Walker
School of Life Sciences
University of Hertfordshire
Hatfield, Hertfordshire, AL10 9AB, UK

For further volumes:
http://www.springer.com/series/7651

Eosinophils

Methods and Protocols

Edited by

Garry M. Walsh

*Division of Applied Medicine, School of Medicine and Dentistry,
Institute of Medical Sciences, University of Aberdeen, Foresterhill, Aberdeen, UK*

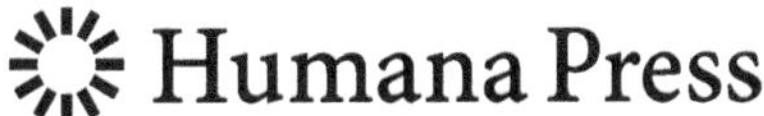 Humana Press

Editor
Garry M. Walsh
Division of Applied Medicine
School of Medicine and Dentistry
Institute of Medical Sciences
University of Aberdeen
Foresterhill, Aberdeen, UK

ISSN 1064-3745 ISSN 1940-6029 (electronic)
ISBN 978-1-4939-1015-1 ISBN 978-1-4939-1016-8 (eBook)
DOI 10.1007/978-1-4939-1016-8
Springer New York Heidelberg Dordrecht London

Library of Congress Control Number: 2014940964

Printed on acid-free paper

Humana Press is a brand of Springer
Springer is part of Springer Science+Business Media (www.springer.com)

Preface

Eosinophils were first described in the blood of various species as "course granule cells" in 1846 by Wharton Jones. The striking hues exhibited by eosinophils when stained with acidophilic dyes were first described in 1879 by Paul Ehrlich who termed them "eosinophils" on the basis of their strong avidity for eosin, and to the present day eosinophils retain a continuing ability to fascinate. However despite the passage of more than 130 years and a considerable body of research endeavour, a complete understanding of the function of these cells in health and disease remains elusive. Some basic characteristics of eosinophils are well established and widely accepted. Like all leukocytes eosinophils develop in the bone marrow from pluripotent progenitors from where they are released into the circulation as phenotypically mature granulocytes. Eosinophils spend only a brief time in the peripheral blood before migrating to the thymus or the gastrointestinal tract, where they reside under homeostatic conditions, while in inflammatory conditions the majority of their functions are exerted in the tissues. Perhaps one of the most fascinating aspects of the eosinophil is how accumulating knowledge has changed the perception of its function from a passive bystander to modulator of inflammation, to potent pro-inflammatory cell loaded with histotoxic substances through to the more recent recognition that it can act as both a positive and a negative regulator of complex events in innate and adaptive immunity. It is a basic evolutionary principle that eosinophils did not develop to induce human pathology. Although there are questions about the long-held belief that eosinophils make a major contribution to immunity against parasitic helminthic worms, recent findings on the antimicrobial and antiviral activities of eosinophils suggest that the pathology in eosinophilic diseases might be a consequence of collateral damage related to host defence or inappropriate accumulation. There therefore remains much to be understood about the properties and functions of the eosinophil. It is timely therefore that the current volume presents a series of comprehensive and clear step-by-step protocols whose goal is to facilitate research into this fascinating cell. Written by acknowledged authorities each protocol is aimed at the beginner in this field with each technique spelt out in very simple terms, assuming no previous knowledge of the method without the need to find information elsewhere. The protocols cover established and more novel in vitro and in vivo methodologies. It is hoped that this book will help extend our knowledge on eosinophil function that may in turn lead to new hypotheses for future examination of this intriguing cell.

Aberdeen, Scotland, UK   *Garry M. Walsh*

Contents

Contributors

PRAVEEN AKUTHOTA • *Division of Pulmonary, Critical Care and Sleep Medicine, Department of Medicine, Beth Israel Deaconess Medical Center, Harvard Medical School, Boston, MA, USA; Division of Allergy and Inflammation, Department of Medicine, Beth Israel Deaconess Medical Center, Harvard Medical School, Boston, MA, USA*

ANA L. ALESSANDRI • *MRC Centre for Inflammation Research, Queen's Medical Research Institute, University of Edinburgh, Edinburgh, UK*

RENATA BAPTISTA-DOS-REIS • *Institute of Biomedical Sciences, Federal University of Rio de Janeiro, Rio de Janeiro, Brazil*

JANENDRA K. BATRA • *Immunochemistry Laboratory, National Institute of Immunology, New Delhi, India; Centre for Molecular Medicine, National Institute of Immunology, New Delhi, India*

STANISLAWA BAZAN-SOCHA • *2nd Department of Internal Medicine, Jagiellonian University Medical College, Krakow, Poland*

MARIE-RENÉE BLANCHET • *Centre de Recherche, Institut Universitaire de Cardiologie et de Pneumologie de Québec, Quebec City, Canada*

APOSTOLOS BOSSIOS • *Krefting Research Centre, Department of Internal Medicine and Clinical Nutrition, Institute of Medicine, The Sahlgrenska Academy, University of Gothenburg, Gothenburg, Sweden*

FABRIZIO BRUSCHI • *Department of Translational Research, and of New Technologies in Medicine and Surgery, Medical School, Università di Pisa, Pisa, Italy*

MIRANDA BUITENHUIS • *Department of Hematology, Erasmus MC, Rotterdam, The Netherlands*

JOSE A. CANCELAS • *Division of Experimental Hematology, Department of Pediatrics, Cincinnati Children's Hospital Medical Center, Cincinnati, OH, USA; Hoxworth Blood Center, University of Cincinnati College of Medicine, Cincinnati, OH, USA*

KELSEY CAPRON • *Division of Allergy & Inflammation, Department of Medicine, Beth Israel Deaconess Medical Center, Harvard Medical School, Boston, MA, USA*

EDWIN R. CHILVERS • *Department of Medicine, Addenbrooke's and Papworth Hospitals, University of Cambridge School of Clinical Medicine, Cambridge, UK*

ANU CHOPRA • *Immunochemistry Laboratory, National Institute of Immunology, New Delhi, India*

ALISON M. CONDLIFFE • *Department of Medicine, Addenbrooke's and Papworth Hospitals, University of Cambridge School of Clinical Medicine, Cambridge, UK*

COLLEEN S. CURRAN • *Department of Cell and Regenerative Biology, University of Wisconsin School of Medicine and Public Health, Madison, WI, USA*

F. DAUBEUF • *Faculté de Pharmacie, Laboratoire d'Innovation Thérapeutique, LabEx MEDALIS, UMR 7200, CNRS-Université de Strasbourg, Illkirch, France*

FRANCIS DAVOINE • *Campus Saint-Jean, University of Alberta, Edmonton, AB, Canada; Pulmonary Research Group, University of Alberta, Edmonton, AB, Canada*

GORDON DENT • *Institute of Science & Technology in Medicine, Keele University, Keele, Staffordshire, UK*

JOSEPH B. DOMACHOWSKE • *Division of Infectious Diseases, Department of Pediatrics, SUNY Upstate Medical University, Syracuse, NY, USA*

DAVID A. DORWARD • *MRC Centre for Inflammation Research, Queen's Medical Research Institute, University of Edinburgh, Edinburgh, UK*

KIMBERLY D. DYER • *Inflammation Immunobiology Section, National Institute of Allergy and Infectious Diseases, National Institutes of Health, Bethesda, MD, USA*

CAROLINE ETHIER • *Pulmonary Research Group, University of Alberta, Edmonton, AB, Canada*

NEDA FARAHI • *Department of Medicine, Addenbrooke's and Papworth Hospitals, University of Cambridge School of Clinical Medicine, Cambridge, UK*

NELLY FROSSARD • *Faculté de Pharmacie, Laboratoire d'Innovation Thérapeutique, LabEx MEDALIS, UMR 7200, CNRS-Université de Strasbourg, Illkirch, France*

ROOPESH SINGH GANGWAR • *Department of Pharmacology and Experimental Therapeutics, Institute for Drug Research, School of Pharmacy, Faculty of Medicine, The Hebrew University of Jerusalem, Jerusalem, Israel*

DANIEL GILLETT • *Nuclear Medicine, Cambridge University Hospitals National Health Service Foundation Trust, Cambridge, UK*

MATTHEW GOLD • *The Biomedical Research Centre, University of British Columbia, Vancouver, BC, Canada*

SARAH HEARD • *Nuclear Medicine, Cambridge University Hospitals National Health Service Foundation Trust, Cambridge, UK*

AKOS HEINEMANN • *Institute of Experimental and Clinical Pharmacology, Medical University of Graz, Graz, Austria*

PINJA ILMARINEN • *The Immunopharmacology Research Group, University of Tampere School of Medicine and Tampere University Hospital, Tampere, Finland*

KENJI ISHIHARA • *Laboratory of Medical Science, Course for School Nurse Teacher, Faculty of Education, Ibaraki University, Ibaraki, Japan*

DAVID B. JACOBY • *Pulmonary and Critical Care Medicine, Oregon Health and Science University, Portland, OR, USA*

ELIZABETH A. JACOBSEN • *Division of Pulmonary Medicine, Department of Biochemistry and Molecular Biology, Mayo Clinic, Scottsdale, AZ, USA*

BOGDAN JAKIELA • *2nd Department of Internal Medicine, Jagiellonian University Medical College, Krakow, Poland*

DIANE F. JELINEK • *Department of Immunology, Mayo Clinic, Rochester, MN, USA*

HANNU KANKAANRANTA • *The Immunopharmacology Research Group, University of Tampere School of Medicine and Tampere University Hospital, Tampere, Finland; Department of Respiratory Medicine, Seinäjoki Central Hospital, Seinäjoki, Finland; Department of Respiratory Medicine, University of Tampere, Tampere, Finland*

OSMO KARI • *Helsinki University Central Hospital, Helsinki, Finland*

KENDAL A. KARPE • *Inflammation Immunobiology Section, National Institute of Allergy and Infectious Diseases, National Institutes of Health, Bethesda, MD, USA*

VIKTORIA KONYA • *Institute of Experimental and Clinical Pharmacology, Medical University of Graz, Graz, Austria*

MASATAKA KORENAGA • *Department of Parasitology, Kochi Medical School, Kochi University, Kochi, Japan*

PAIGE LACY • *Pulmonary Research Group, Department of Medicine, University of Alberta, Edmonton, AB, Canada*

JAMES J. LEE • *Division of Pulmonary Medicine, Department of Biochemistry and Molecular Biology, Mayo Clinic, Scottsdale, AZ, USA*

FRANCESCA LEVI-SCHAFFER • *Department of Pharmacology and Experimental Therapeutics, Institute for Drug Research, Faculty of Medicine, The Hebrew University of Jerusalem, Jerusalem, Israel*

CHRYSTALLA LOUTSIOS • *Department of Medicine, Addenbrooke's and Papworth Hospitals, University of Cambridge School of Clinical Medicine, Cambridge, UK*

CHRISTOPHER D. LUCAS • *MRC Centre for Inflammation Research, Queen's Medical Research Institute, University of Edinburgh, Edinburgh, UK*

KELLY M. MCNAGNY • *The Biomedical Research Centre, University of British Columbia, Vancouver, BC, Canada*

EEVA MOILANEN • *The Immunopharmacology Research Group, University of Tampere School of Medicine and Tampere University Hospital, Tampere, Finland*

VALDIRENE S. MUNIZ • *Institute of Biomedical Sciences, Federal University of Rio de Janeiro, Rio de Janeiro, Brazil*

JACEK MUSIAL • *2nd Department of Internal Medicine, Jagiellonian University Medical College, Krakow, Poland*

JOSIANE S. NEVES • *Institute of Biomedical Sciences, Federal University of Rio de Janeiro, Rio de Janeiro, Brazil*

ZHENYING NIE • *Pulmonary and Critical Care Medicine, Oregon Health and Science University, Portland, OR, USA*

SERGEI I. OCHKUR • *Division of Pulmonary Medicine, Department of Biochemistry and Molecular Biology, Mayo Clinic, Scottsdale, AZ, USA*

MIRIAM PEINHAUPT • *Institute of Experimental and Clinical Pharmacology, Medical University of Graz, Graz, Austria*

CAROLINE M. PERCOPO • *Inflammation Immunobiology Section, National Institute of Allergy and Infectious Diseases, National Institutes of Health, Bethesda, MD, USA*

A. MICHAEL PETERS • *Clinical Imaging Sciences Centre, Brighton and Sussex Medical School, Brighton, UK*

LINSEY PORTER • *Department of Medicine, Addenbrooke's and Papworth Hospitals, University of Cambridge School of Clinical Medicine, Cambridge, UK*

MADELEINE RÅDINGER • *Krefting Research Centre, Department of Internal Medicine and Clinical Nutrition, Institute of Medicine, The Sahlgrenska Academy, University of Gothenburg, Gothenburg, Sweden*

HELENE F. ROSENBERG • *Laboratory of Allergic Diseases, Inflammation Immunobiology Section, National Institute of Allergy and Infectious Diseases, National Institutes of Health, Bethesda, MD, USA*

ADRIANO G. ROSSI • *MRC Centre for Inflammation Research, Queen's Medical Research Institute, University of Edinburgh, Edinburgh, UK*

QUINN R. ROTH-CARTER • *Pulmonary and Critical Care Medicine, Oregon Health and Science University, Portland, OR, USA*

MARC E. ROTHENBERG • *Division of Allergy and Immunology, Department of Pediatrics, Cincinnati Children's Hospital Medical Center, Cincinnati, OH, USA*

K. MATTI SAARI • *Department of Ophthalmology, University of Turku, Turku, Finland*

SIDHARTH SHARMA • *MRC Centre for Inflammation Research, Queen's Medical Research Institute, University of Edinburgh, Edinburgh, UK*

ROSALIND P. SIMMONDS • *Department of Medicine, Addenbrooke's and Papworth Hospitals, University of Cambridge School of Clinical Medicine, Cambridge, UK*

GARRY M. WALSH • *Division of Applied Medicine, School of Medicine & Dentistry, Institute of Medical Sciences, University of Aberdeen, Aberdeen, UK*

PETER F. WELLER • *Division of Allergy & Inflammation, Department of Medicine, Beth Israel Deaconess Medical Center Harvard Medical, School Boston, MA, USA; Division of Infectious Diseases, Department of Medicine, Beth Israel Deaconess Medical Center, Harvard Medical School, Boston, MA, USA*

LIAN WILLETTS • *Pulmonary Research Group, Department of Medicine, University of Alberta, Edmonton, AB, Canada*

TINA W. WONG • *Department of Immunology, Mayo Clinic, Rochester, MN, USA*

YOSHIYUKI YAMADA • *Division of Allergy and Immunology, Gunma Children's Medical Center, Shibukawa, Gunma, Japan*

JOANNA ZUK • *2nd Department of Internal Medicine, Jagiellonian University Medical College, Krakow, Poland*

Chapter 1

Eosinophil Overview: Structure, Biological Properties, and Key Functions

Paige Lacy, Helene F. Rosenberg, and Garry M. Walsh

Abstract

The eosinophil is an enigmatic cell with a continuing ability to fascinate. A considerable history of research endeavor on eosinophil biology stretches from the present time back to the nineteenth century. Perhaps one of the most fascinating aspects of the eosinophil is how accumulating knowledge has changed the perception of its function from passive bystander, modulator of inflammation, to potent effector cell loaded with histotoxic substances through to more recent recognition that it can act as both a positive and negative regulator of complex events in both innate and adaptive immunity. This book consists of 26 chapters written by experts in the field of eosinophil biology that provide comprehensive and clearly written protocols for techniques designed to underpin research into the function of the eosinophil in health and disease.

Key words Eosinophil, Accumulation, Apoptosis, Degranulation, Animal models

1 Introduction

Eosinophil involvement in inflammatory conditions affecting the skin, gastrointestinal tract, and upper and lower airways is well documented [1]. Although asthma is recognized as a heterogeneous condition, eosinophilic asthma is a recently described phenotype of the disease characterized by increased blood or sputum eosinophils [2] whose numbers correlate with disease severity [3]. Infiltrating tissue eosinophils release their potent pro-inflammatory arsenal including granule-derived basic proteins, lipid mediators, cytokines, and chemokines. These contribute to airway inflammation and lung tissue remodelling that includes epithelial cell damage and loss, airway thickening, fibrosis, and angiogenesis [4]. More recent evidence suggests that in addition to their role as degranulating effector cells, eosinophils have the capacity to act as antigen-presenting cells resulting in T cell proliferation and activation thereby propagating inflammatory responses [5, 6].

Garry M. Walsh (ed.), *Eosinophils: Methods and Protocols*, Methods in Molecular Biology, vol. 1178, DOI 10.1007/978-1-4939-1016-8_1, © Springer Science+Business Media New York 2014

2   Accumulation and Fate

In healthy individuals, eosinophils are present in the circulation in low numbers and are rarely found in the lung, being mostly confined to the tissues surrounding the gut. Eosinophil accumulation during inflammatory events is complex, involving their maturation in and release from the bone marrow, adhesion to and transmigration through the post-capillary endothelium, followed by their chemotaxis to and activation/degranulation at inflammatory foci [7]. The processes controlling eosinophil accumulation are of obvious importance and represent potential therapeutic targets for antagonism of their accumulation in allergic-based disease [8]. Asthma pathology is characterized by excessive leukocyte infiltration that leads to tissue injury. Cell adhesion molecules, i.e., selectins, integrins, and members of the immunoglobulin superfamily control leukocyte extravasation, migration within the interstitium, cellular activation, and tissue retention. Numerous animal studies have demonstrated essential roles for these cell adhesion molecules in lung inflammation including L-selectin, P-selectin, and E-selectin, ICAM-1, VCAM-1 together with many of the $\beta1$ and $\beta2$ integrins. These families of adhesion molecules have therefore been under intense investigation to inform the development of novel therapeutics [9]. Furthermore, a number of in vitro studies of currently available drugs have shown these to be potential antagonists of eosinophil adhesion under physiological flow conditions [10–12].

The ultimate fate of eosinophils is also important, apoptosis and the disposal of apoptotic cells by phagocytic removal (efferocytosis) is a vital aspect of inflammation resolution in all multicellular organisms. Eosinophils have a limited life-span in the circulation of 8–18 h, which is extended to 3–4 days in tissues. Similar to neutrophils, they are terminally end-differentiated cells programmed to undergo apoptosis in the absence of viability-enhancing stimuli [13]. Eosinophil persistence in the tissues is enhanced by the presence of several asthma-relevant cytokines that prolong eosinophil survival by inhibition of apoptosis. The roles of interleukin (IL)-3, IL-5, IL-9, IL-13, IL-15, and granulocyte/macrophage colony-stimulating factor (GM-CSF) in this regard are well established, [14–16] and there is ample evidence that all are present in the asthmatic lung in significant quantities [17].

Thymic stromal protein (TSLP), IL-25, and IL-33 represent a triad of cytokines released by airway epithelial cells in response to various environmental stimuli or by cellular damage. They act in concert to drive Th2 polarization through overlapping mechanisms causing remodelling and pathological changes in the airway walls, suggesting pivotal roles in the pathophysiology of asthma. All three have been shown to have a number of effects on eosinophil function including enhancement of their receptor expression, adhesion, and viability through inhibition of apoptosis [18–20]. Eosinophil interactions with the proteins of the extracellular matrix are likely to contribute to their persistence within the tissues. For example, integrin-mediated eosinophil adhesion to fibronectin results in the autocrine production of viability-enhancing cytokines GM-SCF, IL-3, and IL-5 [21, 22]. These interactions between multiple cytokines and extracellular matrix components antagonize eosinophil programmed cell death thereby prolonging their longevity for weeks. Thus, a balance in the tissue microenvironment between pro- and anti-apoptotic signals is likely to greatly influence the load of eosinophils in the tissues.

3 Secretion and Receptors

Eosinophils express a wide repertoire of granule proteins, cytokines, growth factors, and chemokines that are secreted in response to receptor stimulation [23]. These are synthesized at early stages of eosinophil maturation in the bone marrow and are packaged into various intracellular organelles, including the eosinophil crystalloid granule [24, 25]. During activation, eosinophils generate an elaborate tubulovesicular network that is composed of small secretory vesicles and elongated tubules, which appear to carry the contents of the crystalloid granule to the cell surface [26–28]. Both the crystalloid granule, and the tubulovesicular network that forms during eosinophil activation, are remarkable and only recently characterized features of this enigmatic cell.

The crystalloid granule in eosinophils is comprised of two compartments: a core and a surrounding matrix [29]. Both the core and matrix are enriched in highly cationic proteins, principally major basic protein (MBP) [30]. Electron microscopy images of sectioned eosinophils display the strikingly electron-dense crystalline cores in crystalloid granules, visible in eosinophils from many different mammalian species [31]. In the matrix that envelopes the MBP-rich core, eosinophil peroxidase (EPX), eosinophil-derived neurotoxin (EDN), and eosinophil cationic protein (ECP) are found in high concentrations, along with many other granule proteins, including cytokines [30]. Typically, eosinophils do not release granule products during transit through the bloodstream, and these cells are relatively benign even as they marginate into tissues, predominantly the gut in healthy individuals [24, 25]. However, in diseases such as allergy and atopic asthma, eosinophils undergo a high degree of proliferation, and may be found degranulating in nasal and airway mucosa [32]. Degranulation is a general term that describes an activated phenotype ranging from piecemeal degranulation to degradation of cells and cytolysis (necrosis) [33]. When eosinophils encounter secretagogues, they will release the contents of their crystalloid granules by mobilizing granules and secretory vesicles to the cell surface, inducing granule-membrane fusion in a regulated manner; hence the term, "regulated exocytosis" [33, 34].

In the case of cytolysis, eosinophils release intact crystalloid granules with their lipid bilayer membranes still surrounding their core and matrix components, and whole granules infiltrating tissues may be readily visible upon appropriate staining of tissue sections [35]. Mechanisms that may control eosinophil cytolysis, or whether any mechanisms are involved at all, are of current research interest.

A wide range of pro-inflammatory mediators are capable of activating eosinophils. Eosinophils express and present on their cell surface a large variety of receptors allowing them to interact with, and respond to, their environmental milieu [36]. However, in in vitro experiments, it is difficult to induce eosinophil degranulation by soluble secretagogues, and they frequently require potent or multiple stimuli to evoke significant secretory responses. This is likely related to the observation that eosinophils do not degranulate readily in the blood, but rather release their granule contents only after they transmigrate into tissues and become activated by inflammatory reactions. At some types of inflammatory foci, eosinophils appear to undergo degranulation in response to both soluble and immobilized stimuli that activate multiple receptors [35]. Only a minority of these receptors are capable of directly evoking secretion from eosinophils in vitro. Secretagogue-binding receptors include those to complement factors (C5aR), immunoglobulins (FcαRc, FcγRcs), platelet activating factor (PAF), and fungal extracts (such as Alternaria acting on protease-activated receptor-2, PAR-2) [33, 37].

Receptors are generally classified by their signaling mechanisms, such as G protein-coupled receptors that activate dissociation of α and βγ subunits of heterotrimeric G proteins, and immunoglobulin- or cytokine-binding families that activate a cascade of tyrosine kinase phosphorylation. Eosinophils have been demonstrated to express many of the signaling components necessary for receptor activation of cellular events [33]. Perhaps somewhat surprisingly, eosinophils do not undergo degranulation in response to the potent eosinophil differentiation and maturation-inducing cytokines, IL-3, IL-5, or GM-CSF, when these are applied individually. These three cytokines must be combined together in a "cytokine cocktail" in order to elicit degranulation in human eosinophils [38]. This is likely associated with the relatively quiescent state of eosinophils during their proliferation and maturation in the bone marrow in response to these cytokines.

Following binding and activation of specific receptors, secretagogues induce the mobilization of granules through the cytoplasm of the eosinophil, which may be associated with the formation of large tubulovesicular structures containing small secretory vesicles and elongated tubules that may extend from crystalloid granules [26, 28, 39]. The tubulovesicular structure appears in the cytoplasm in correlation with piecemeal degranulation, where membrane-bound vesicles bud off from crystalloid granules and selectively shuttle specific granule contents to the plasma membrane for release. The tubulovesicular network is responsible for trafficking cytokines and chemokines such as IL-4 and CCL5/RANTES [40, 41]. The movement of granules and vesicles through the cells is controlled by actin cytoskeleton remodeling. Actin remodeling in eosinophils is regulated by a family of guanosine triphosphatases (GTPases), particularly Rac2 [42]. When vesicles and granules approach the inner leaflet of the lipid bilayer in the plasma membrane, they bind to specific intracellular receptors known as SNAREs (soluble N-ethylmaleimide-sensitive attachment protein receptors) which facilitate their docking and fusion with the cell membrane. This is followed by membrane fusion, in which the internal surface of the granule membrane becomes exposed to the outside of the cell membrane [43, 44]. Concurrently with this, vesicle fusion is mediated by another membrane-bound GTPase, Rab27a, which conveys the secretagogue signal through to SNARE binding and ensures that granule membranes come into close proximity with cell membrane lipid bilayer [45]. Eosinophils exhibit granule polarization towards their leading edges during shape change and degranulation [42, 45], suggesting that they may have the ability to focus their granule contents onto target surfaces, as previously observed in vitro using opsonized helminthic parasites [46].

4 Clinical Overview

A substantial body of clinical evidence has demonstrated that eosinophils degranulate upon recruitment and activation at inflammatory foci in tissue biopsies from many different diseases, including allergy and asthma [24, 25, 32]. Eosinophil degranulation is thought to be an essential component of the late phase mucosal tissue response to allergen challenge. Evidence of tissue eosinophil degranulation has been detected in allergic rhinitis, cutaneous allergic reactions, and atopic asthma, which in many cases correlates with a deteriorating clinical outcome [47].

Furthermore, eosinophils and their granule products are elevated in specific types of respiratory virus, fungal, and parasitic infections [37, 48–50]. Infectious diseases involving helminthic parasite infestation or respiratory viruses have been shown to be associated with eosinophilia and degranulation from tissue eosinophils. While early studies suggested that eosinophils were essential for controlling or containing helminthic parasite infections, new evidence has emerged suggesting that in contrast to these earlier studies, eosinophils have little effect on helminthic larval transmission and survival in the host, at least in eosinophil-deleted mouse models of parasitic infection [51]. Recent discoveries show that activated eosinophils may have an important role in maintaining host survival in life-threatening respiratory viral infections [52]. Thus, identification of signaling steps occurring in eosinophil degranulation is essential for developing novel targets for therapeutic strategies.

5　Functional Studies in Animal Models

Numerous animal models have been developed to model eosinophil-driven inflammation and they have been instrumental in furthering our understanding of the role of eosinophils in disease. While there are certain advantages inherent in working with guinea pigs [53], the availability of sophisticated genetic and molecular tools has led to a preference for inbred strains of mice (particularly BALB/c and C57BL/6) for most in vivo studies of eosinophil biology. However, it is important to emphasize that mouse models have limitations in general, and for the study of eosinophils in particular. Specifically, one must recognize that no single experiment carried out in an inbred mouse strain can recapitulate all facets and features of human health and disease. Likewise, while clearly recognizable and generally of similar nature, the mouse eosinophil has distinct features that differentiate it from its human counterpart. A very complete review of the unique biology of the mouse eosinophil has recently been published by Lee and colleagues [54]. The following is a very brief overview of hypereosinophilic and eosinophil-deficient mice, with an emphasis on the most commonly used and most recently described models. More information can be found in recent reviews [23, 55].

There are two unique strains of transgenic mice that display systemic hypereosinophilia secondary to overexpression of the cytokine interleukin-5 (IL-5). In the first, described by Dent and colleagues [56], the IL-5 transgene is expressed under the control of the CD2 antigen promoter. The second, described by Macias and colleagues; strain NJ.1638 [57], the IL-5 transgene is expressed by the T cell CD3delta promoter/enhancer. A third set of strains, described by Ochkur and colleagues [58], display dramatic hypereosinophilia, accomplished via addition of a transgene for either human or mouse eotaxin-2, the latter under the control of the lung-specific Clara-cell promoter, CC10 to the IL-5 transgenic NJ.1638. In these mice, peripheral eosinophils are recruited to the lung where they undergo extensive activation and degranulation in situ.

IL-5 gene-deleted mice [59] and mice devoid of the receptor for IL-5 [60] cannot generate eosinophilia in response to (Th2) allergic stimuli or parasitic infection, but these mice are not eosinophil-deficient, and maintain near homeostatic levels in the blood and bone marrow. However, there are now several strains of mice that are predominantly or fully eosinophil-deficient. The first eosinophil-deficient strain to emerge was the ΔdblGATA, reported by Yu and colleagues [61] as a serendipitous result of deletion of a palindromic enhancer element in the hematopoietic promoter of GATA-1. These mice are fully eosinophil-deficient at homeostasis and remain so in response to Th2 stimuli, with little to no impact on other hematopoietic lineages. However, a recent report suggests that these mice may have a functional basophil deficiency [62] which requires further exploration. Another strain, the eosinophil-deficient PHIL mice [63] were generated as a direct result of eosinophil peroxidase (EPX) promoter-directed cytosuicide during hematopoiesis in the bone marrow. Lee and colleagues [64, 65] have recently developed an inducible version of this strain (iPHIL), and have also noted that mice devoid of two major granule proteins, MBP and EPX, are likewise predominantly eosinophil-deficient. As a final note, Doyle and colleagues [66] have recently described the generation of a strain of mice that express Cre recombinase, similarly under the control of the EPX promoter. When crossed with appropriately "floxed" mouse strains, specific sequences (e.g., coding sequences, stop codons) can be deleted solely and uniquely within the eosinophil lineage. As already shown in this manuscript, crossing EoCre with a mouse strain that includes a "floxed" stop codon releasing Rosa26-directed diphtheria-toxin (DT) alpha, another unique eosinophil-deficient lineage was created. Similarly, a cross with a GFP-reporter strain permits Cre-dependent, lineage-specific labeling of eosinophils for isolation and in vivo trafficking studies. The possibilities are virtually limitless [67].

6   Role in Innate and Adaptive Immunity

While eosinophils clearly respond to signals from other leukocytes, most notably cytokines from Th2 cells (i.e. IL-5), it has become clear that eosinophils in turn release cytokines and granule proteins that provide signals that promote local immune regulation and have impact on the function of other leukocyte lineages [68, 69]. Eosinophils have been implicated in directing the functions of both B and T lymphocytes. Among them, Weller and colleagues [70] documented the expression of MHC class II, and co-stimulatory molecules CD80 and CD86 on human eosinophils and determined that eosinophils could likewise process antigen and direct antigen-specific T cell proliferation and cytokine release. Eosinophils can also promote humoral immune responses by promoting production of antigen-specific IgM [71] and supporting plasma cell growth and development in the bone marrow [72].

Eosinophils also interact directly with innate immune cells, and have a role in supporting the viability of alternatively activated macrophages in adipose tissue [73] promote migration and activation of myeloid dendritic cells [74], participate in extensive bidirectional signaling with tissue resident mast cells [75] and elicit production and release of pro-inflammatory mediators from isolated peripheral blood neutrophils [76].

While the earlier literature described anti-parasite activities of eosinophil granule proteins in experiments carried out in vitro, the role of eosinophils as providing direct host defense against these pathogens in vivo remains uncertain (reviewed in ref. 77). More recently, the focus on eosinophils has been on the immunomodulatory nature of these cells in this setting. As but one example, Appleton and colleagues [78, 79] have reported that infection of wild-type mice with the nematode, *Trichinella spiralis*, results in eosinophil recruitment to muscle and supports generation of nurse cells; *T. spiralis* larvae are not killed by eosinophils, but paradoxically, do not survive in eosinophil-deficient mice; results suggest that this is largely due to the resulting Th2 imbalance and overabundance of nitric oxide production in local macrophages.

As mentioned above, eosinophils are recruited to the airways as a prominent feature of the asthmatic inflammatory response where they are broadly perceived as promoting pathophysiology. Respiratory virus infections, notably rhinovirus and respiratory syncytial virus, exacerbate established asthma. Among the recent concepts under exploration is the role of eosinophils in promoting antiviral host defense in this setting (reviewed in ref. 80). Toward this end, Percopo and colleagues [52] have recently found that activated eosinophils from both *Aspergillus* antigen and cytokine-driven mouse asthma models are profoundly antiviral and promote survival in response to a superimposed and otherwise lethal respiratory virus infection. Finally, Lehrer and colleagues [81] were among the first to document the bactericidal activities of eosinophil cationic granule proteins in experiments carried out in vitro. Torrent and colleagues [82] have since characterized a specific affinity between ECP and bacterial peptidoglycan and lipopolysaccharides. More recently, Yousefi and colleagues [83] showed that eosinophils responded to lipopolysaccharide from gram-negative bacteria by releasing mitochondrial DNA complexed with cationic proteins, forming extracellular traps similar to those characterized for neutrophils. However, the question of a role for eosinophils in providing host defense against bacterial pathogens in vivo remains controversial [83, 84]. It remains to be seen whether eosinophils serve as host defense against bacteria, or perhaps interact primarily with non-pathogenic bacteria. This hypothesis is particularly attractive, given the predominance of resident eosinophils in the intestines, and the possibility of a more complex role involving eosinophils with commensal bacteria in the gut [85, 86].

7 Conclusion

Our understanding of the immunological role of the eosinophil is continually evolving, from earlier dogma that emphasized a role in combating helminthic parasitic infections and as a key effector cell in allergic inflammation to more recent discoveries suggesting important roles in immunomodulation. Other emerging roles include life-saving functions against numerous pathogens such as respiratory viruses and in interactions with nerves that impact on the pathology of many diseases [87]. This book provides a comprehensive series of protocols designed to address both the more established and more recent aspects of the functional properties of this truly fascinating and enigmatic cell.

References

1. Blanchard C, Rothenberg ME (2009) Biology of the eosinophil. Adv Immunol 101:81–121

2. Walsh GM (2013) Profile of reslizumab in eosinophilic disease and its potential in the treatment of poorly controlled eosinophilic asthma. Biologics 7:7–11

3. Bousquet J, Chanez P, Lacoste JY, Barneon G, Ghavanian N, Enander I, Venge P, Ahlstedt S, Simony-Lafontaine J, Godard P et al (1990) Eosinophilic inflammation in asthma. N Engl J Med 323:1033–1039

4. Nissim Ben Efraim AH, Levi-Schaffer F (2008) Tissue remodeling and angiogenesis in asthma: the role of the eosinophil. Ther Adv Respir Dis 2:163–171

5. Akuthota P, Wang H, Weller PF (2010) Eosinophils as antigen presenting cells in allergic upper airway disease. Curr Opin Allergy Clin Immunol 10(1):14–19

6. Walsh ER, August A (2010) Eosinophils and allergic airway disease: there is more to the story. Trends Immunol 31:39–44

7. Wardlaw AJ (1999) Molecular basis for selective eosinophil trafficking in asthma: a mulitstep paradigm. J Allergy Clin Immunol 104:917–926

8. Walsh GM (2010) Antagonism of eosinophil accumulation in asthma. Recent Pat Inflamm Allergy Drug Discov 4:210–213

9. Matsumoto K, Bochner BS (2012) Adhesion molecules. In: Lee JJ, Rosenberg HF (eds) Eosinophils in health and disease. Elsevier, New York, NY

10. Robinson AJ, Kashanin D, O'Dowd F, Williams V, Walsh GM (2008) Montelukast inhibition of resting and GM-CSF-stimulated eosinophil adhesion to VCAM-1 under flow conditions appears independent of CysLT1 antagonism. J Leukoc Biol 83:1522–1529

11. Wu P, Mitchell S, Walsh GM (2005) A new antihistamine levocetirizine inhibits eosinophil adhesion to vascular cell adhesion molecule-1 under flow conditions. Clin Exp Allergy 35:1073–1079

12. Robinson AJ, Kashanin D, O'Dowd F, Fitzgerald K, Williams V, Walsh GM (2009) Fluvastain and lovastatin inhibit GM-CSF-stimulated human eosinophil adhesion to intercellular adhesion molecule-1 under flow conditions. Clin Exp Allergy 39:1866–1874

13. Walsh GM (2013) Eosinophil apoptosis and clearance in asthma. J Cell Death 6:17–25

14. Gounni AS, Gregory B, Nutku E, Aris F, Latifa K, Minshall E et al (2000) Interleukin-9 enhances interleukin-5 receptor expression, differentiation, and survival of human eosinophils. Blood 96:2163–2171

15. Luttmann W, Knoechel B, Foerster M, Matthys H, Virchow JC Jr, Kroegel C (1996) Activation of human eosinophils by IL-13. Induction of CD69 surface antigen, its relationship to messenger RNA expression, and promotion of cellular viability. J Immunol 157:1678–1683

16. Hoontrakoon R, Chu HW, Gardai SJ, Wenzel SE, McDonald P, Fadok VA, Henson PM, Bratton DL (2002) Interlukin-15 inhibits spontaneous apoptosis in human eosinophils via autocrine production of granulocyte macrophage-colony stimulating factor and nuclear factor-kappaB activation. Am J Respir Cell Mol Biol 26:404–412

17. Leung DYM (1998) Molecular basis of allergic disease. Mol Genet Metab 63:177

18. Cheung PF, Wong CK, Ip WK, Lam CW (2006) IL-25 regulates the expression of adhesion molecules on eosinophils: mechanism of eosinophilia in allergic inflammation. Allergy 61:878–885

19. Suzukawa M, Koketsu R, Iikura M, Nakae S, Matsumoto K, Nagase H, Saito H, Matsushima K, Ohta K, Yamamoto K, Yamaguchi M (2008) Interleukin-33 enhances adhesion, CD11b expression and survival in human eosinophils. Lab Invest 88:1245–1253

20. Wong C, Hu S, Cheung P, Lam C (2010) Thymic stromal lymphopoietin induces chemotactic and pro-survival effects in eosinophils: implications in allergic inflammation. Am J Respir Cell Mol Biol 43:305–315

21. Anwar ARE, Moqbel R, Walsh GM, Kay AB, Wardlaw AJ (1993) Adhesion to fibronectin prolongs eosinophil survival. J Exp Med 177:839–843

22. Walsh GM, Symon FA, Wardlaw AJ (1995) Human eosinophils preferentially survive on tissue fibronectin compared with plasma fibronectin. Clin Exp Allergy 25:1128–1136

23. Rosenberg HF, Dyer KD, Foster PS (2013) Eosinophils: changing perspectives in health and disease. Nat Rev Immunol 13:9–22

24. Hogan SP, Rosenberg HF, Moqbel R et al (2008) Eosinophils: biological properties and role in health and disease. Clin Exp Allergy 38:709–750

25. Rothenberg ME, Hogan SP (2006) The eosinophil. Annu Rev Immunol 24:147–174

26. Dvorak AM, Furitsu T, Letourneau L et al (1991) Mature eosinophils stimulated to develop in human cord blood mononuclear cell cultures supplemented with recombinant human interleukin-5. Part I. Piecemeal degranulation of specific granules and distribution of Charcot-Leyden crystal protein. Am J Pathol 138:69–82

27. Melo RC, Spencer LA, Perez SA et al (2005) Human eosinophils secrete preformed, granule-stored interleukin-4 through distinct vesicular compartments. Traffic 6:1047–1057

28. Melo RC, Weller PF (2010) Piecemeal degranulation in human eosinophils: a distinct secretion mechanism underlying inflammatory responses. Histol Histopathol 25:1341–1354

29. Lacy P, Moqbel R (2000) Eosinophil cytokines. Chem Immunol 76:134–155

30. Peters MS, Rodriguez M, Gleich GJ (1986) Localization of human eosinophil granule major basic protein, eosinophil cationic protein, and eosinophil-derived neurotoxin by immuno-electron microscopy. Lab Invest 54:656–662

31. Lewis DM, Lewis JC, Loegering DA et al (1978) Localization of the guinea pig eosinophil major basic protein to the core of the granule. J Cell Biol 77:702–713

32. Lacy P, Adamko DJ, Moqbel R (2013) The human eosinophil. In: Greer JP, Arber DA, Glader B, List AF, Means RT, Paraskevas F, Rogers GM, Foerster J (eds) Wintrobe's Clinical hematology. Lippincott Williams & WIlkins, Philadelphia, PA, pp 214–235

33. Lacy P, Moqbel R (2013) Signaling and degranulation. In: Lee JJ, Rosenberg HF (eds) Eosinophils in health and disease. Elsevier, New York, NY, pp 206–219

34. Lacy P, Stow JL (2011) Cytokine release from innate immune cells: association with diverse membrane trafficking pathways. Blood 118:9–18

35. Erjefalt JS, Persson CG (2000) New aspects of degranulation and fates of airway mucosal eosinophils. Am J Respir Crit Care Med 161:2074–2085

36. Driss V, Legrand F, Capron M (2013) Eosinophil receptor profile. In: Lee JJ, Rosenberg HF (eds) Eosinophils in heatlh and disease. Elsevier, New York, NY, pp 30–38

37. Kita H (2013) Antifungal immunity by eosinophils: mechanisms and implications in human diseases. In: Lee JJ, Rosenberg HF (eds) Eosinophils in health and disease. Elsevier, New York, NY, pp 291–299

38. Adamko DJ, Wu Y, Gleich GJ et al (2004) The induction of eosinophil peroxidase release: improved methods of measurement and stimulation. J Immunol Methods 291:101–108

39. Melo RC, Perez SA, Spencer LA et al (2005) Intragranular vesiculotubular compartments are involved in piecemeal degranulation by activated human eosinophils. Traffic 6:866–879

40. Lacy P, Mahmudi-Azer S, Bablitz B et al (1999) Rapid mobilization of intracellularly stored RANTES in response to interferon-γ in human eosinophils. Blood 94:23–32

41. Spencer LA, Melo RC, Perez SA et al (2006) Cytokine receptor-mediated trafficking of preformed IL-4 in eosinophils identifies an innate immune mechanism of cytokine secretion. Proc Natl Acad Sci U S A 103:3333–3338

42. Lacy P, Willetts L, Kim JD et al (2011) Agonist activation of F-actin-mediated eosinophil shape change and mediator release is dependent on Rac2. Int Arch Allergy Immunol 156:137–147

43. Lacy P, Logan MR, Bablitz B et al (2001) Fusion protein vesicle-associated membrane protein 2 is implicated in IFNγ-induced piecemeal degranulation in human eosinophils from

atopic individuals. J Allergy Clin Immunol 107:671–678

44. Logan MR, Lacy P, Bablitz B et al (2002) Expression of eosinophil target SNAREs as potential cognate receptors for vesicle-associated membrane protein-2 in exocytosis. J Allergy Clin Immunol 109:299–306

45. Kim JD, Willetts L, Ochkur S et al (2013) An essential role for Rab27a GTPase in eosinophil exocytosis. J Leukoc Biol 94:1265–1274

46. McLaren DJ, Ramalho-Pinto FJ, Smithers SR (1978) Ultrastructural evidence for complement and antibody-dependent damage to schistosomula of Schistosoma mansoni by rat eosinophils in vitro. Parasitology 77:313–324

47. Foster PS, Rosenberg HF, Asquith KL et al (2008) Targeting eosinophils in asthma. Curr Mol Med 8:585–590

48. Gentil K, Hoerauf A, Layland LE (2013) Eosinophil-mediated responses toward helminths. In: Lee JJ, Rosenberg HF (eds) Eosinophils in health and disease. Elsevier, New York, NY, pp 303–312

49. Nutman TB (2013) Immune responses in helminth infections. In: Lee JJ, Rosenberg HF (eds) Eosinophils in health and disease. Elsevier, New York, NY, pp 312–320

50. Rosenberg HF, Dyer KD, Domachowske JB (2013) Interactions of eosinophils with respiratory virus pathogens. In: Lee JJ, Rosenberg HF (eds) Eosinophils in health and disease. Elsevier, New York, NY, pp 281–290

51. Swartz JM, Dyer KD, Cheever AW et al (2006) Schistosoma mansoni infection in eosinophil lineage-ablated mice. Blood 108:2420–2427

52. Percopo CM, Dyer KD, Ochkur SI et al (2014) Activated mouse eosinophils protect against lethal respiratory virus infection. Blood 123(5): 743–752

53. Evans RL, Nials AT, Knowles RG, Kidd EJ, Ford WR, Broadley KJ (2012) A comparison of antiasthma drugs between acute and chronic ovalbumin-challenged guinea-pig models of asthma. Pulm Pharmacol Ther 25:453–464

54. Lee JJ, Jacobsen EA, Ochkur SI, McGarry MP, Condjella RM, Doyle AD, Luo H, Zellner KR, Protheroe CA, Willetts L, Lesuer WE, Colbert DC, Helmers RA, Lacy P, Moqbel R, Lee NA (2012) Human versus mouse eosinophils: "that which we call an eosinophil, by any other name would stain as red". J Allergy Clin Immunol 130:572–584

55. Lee NA (2012) Mouse models manipulating eosinophilopoiesis. In: Lee JJ, Rosenberg HF (eds) Eosinophils in health and disease. Elsevier, Waltham, MA, pp 111–120

56. Dent LA, Strath M, Mellor AL, Sanderson CJ (1990) Eosinophilia in transgenic mice expressing interleukin 5. J Exp Med 172:1425–1431

57. Macias MP, Fitzpatrick LA, Brenneise I, McGarry MP, Lee JJ, Lee NA (2001) Expression of IL-5 alters bone metabolism and induces ossification of the spleen in transgenic mice. J Clin Invest 107:949–959

58. Ochkur SI, Jacobsen EA, Protheroe CA, Biechele TL, Pero RS, McGarry MP, Wang H, O'Neill KR, Colbert DC, Colby TV, Shen H, Blackburn MR, Irvin CC, Lee JJ, Lee NA (2007) Co-expression of IL-5 and eotaxin-2 in mice creates an eosinophil-dependent model of respiratory inflammation with characteristics of severe asthma. J Immunol 78:7879–7889

59. Kopf M, Brombacher F, Hodgkin PD, Ramsay AJ, Milbourne EA, Dai WJ, Ovington KS, Behm CA, Köhler G, Young IG, Matthaei KI (1996) IL-5-deficient mice have a developmental defect in CD5+ B-1 cells and lack eosinophilia but have normal antibody and cytotoxic T cell responses. Immunity 4:15–24

60. Yoshida T, Ikuta K, Sugaya H, Maki K, Takagi M, Kanazawa H, Sunaga S, Kinashi T, Yoshimura K, Miyazaki J, Takaki S, Takatsu K (1996) Defective B-1 cell development and impaired immunitiy against Angiostrongylus cantonensis in IL-5R alpha-deficient mice. Immunity 4:483–494

61. Yu C, Cantor AB, Yang H, Browne C, Wells RA, Fujiwara Y, Orkin SH (2002) Targeted deletion of a high-affinity GATA-binding site in the GATA-1 promoter leads to selective loss of the eosinophil lineage in vivo. J Exp Med 195:1387–1395

62. Nei Y, Obata-Ninomiya K, Tsutsui H, Ishiwata K, Miyasaka M, Matsumoto K, Nakae S, Kanuka H, Inase N, Karasuyama H (2013) GATA-1 regulates the generation and function of basophils. Proc Natl Acad Sci U S A 110: 18620–18625

63. Lee JJ, Dimina D, Macias MP, Ochkur SI, McGarry MP, O'Neill KR, Protheroe C, Pero R, Nguyen T, Cormier SA, Lenkiewicz E, Colbert D, Rinaldi L, Ackerman SJ, Irvin CG, Lee NA (2004) Defining a link with asthma in mice congenitally deficient in eosinophils. Science 305:1773–1776

64. Jacobsen EA, Lesuer WE, Willetts L, Zellner KR, Mazzolini K, Antonios N, Beck B, Protheroe C, Ochkur SI, Colbert D, Lacy P, Moqbel R, Appleton J, Lee NA, Lee JJ (2014) Eosinophil activities modulate the immune/ inflammatory character of allergic respiratory responses in mice. Allergy 69(3):315–327. doi:10.1111/all.12321

65. Doyle AD, Jacobsen EA, Ochkur SI, McGarry MP, Shim KG, Nguyen DT, Protheroe C, Colbert D, Kloeber J, Neely J, Shim KP, Dyer KD, Rosenberg HF, Lee JJ, Lee NA (2013) Expression of the secondary granule proteins major basic protein 1 (MBP-1) and eosinophil peroxidase (EPX) is required for eosinophilopoiesis in mice. Blood 122:781–790

66. Doyle AD, Jacobsen EA, Ochkur SI, Willetts L, Shim K, Neely J, Kloeber J, Lesuer WE, Pero RS, Lacy P, Moqbel R, Lee NA, Lee JJ (2013) Homologous recombination into the eosinophil peroxidase locus generates a strain of mice expressing Cre recombinase exclusively in eosinophils. J Leukoc Biol 94:17–24

67. Rosenberg HF (2013) Mouse eosinophils expressing Cre recombinase: endless "flox"ibilities. J Leukoc Biol 94:3–4

68. Lee JJ, Jacobsen EA, McGarry MP, Schleimer RP, Lee NA (2010) Eosinophils in health and disease: the LIAR hypothesis. Clin Exp Allergy 40:563–575

69. Akuthota P, Wang HB, Spencer LA, Weller PF (2008) Immunoregulatory roles of eosinophils: a new look at a familiar cell. Clin Exp Allergy 38:1254–1263

70. Wang HB, Ghiran I, Matthaei K, Weller PF (2007) Airway eosinophils: allergic inflammation recruited professional antigen presenting cells. J Immunol 179:7585–7592

71. Wang HB, Weller PF (2008) Pivotal Advance: eosinophils mediate early alum adjuvant elicited B cell priming and IgM production. J Leukoc Biol 83:817–821

72. Chu VT, Fröhlich A, Steinhauser G, Scheel T, Roch T, Fillatreau S, Lee JJ, Löhning M, Berek C (2011) Eosinophils are required for the maintenance of plasma cells in the bone marrow. Nat Immunol 12:151–159

73. Wu D, Molofsky AB, Liang HE, Ricardo-Gonzalez RR, Jouihan HA, Bando JK, Chawla A, Locksley RM (2011) Eosinophils sustain adipose alternatively activated macrophages associated with glucose homeostasis. Science 332:243–247

74. Yang D, Chen Q, Su SB, Zhang P, Kurosaka K, Caspi RR, Michalek SM, Rosenberg HF, Zhang N, Oppenheim JJ (2008) Eosinophil-derived neurotoxin acts as an alarmin to activated the TLR2-MyD88 signal pathway in dendritic cells and enhances Th2 immune responses. J Exp Med 205:79–90

75. Minai-Fleminger Y, Levi-Schaffer F (2009) Mast cells and eosinophils: the two key effector cells in allergic inflammation. Inflamm Res 58:631–638

76. Haskell MD, Moy JN, Gleich GJ, Thomas LL (1995) Analysis of signaling events associated with activation of neutrophil superoxide anion production by eosinophil granule major basic protein. Blood 86:4627–4637

77. Klion AD, Nutman TB (2004) The role of eosinophils in host defense against helminth parasites. J Allergy Clin Immunol 113: 30–37

78. Fabre V, Beiting DP, Bliss SK, Gebreselassie NG, Gagliardo LF, Lee NA, Lee JJ, Appleton JA (2009) Eosinophil deficiency compromises parasite survival in chronic nematode infection. J Immunol 182:1577–1583

79. Gebreselassie NG, Moorhead AR, Fabre V, Gagliardo LF, Lee NA, Lee JJ, Appleton JA (2012) Eosinophils preserve parasitic nematode larvae by regulating local immunity. J Immunol 188:417–425

80. Rosenberg HF, Dyer KD, Domachowske JB (2009) Respiratory viruses and eosinophils: exploring the connections. Antiviral Res 83:1–9

81. Lehrer RI, Szklarek D, Barton A, Ganz T, Hamann KJ, Gleich GJ (1989) Antibacterial properties of eosinophil major basic protein and eosinophil cationic protein. J Immunol 142:4428–4434

82. Torrent M, Navarro S, Moussaoui M, Nogues MV, Boix E (2008) Eosinophil cationic protein high affinity binding to bacteria-wall lipopolysaccharides and peptidoglycans. Biochemistry 47:3544–3555

83. Yousefi S, Gold JA, Andina N, Lee JJ, Kelly AM, Kozlowski E, Schmid I, Straumann A, Reichenbach J, Gleich GJ, Simon HU (2008) Catapult-like release of mitochondrial DNA by eosinophils contributes to antibacterial defense. Nat Med 14:949–953

84. Linch SN, Danielson ET, Kelly AM, Tamakawa RA, Lee JJ, Gold JA (2012) Interleukin 5 is protective during sepsis in an eosinophil-independent manner. Am J Respir Crit Care Med 186:246–254

85. Herbst T, Sichelstiel A, Schar C, Yadava K, Burki K, Cahenzli J, McCoy K, Marsland BJ, Harris NL (2011) Dysregulation of allergic airway inflammation in the absence of microbial colonization. Am J Respir Crit Care Med 184:198–205

86. Bisgaard H, Li N, Bonnelykke K, Chawes BL, Skov T, Paludan-Muller G, Stokholm J, Smith B, Krogfelt KA (2011) Reduced diversity of the intestinal microbiotal during infancy is associated with increased risk of allergic disease at school age. J Allergy Clin Immunol 128: 646–652

87. Raap U, Wardlaw AJ (2008) A new paradigm of eosinophil granulocytes: neuroimmune interactions. Exp Dermatol 17(9):731–738

Chapter 2

Eosinophil Purification from Peripheral Blood

Praveen Akuthota, Kelsey Capron, and Peter F. Weller

Abstract

Eosinophils are granulocytes integral to allergic inflammation and parasitic responses and comprise 1–4 % of the circulating leukocytes in human beings under normal conditions. Isolation of human eosinophils allows for ex vivo and in vitro experimentation, providing a valuable tool for the study of allergic mechanisms. Here, we describe a technique for the isolation of human eosinophils by negative selection from whole blood obtained by venipuncture.

Key words Eosinophils, Cell separation/instrumentation, Cell separation/methods, Granulocytes, Humans

1 Introduction

Negative selection methods have allowed investigators to obtain purified populations of eosinophils from both normal and eosinophilic human donors [2–4]. The resulting availability of human eosinophils has directly led to a wide range of ex vivo and in vitro studies that have greatly enhanced understanding of human eosinophil immunobiology [1, 5].

In this protocol, we describe the use of a commercially available negative selection system from StemCell Technologies. Prior to employing magnetic negative selection, an enriched granulocyte population is obtained from whole blood obtained by venipuncture through a series of steps. Red blood cells are first depleted by dextran sedimentation. After depletion of red blood cells, an enriched granulocyte population is then obtained by density gradient separation. Granulocytes are then incubated with an antibody cocktail against multiple surface antigens found on specific non-eosinophil blood components, including neutrophils (CD16), monocytes (CD14), lymphocytes (CD2), natural killer cells (CD56), and red blood cells (glycophorin A), allowing for efficient negative selection. These antibodies also specifically bind to the dextran-based magnetic colloid with which the

Garry M. Walsh (ed.), *Eosinophils: Methods and Protocols*, Methods in Molecular Biology, vol. 1178,
DOI 10.1007/978-1-4939-1016-8_2, © Springer Science+Business Media New York 2014

granulocyte suspension is subsequently incubated [6]. When the cell suspension is passed through a magnetized steel mesh column, the antibody-bound non-eosinophil blood cells are trapped in the column. The purified eosinophil population flows through unhindered and is collected.

Of note, other commercially available negative selection products are available, including products from Miltenyi Biotec and R&D Systems. We have chosen to describe eosinophil isolation using the column-based StemCell system based on the routine use of this product in our laboratory. Non-column-based negative selection systems are also available.

2 Materials

All reagents and equipment coming into contact with live cells must be sterile, and proper sterile technique should be followed accordingly.

2.1 Blood Donation

1. Human blood donor (*see* **Note 1**).

2. Butterfly needle (with Luer-lock compatibility) for venipuncture, 19-gauge.

3. Sterile Luer-lock syringes, 60 ml (1–8 syringes depending on volume of blood drawn, *see* **Note 2**).

4. Alcohol wipe.

5. Gauze.

6. Rubber tourniquet.

7. Adhesive bandage.

8. Sodium citrate: 3.2 % (w/v) solution in water (*see* **Note 3**).

2.2 Eosinophil Purification

1. Dextran 70 (Pharmacosmos, Denmark): 6 % (w/v) solution in 0.9 % sodium chloride (*see* **Note 4**).

2. Ficoll-Paque Premium.

3. Hanks' Buffer Salt Solution, without calcium or magnesium (HBSS).

4. Ovalbumin for Separation Medium (*see* **Note 5**).

5. Parafilm.

6. Conical polypropylene centrifuge tubes, 50 ml.

7. Sterile disposable transfer pipets.

8. Turk Blood Diluting Fluid (Ricca Chemical Company).

9. Hemocytometer for cell counting.

10. Magnet for cell separation (*see* **Note 6**).

11. Cell separation magnetic column (StemCell Technologies, size will depend size of granulocyte input).

12. Three-way Luer-lock stopcock.

13. Sterile Luer-lock syringe, 10 ml.

14. Negative selection antibody cocktail (StemCell Technologies).

15. Magnetic colloid (StemCell Technologies).

16. Hema 3 Staining Kit (Fisher Scientific).

3 Methods

3.1 Blood Draw

1. Bring sodium citrate solution, dextran, and Ficoll-Paque to room temperature.

2. Fill 60 ml syringes each with 10 ml of sodium citrate solution in a tissue culture hood. One syringe should be used for each 40 ml of blood drawn (up to 320 ml, *see* **Note 2**).

3. Apply tourniquet to the arm of the donor and wipe the antecubital fossa with an alcohol pad. Allow alcohol to dry prior to venipuncture.

4. Attach 60 ml syringe to a 19-gauge butterfly needle and draw blood from an antecubital vein by venipuncture.

5. Fill each syringe with 40 ml of blood by applying gentle negative pressure with the plunger of the syringe. (This will bring the total volume in each syringe to 50 ml). Pinch off the butterfly when switching to subsequent Luer-lock syringes to avoid blood spillage.

6. Remove tourniquet after filling final syringe.

7. Remove butterfly needle and apply pressure with gauze to achieve hemostasis.

8. Apply adhesive bandage to venipuncture site.

3.2 Eosinophil Purification

1. Move syringes to a tissue culture hood and add 10 ml of dextran solution to each syringe. Dextran can be drawn into the syringes using a fresh Luer-lock butterfly needle, taking care to maintain sterility of the needle tip and the dextran solution. Introduction of any air bubbles into the syringes should also be avoided to the greatest extent possible as well.

2. Gently mix syringes by holding a piece of Parafilm over the open Luer-lock end and inverting ten times.

3. Place syringes standing upright in the hood in a compatible rack and allow red blood cells to settle for approximately 40 min. Approximately 20–25 ml of red blood cell-depleted straw-colored fluid will form as the upper layer (*see* **Note 7**).

4. Remove the needle from a new butterfly infusion set and attach to the first syringe. Keeping the syringe upright and taking care not to disturb the interface between the two layers, collect the straw-colored layer by pushing through the tubing and into a 50 ml conical tube. Take care to not collect any material from the red cell layer to minimize red cell contamination. Discard red cell layer in an appropriate biohazard container. Repeat for each syringe (Fractions from separate syringes may be combined in the collection process in order to minimize the number of conical tubes needed at this step).

5. Fill fresh 50 ml conical tubes each with 23 ml of Ficoll-Paque Premium. The number of tubes used will depend on the amount of straw-colored layer collected. Using a serological pipette, carefully layer the straw-colored fluid over the Ficoll-Paque in an approximately 1:1 ratio (about 20–25 ml per conical tube). Take care to minimize any disturbance in the interface between the two layers when pipetting.

6. Carefully transfer the conical tubes to the centrifuge and centrifuge for 20 min at $300 \times g$ at room temperature. Use the lowest acceleration and deceleration setting (no brake) available on the centrifuge (For subsequent centrifugation steps, mid-range acceleration and deceleration settings may be used).

7. Granulocytes, consisting of eosinophils and neutrophils, will be pelleted at the bottom of the conical tube at the bottom of the Ficoll-Paque layer. Immediately above the Ficoll-Paque layer will be a pale whitish interface consisting of mononuclear cells, with a true plasma layer formed above the monocyte layer (Fig. 1).

8. Aspirate the plasma layer using a vacuum apparatus with a clean pipette tip (The same tip may be used for the plasma layer for all tubes if care is made maintain sterility between tubes). Using a fresh pipette tip, then aspirate the mononuclear cell layer. Again using a fresh pipette tip, aspirate the Ficoll layer

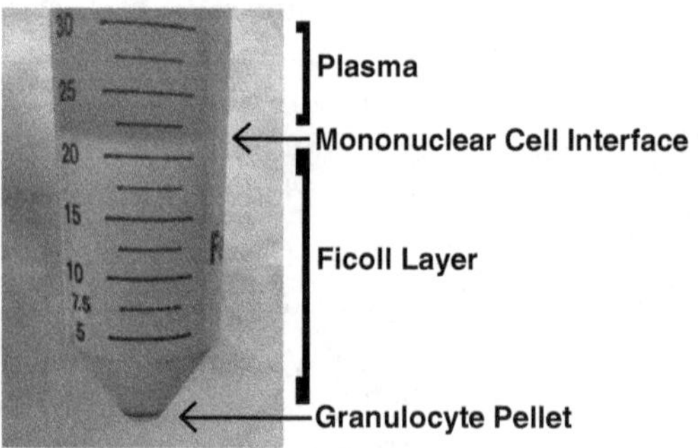

Fig. 1 Appearance of conical tube after Ficoll-Paque density gradient separation

down to the granulocyte pellet, taking care to not contact the pellet with the pipette tip.

9. Using a transfer pipette, resuspend the granulocyte pellet with 1 ml of ice-cold sterile HBSS. Minimize contact of the transfer pipette with the walls of the conical tube in the interest of avoiding contamination with mononuclear cells that may be adherent to the wall of the tube. From this point forward, all steps will be done on ice.

10. Transfer and combine the resuspended pellets to a new 50 ml conical tube containing 30 ml of ice-cold sterile HBSS. In order to maximize cell recovery, the bottom of the tubes containing granulocyte pellets may be washed with an additional 1 ml HBSS which is then transferred to the new conical tube. Bring the total volume of the new conical tube up to 50 ml with ice-cold sterile HBSS after granulocyte transfer.

11. Centrifuge at $300 \times g$ for 5 min at 4 °C. Remove supernatant and discard, resuspend pellet, and refill tube to 50 ml with ice-cold HBSS (*see* **Note 8**).

12. Count granulocytes using a hemocytometer. Dilute the aliquot of granulocyte suspension used for counting 1:1 in Turk Blood Diluting Fluid prior to counting in order to lyse red blood cells (*see* **Note 9**).

13. Centrifuge at $300 \times g$ for 5 min at 4 °C. Remove supernatant and discard.

14. Resuspend granulocyte pellet in 1 ml of separation medium per 50×10^6 granulocytes (from count obtained in **step 20**).

15. Add 100 µl of negative selection antibody cocktail per ml of cell suspension in separation medium. Incubate for 20 min on ice.

16. Add 60 µl of magnetic colloid per ml of cell suspension. Incubate for 20 min on ice with periodic manual gentle agitation to prevent settling of the magnetic colloid.

17. During the incubation with magnetic colloid, set up the negative selection column. Attach a three-way Luer lock stopcock to the end of the column, and prime the column with about 12 ml of separation medium through the side port of the three-way stopcock using a 10 ml Luer lock syringe. Attach a 21-guage needle to unoccupied end of the stopcock. Open the stopcock to the needle and allow the liquid level to drop to just above the level of the metallic mesh and close stopcock. Insert column into the magnet, which should be located in either a cold room or a refrigerated cabinet.

18. Load the top of the column with the cell suspension and open the stopcock, collecting the effluent in a 50 ml conical tube. Continue to add cell suspension followed by 20 ml of separation

medium to the top of the column without allowing any of the metal mesh to run dry until all the liquid has passed through the column (*see* **Note 10**). The effluent will contain the purified eosinophil population.

19. Count eosinophils in the effluent using a hemocytometer (*see* **Note 11**).

20. Centrifuge eosinophils at $300 \times g$ for 5 min at 4 °C. Discard supernatant and resuspend in desired volume of HBSS. Purified eosinophils are ready for experimental use.

4   Notes

1. A human blood donor is required for this protocol. Blood must be drawn by trained personnel after informed consent is obtained under the auspices of a study approved by the investigator's Institutional Review Board (or equivalent).

2. We recommend that no more than 320 ml of blood is drawn from a human volunteer at a time. Though adjustments may be made depending on the volume of blood drawn, male volunteers should not donate blood more frequently than every 2 months, while female volunteers should not donate blood more frequently than every 3 months. The primary purpose of this restriction is to avoid anemia.

3. We use commercially available 4 % (w/v) sodium citrate solution (Sigma Aldrich) that is diluted to 3.2 % in sterile water in a tissue culture hood. Sterile water is added to 4 % sodium citrate in a ratio of 1:4 to arrive at the desired concentration. The solution should be stored at 4 °C and brought to room temperature prior to use in this protocol. Alternatively, sodium citrate solution can be made by combining 37.3 g of sodium citrate powder and 8 g of citric acid in 500 ml of distilled water. Adjust pH to 5.2 with sodium hydroxide, filter sterilize (0.22 μm pore size), and store at 4 °C.

4. The 6 % dextran 70 solution is used for red blood cell sedimentation. Alternatively, 6 % hetastarch may be used in a buffered formulation available from StemCell Technologies. However, the use of hetastarch may affect eosinophil granule morphology [7].

5. Separation medium consists of 0.5 % (w/v) of Grade V ovalbumin in HBSS without calcium or magnesium. A 5× stock solution of 2.5 % (w/v) ovalbumin in HBSS may be made and stored in aliquots at –20 °C.

6. Our laboratory uses a magnet from StemCell Technologies that can fit their 0.5-in. or 0.6-in. columns.

7. This is not truly plasma because it contains cellular components, including eosinophils and other leukocytes.

8. Because the negative selection protocol efficiently removes red blood cells under most circumstances, we do not recommend routine red blood cell lysis with hypotonic saline. However, if lysis must be performed to ensure an eosinophil population completely devoid of red blood cells, it can occur at this point prior to resuspension of the granulocyte pellet in HBSS. We recommend hypotonic saline lysis and recommend against the use of ammonium chloride, as exposure to ammonium chloride will effect eosinophil functional responses [8, 9]. Resuspend the granulocyte pellet in 20–25 ml of 0.2 % sodium chloride. Within 30 s, add an equal volume of 1.6 % sodium chloride. Centrifuge at $300 \times g$ for 5 min at 4 °C. Discard supernatant and wash pellet in 50 ml of HBSS. Repeat centrifugation and wash before proceeding with the remainder of the protocol.

9. This dilution must be accounted for in calculating the number total granulocytes. The cell suspension may be made more dilute if necessary to facilitate counting on the hemocytometer.

10. The size of the column used will depend on the number of granulocytes counted. The 0.5-inch column is designed to process $50–300 \times 10^6$ granulocytes; the 0.6-inch column is designed to process $100–1,500 \times 10^6$ granulocytes.

11. We also recommend assessment of eosinophil purity by examination of a cytocentrifuge slide prepared with Hema 3 staining (similar to Wright-Giemsa staining) and assessment of viability by Trypan Blue staining. Eosinophils will demonstrate purple bilobed (or multilobed) nuclei with pink granular cytoplasmic staining with the Hema 3 stain (Fig. 2).

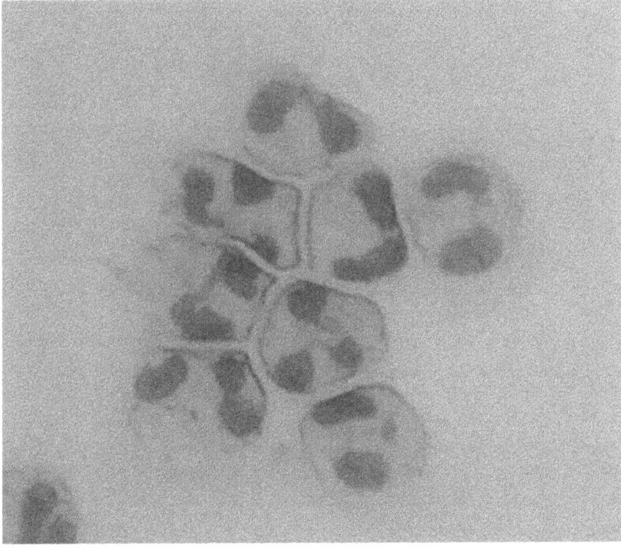

Fig. 2 Cytocentrifuge slide of purified eosinophils prepared with Hema 3 staining, 40× objective

Acknowledgments

This work was supported by a HOPE Pilot Grant from the American Partnership for Eosinophilic Disorders (to PA) and National Institutes of Health grants R01AI051645 and R37AI020241 (to PFW).

References

1. Rosenberg H, Dyer K, Foster P (2013) Eosinophils: changing perspectives in health and disease. Nat Rev Immunol 13:9–22

2. Hansel T, Pound J, Thompson R (1990) Isolation of eosinophils from human blood. J Immunol Methods 127:153–164

3. Hansel T, de Vries I, Iff T et al (1991) An improved immunomagnetic procedure for the isolation of highly purified human blood eosinophils. J Immunol Methods 145:105–110

4. Miltenyi S, Müller W, Weichel W et al (1990) High gradient magnetic cell separation with MACS. Cytometry 11:231–238

5. Rothenberg M, Hogan S (2006) The eosinophil. Annu Rev Immunol 24:147–174

6. Lansdorp P, Thomas T (1990) Purification and analysis of bispecific tetrameric antibody complexes. Mol Immunol 27:659–666

7. Jackson M, Millar A, Dawes J et al (1989) Neutrophil activation during cell separation procedures. Nucl Med Commun 10:901–904

8. Ide M, Weiler D, Kita H et al (1994) Ammonium chloride exposure inhibits cytokine-mediated eosinophil survival. J Immunol Methods 168: 187–196

9. Wang H, Ghiran I, Matthaei K et al (2007) Airway eosinophils: allergic inflammation recruited professional antigen-presenting cells. J Immunol 179:7585–7592

Chapter 3

Eosinophil Purification from Human Bone Marrow

Tina W. Wong and Diane F. Jelinek

Abstract

Eosinophils are innate immune cells that are best known for their involvement in host defense against parasitic infections and in asthma and allergic diseases. In vitro characterization of the function of human eosinophils has traditionally relied on the purification of these cells from the peripheral blood as reviewed in Chapter 2. Here, we describe a newly developed protocol for the purification of eosinophils from human bone marrow.

Key words Bone marrow eosinophils, Purification, Human bone marrow, Cell isolation

1 Introduction

Eosinophils are innate immune cells that play a role in anti-helminthic host defense and in allergic diseases such as asthma. The in vitro study of human eosinophils along with the characterization of their biological functions is most commonly achieved via their purification from peripheral blood using anti-CD16-conjugated-magnetic beads as described in Chapter 2.

In recent years, eosinophils have been demonstrated to play additional roles beyond those described above. For example, eosinophils can serve as professional antigen presenting cells during an immune response as well as modulate other components of the innate and adaptive immune system [1, 2]. Additionally, recent work in the mouse showed a role for eosinophils in plasma cell retention in the bone marrow [3, 4]. However, to date, it remains unclear whether eosinophils involved in bone marrow plasma cell homeostasis are a distinct subset of eosinophils that differ intrinsically in their biology from those found in the peripheral blood.

Eosinophils make up approximately 1–4 % of the cellular compartment within human bone marrow [5, 6]. The purification of these cells from the bone marrow cannot be achieved via the same methodologies as used with peripheral blood because the absence or low-level expression of CD16 by immature neutrophils renders the

Garry M. Walsh (ed.), *Eosinophils: Methods and Protocols*, Methods in Molecular Biology, vol. 1178,
DOI 10.1007/978-1-4939-1016-8_3, © Springer Science+Business Media New York 2014

anti-CD16 negative selection protocol ineffective for the isolation of eosinophils from whole bone marrow [7]. While positive selection methodologies exist for the isolation of highly pure eosinophils from a mixed bone marrow population, e.g., antibody labeling of eosinophil-specific surface markers followed by FACS sorting, the use of these antibodies often leads to eosinophil activation and subsequent cell death [8]. Thus, in order to study these cells and compare them to those purified from the peripheral blood, we devised a novel method for the purification of untouched eosinophils from human bone marrow [7]. In principle, this purification protocol relies on the initial separation of granulocytes (i.e., immature and mature neutrophils and eosinophils) from whole human bone marrow followed by the use of the eosinophil survival factor, IL-5, to maintain the viability of bone marrow eosinophils in an 8-day in vitro culture during which neutrophils undergo apoptosis in the absence of neutrophil survival factors.

2   Materials

Prepare all solutions using sterile-filtered ultrapure water. Store all reagents at 4 °C unless indicated otherwise.

1. 56 % Percoll: Add 140 mL and 25 mL 10× phosphate-buffered saline (PBS) to 85 mL water. Mix well and store at 4 °C.

2. 1× PBS.

3. 2× PBS: Dilute 10× PBS fivefold to make 2× PBS.

4. Cold sterile water.

5. $RPMI_{eos}$: RPMI 1640 supplemented with 100 U/mL penicillin G, 10 µg/mL streptomycin, 3 µg/mL ι-glutamine, 50 µM β-mercaptoethanol, 20 % heat-inactivated fetal calf serum (FCS), and 1 ng/mL human recombinant IL-5.

6. 75 cm^2 tissue culture flask.

7. 10 cm tissue culture dish.

8. 15- and 50-mL conical tubes.

3   Methods

A summary of the purification protocol is depicted as a flowchart in Fig. 1. Perform all steps in a sterile tissue culture room or a designated sterile ventilated tissue culture hood.

1. Dilute 40 mL whole bone marrow aspirate 1:2 in 1× PBS. This yields a total volume of 120 mL.

2. Divide diluted bone marrow sample into three 50-mL conical tubes (i.e., 40 mL sample per tube). Underlay each sample with 10 mL 56 % Percoll (*see* **Note 1**).

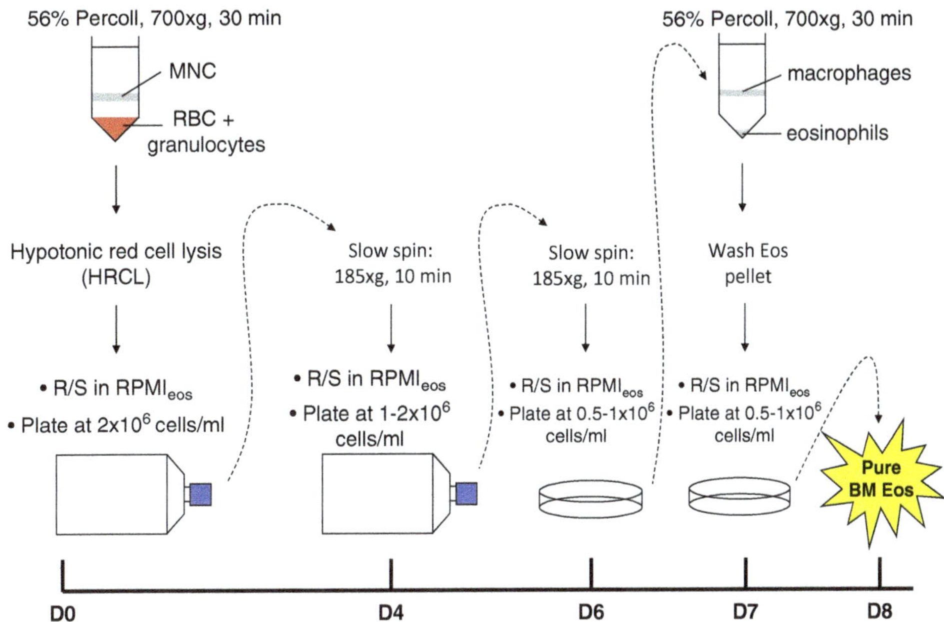

Fig. 1 Schematic of the optimized protocol for the purification of human bone marrow eosinophils (reproduced from [7] with permission from Elsevier)

3. Centrifuge samples in a swing-bucket rotor at $700 \times g$ for 30 min at room temperature. At the end of the centrifugation, allow rotor to decelerate with no brake (*see* **Note 2**).

4. Carefully aspirate off the plasma, mononuclear cell layer, and Percoll to within 0.5 cm of the red blood cell–granulocyte pellet (*see* Fig. 2 and **Note 3**).

5. With a clean pipette, transfer red blood cell–granulocyte pellet to new 50-mL conical tubes (*see* **Note 4**).

6. Perform hypotonic lysis of red blood cells as follows:

    (a) Add 20 mL cold sterile water to the first 50-mL conical tube containing red blood cells–granulocytes. Mix the sample with a 10 mL pipette by pipetting up and down three times.

    (b) *Immediately* add 20 mL cold 2× PBS to the tube to stop the lysis. Mix well by inversion and place tube on ice (*see* **Note 5**).

    (c) Repeat the lysis procedure for each tube of red blood cells–granulocytes.

    (d) Centrifuge tubes at $200 \times g$ for 10 min at 4 °C.

    (e) Aspirate supernatant without disturbing the cell pellet (*see* **Note 6**).

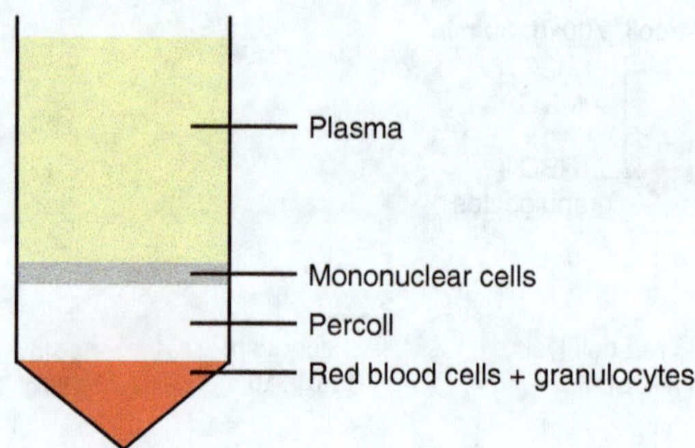

Fig. 2 Diagrammatic representation of bone marrow sample tube post density gradient centrifugation with 56 % Percoll

(f) Combine the cell pellets from the three tubes into a single 50-mL conical tube.

(g) Repeat **steps a–e** two to three more times until granulocyte pellet is no longer red.

7. At this point, the tube should contain granulocytes free of red blood cells. Resuspend the cells in 25 mL RPMI$_{eos}$.

8. Calculate the cell concentration (i.e., number of cells per mL). To determine total cell recovery, multiply by 25 (*see* **Note 7**).

9. Transfer the cells to a 75 cm² flask and adjust the volume with RPMI$_{eos}$ to achieve a final culture concentration of 2×10^6 cells/mL. If the culture exceeds 50 mL in volume, split the culture into multiple flasks so that each flask contains no more than 50 mL.

10. Incubate the cells undisturbed for 4 days at 37 °C, with flasks lying flat, in a humidified 5 % CO_2 incubator (*see* **Note 8**).

11. On day 4 of culture, collect the cells by first gently tilting the flasks from side to side to resuspend the cells followed by transferring into 50-mL conical tubes. Centrifuge the cells at $185 \times g$ for 10 min at 4 °C (*see* **Notes 9** and **10**).

12. Aspirate off supernatant and resuspend the pelleted viable cells with fresh RPMI$_{eos}$ to $1–2 \times 10^6$ cells/mL (*see* **Note 11**).

13. Plate the cells in new 75 cm² flask and incubate with flask lying flat for another 2 days. As before, culture volume per flask should not exceed 50 mL.

14. On day 6, once again collect the cells from flask as described in **step 11** and centrifuge the cells at $185 \times g$ for 10 min at 4 °C.

15. Aspirate off supernatant and resuspend cell pellet with fresh RPMI$_{eos}$ to $0.5–1 \times 10^6$ cells/mL.

16. Plate the cells in a 10 cm tissue culture dish. If culture volume exceeds 10 mL, split the cells into multiple dishes with a maximum volume of 10 mL per dish. Incubate the cells for another day (*see* **Note 12**).

17. On day 7, perform density gradient centrifugation as described previously using 56 % Percoll and centrifuging at $700 \times g$ for 30 min at room temperature with no brake (*see* **Notes 13** and **14**).

18. Aspirate off all layers up to the granulocyte pellet as done in **step 4**. Transfer cell pellet to a new 15 mL tube.

19. Wash the cells by resuspending pellet in 10 mL 1× PBS and centrifuging at $185 \times g$ for 10 min at 4 °C.

20. Remove supernatant and resuspend the cells in $RPMI_{eos}$ to 0.5–1×10^6 cells/mL.

21. Plate the cells in new tissue culture dish and place in humidified 5 % CO_2 incubator.

22. On day 8, the culture now contains pure eosinophils that have initially been obtained from human bone marrow (*see* **Note 15**).

4   Notes

1. Underlaying samples with Percoll is achieved by inserting a 10 mL pipette containing the Percoll to the bottom of the 50-mL conical tube and *slowly* letting out the Percoll from the pipette. The density difference between the Percoll and the bone marrow sample will result in a clear separation of the two if performed properly. If the underlay is performed too fast, the Percoll and the sample may intermix and a clean separation between the layers may not be seen.

2. After centrifuging, layers will appear as follows from top to bottom: plasma (lightly gold), mononuclear cells/buffy coat (white), Percoll (clear), red blood cells and granulocytes (red). The use of brakes will result in an undesired mixing of the different layers achieved by the centrifugation (*see* Fig. 2).

3. Aspiration apparatus can be set up by connecting a side-arm flask to vacuum and a sterile Pasteur pipette. To most effectively aspirate off all layers up to the red blood cell–granulocyte pellet with the least amount of residual mononuclear cell contamination, insert the pipette directly to just above the mononuclear cell layer and circle the pipette around the interphase. Once the mononuclear cell layer has been aspirated completely, continue to aspirate off the remaining plasma and most of the Percoll layer.

4. The goal of this step is to minimize contamination with mononuclear cells as they may stick to the side of the 50-mL conical tubes. Thus, when performing this step, take extra caution to prevent the pipette tip from touching the side of the 50-mL conical tube.

5. A delay in this step will result in increased duration of the granulocytes' exposure to hypotonic shock and thus lead to undesirable cell death.

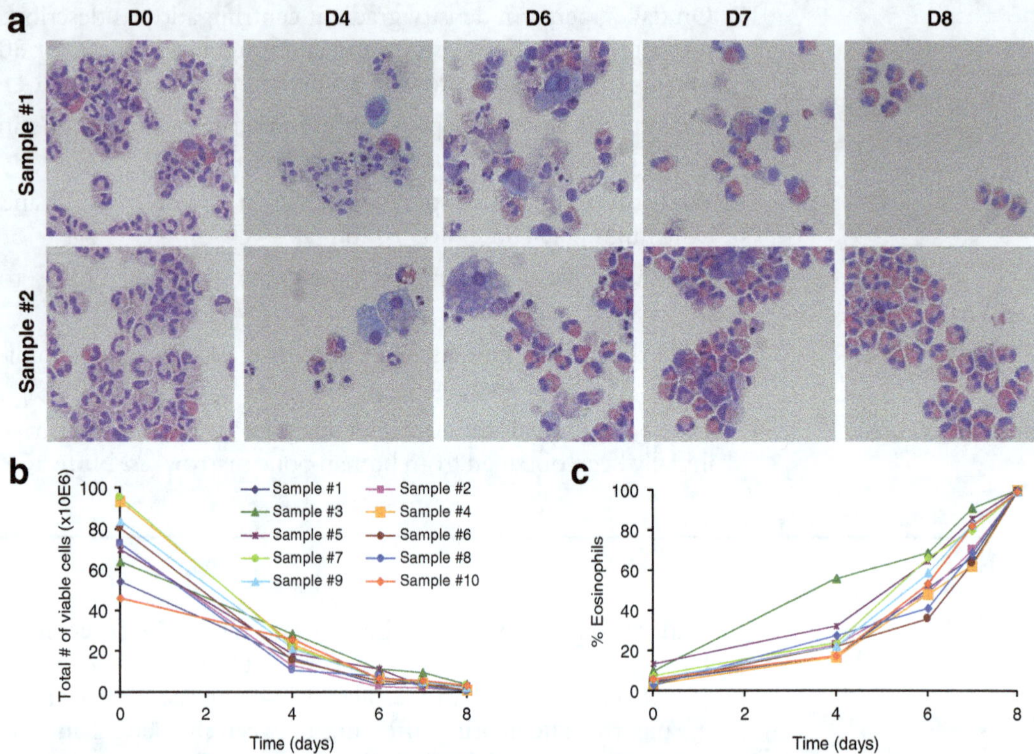

Fig. 3 8-day in vitro culture system yields highly pure eosinophils from human bone marrow. (**a**) Cytospin preparations were made at various time points throughout the 8-day culture system from two different patient samples. (**b**) The number of viable cells from 10 separate patient samples was counted during the 8-day culture. Differences in the initial (day 0) cell counts reflect differences in the bone marrow aspirate volume collected from the patients combined with variability in percentages of granulocytes amongst different bone marrow samples. Cell viability was assessed by trypan blue staining. (**c**) The percent eosinophils in the cultures on day 0, 4, 6, 7, and 8 for these 10 samples were calculated based on modified Wright-stained cytospin preparations (reproduced from [7] with permission from Elsevier)

6. In the first lysis step, the pellet is difficult to visualize due to the opacity of the red supernatant. Thus, for this initial lysis, aspirate supernatant to the shoulder of the conical tubes.

7. Concentration of cells in the tube can be counted via a number of methods, such as using an automated cell counter or a hemocytometer.

8. During the initial 4 day culture period, most of the neutrophils will undergo apoptosis (*see* Fig. 3).

9. Eosinophils are non-adherent cells, and thus, gentle tilting/ swirling of the flask will suffice to mix cells in culture for collection into conical tubes. Avoid vigorous pipetting up and down in attempt to lift off adherent cells on the side of the flasks; any adherent cells that may grow out in the culture represent non-eosinophilic cells and thus need not be transferred.

10. This slow spin at $185 \times g$ allows for the removal of dead cell debris, which does not pellet with the live cells.

11. Neutrophils represent 87–97 % of the granulocytes in the bone marrow. Thus, as a result of neutrophil death in the first 4 days of culture, the culture size will become dramatically reduced.

12. Macrophages are adherent cells in culture dishes. Changing culture flasks/dishes allows for removal of any macrophages that may have grown out from the cultures as a result of the GM-CSF secreted by eosinophils (*see* Fig. 3).

13. Density gradient centrifugation on day 7 allows for the thorough removal of macrophages from the culture.

14. At this point the culture size has reduced significantly from day 0 and is typically small enough that the density gradient centrifugation here can be performed in a single 15-mL conical tube rather than the 50-mL conical tubes. To do so, place cells (up to 9 mL) in a 15-mL conical tube and underlay with 3 mL Percoll. If the cell culture volume exceeds 9 mL, use additional 15-mL conical tubes for this step and recombine granulocyte pellets from all tubes after centrifugation.

15. The purity of the eosinophil culture at day 8 as assessed by morphology is typically between 98.8 and 100 % (*see* Fig. 3).

Acknowledgments

This work was supported by the NIH Predoctoral Immunology Training Grant (T32 AI07425). TWW thanks the Mayo Medical School, Mayo Graduate School, and the Mayo Clinic Medical Scientist Training Program for providing an outstanding training environment.

References

1. Akuthota P, Wang HB, Spencer LA et al (2008) Immunoregulatory roles of eosinophils: a new look at a familiar cell. Clin Exp Allergy 38(8): 1254–1263

2. Rosenberg HF, Dyer KD, Foster PS (2013) Eosinophils: changing perspectives in health and disease. Nat Rev Immunol 13(1):9–22

3. Chu VT, Frohlich A, Steinhauser G et al (2011) Eosinophils are required for the maintenance of plasma cells in the bone marrow. Nat Immunol 12(2):151–159

4. Chu VT, Berek C (2012) Immunization induces activation of bone marrow eosinophils required for plasma cell survival. Eur J Immunol 42(1): 130–137

5. Terstappen LW, Levin J (1992) Bone marrow cell differential counts obtained by multidimensional flow cytometry. Blood Cells 18(2): 311–330

6. Fauci A, Braunwald E, Kasper D et al (2009) Harrison's manual of medicine, 17th edn. McGraw-Hill Companies, New York, NY

7. Wong TW, Jelinek DF (2013) Purification of functional eosinophils from human bone marrow. J Immunol Methods 387(1–2): 130–139

8. Kato M, Abraham RT, Okada S et al (1998) Ligation of the beta2 integrin triggers activation and degranulation of human eosinophils. Am J Respir Cell Mol Biol 18(5):675–686

Chapter 4

CD34+ Eosinophil-Lineage-Committed Cells in the Mouse Lung

Apostolos Bossios and Madeleine Rådinger

Abstract

Several studies suggest that eosinophil progenitor cells are capable of extramedullary proliferation but also enhance chronic inflammation via their own production of inflammatory and chemotactic mediators, thus augmenting the degree of inflammation by recruitment of more progenitors or mature effector cells, such as eosinophils at the site of inflammation. In this chapter, we provide methods focused on detecting eosinophil progenitor cells in the lung of allergen-challenged mice and how to monitor their proliferation capacity.

Key words Allergy, Asthma, Bone marrow, Lung, Eosinophil progenitors, In situ hematopoiesis, CD34, IL-5Ra, CCR3, Fluorescence-activated cell (FACS)

1   Introduction

Allergic asthma, rhinitis, and chronic rhinosinusitis are often characterized by eosinophilic inflammation. Eosinophil development is viewed to primarily occur under the influence of interleukin (IL)-5, IL-3, and GM-CSF, and eosinophilopoiesis is mainly restricted to the bone marrow compartment, although eosinophilopoiesis may also occur to some degree in the spleen, thymus, and lymph nodes. One characteristic of hematopoietic progenitors is that they express the CD34 antigen on their surface and that they have the ability to form colony forming units (CFU) in cultures [1–3].

In the murine bone marrow, eosinophil lineage-committed progenitors are currently defined as $IL\text{-}5R\alpha^{+}Lin^{-}Sca\text{-}1^{-}CD34^{+}$ c-KIT $(CD117)^{lo}$ cells [4].

In allergic diseases, the bone marrow releases a greater quantity of eosinophil progenitor cells that migrate to sites of allergic inflammation. Furthermore, evidence from recent studies suggest that

Financial support for work in the authors' laboratory was provided by the VBG-GROUP Centre for Asthma and Allergy research, Herman Krefting Foundation against Asthma and Allergy, Swedish Heart-Lung Foundation.

Garry M. Walsh (ed.), *Eosinophils: Methods and Protocols*, Methods in Molecular Biology, vol. 1178,
DOI 10.1007/978-1-4939-1016-8_4, © Springer Science+Business Media New York 2014

29

eosinophil progenitor cells are not only capable of extramedullary proliferation but can also enhance chronic inflammation via their own production of inflammatory and chemotactic mediators, thus augmenting the degree of inflammation by recruitment of more progenitors or mature effector cells at sites of inflammation. Indeed, several human studies have identified CD34$^+$IL-5Ra$^+$ cells in lung tissue from patients with asthma as eosinophil progenitors [5–7]. In murine lungs eosinophil-lineage-committed progenitors are defined as CD34$^+$CD45$^+$IL-5Ra$^+$ cells [8–10]. In addition, other expressed surface markers such as CCR3 and Siglec-F have also been described [10, 11].

In this chapter we have described protocols developed and optimized in our laboratory, which will allow researchers to detect eosinophil-lineage-committed progenitors in the lung of allergen-challenged mice, and to monitor the proliferation capacity of these eosinophil progenitors.

2   Materials

2.1   Preparing Lung Tissue Cells

1. Ovalbumin (OVA) for sensitization and challenge of mice.
2. Wild type C57BL/6 or Balb/c mice (6–8-week-old male) sensitized and exposed to OVA.
3. Aluminum hydroxide for sensitization.
4. RPMI-1640.
5. Phosphate Buffer Saline (PBS).
6. Fetal calf serum (FCS).
7. Sterile gauze.
8. Sterile petri dish.
9. Sterile scalpel.
10. Lung isolation media: RPMI-1640 supplemented with 10 % FCS, Collagenase (5.25 mg/ml), and DNase (3 mg/ml).
11. 40-μm nylon filters.
12. Percoll.

2.2   Magnetic Separation for Isolation and Culturing of CD34+ Cells

1. MACS separation buffer: Degassed 0.5 % BSA/PBS supplemented with 2 mM EDTA.
2. Biotin-conjugated rat anti-mouse CD34 monoclonal antibody.
3. MACS Streptavidin MicroBeads, LS Column, MACS Magnet (all from Miltenyi Biotec).
4. CD34 culture medium: RPMI-1640 supplemented with 0.9 % methylcellulose, 20 % FCS, 1 % penicillin–streptomycin, 2 mM L-glutamine, and 50 mM β-mercaptoethanol.

5. Mouse Interleukin-5 (mIL-5), resuspend in 0.1 % BSA/PBS at 5 µg/ml and use at 10 µg/ml. Store aliquots at –80 °C.

6. 12 well tissue culture plates.

2.3 Immunostaining of Eosinophil-Lineage-Committed Cells

1. 5 ml polystyrene round bottom tubes for flow cytometer.

2. 15 and 50 ml conical tubes.

3. Eppendorf sterile tubes (1.5 ml) (for antibody master mix).

4. Blocking Fc Solution: PBS with 4 % mouse serum.

5. Staining buffer: PBS with 1 % FCS.

6. PFA solution: 4 % paraformaldehyde in PBS. Dissolve carefully in 60 °C water bath for 1 h. Can be kept refrigerated at 4 °C for 1 month.

7. Fluorescence-conjugated antibodies against surface molecules of interest (CD45, CD34, IL-5Ra, CCR3, and the corresponding isotype controls), viability/DNA dyes (i.e., 7-AAD) according to provision of available flow cytometry (*see* **Note 1**).

2.4 Monitoring In Situ Proliferation of Eosinophil-Lineage-Committed Cells in the Lung by Flow Cytometry

1. Wild type C57BL/6 or Balb/c mice (6–8-week-old male) sensitized and exposed to OVA.

2. OVA and aluminum hydroxide for sensitization.

3. 5-Bromo-2′-deoxyuridine (BrdU).

4. Fluorescence-conjugated antibodies against surface molecules of interest, BrdU-staining kit that includes DNase and a DNA stain, i.e., 7-AAD.

5. BD Cytofix/Cytoperm: Ready to use (BD Biosciences).

6. BD Perm/Wash Buffer: Dilute the stock 1:10 with double distilled H_2O.

7. BD Cytoperm plus Buffer Ready to use.

2.5 Equipment

1. Refrigerated centrifuge.

2. Flow Cytometer and flow cytometry analysis software.

3. Vortex.

4. Various pipettes.

5. Water bath.

6. MACS Magnet (Miltenyi).

7. Laminar Flow Hood.

8. 37 °C, 5 % CO_2 humidified incubator.

9. Hemacytometer.

10. Light microscope.

3 Methods

3.1 CD34⁺ Lung Colony Assay

In order to obtain sufficient CD34⁺ cells in the lung, mice are sensitized and exposed to allergen (OVA—*see* Chapter 25).

3.2 Preparing Lung Tissue Cells

1. Euthanize mice according to your approved animal care procedures.

2. Take blood from right ventricle and save for serum analysis (*see* **Note 2**).

3. Lavage the mice with 0.5 ml ice-cold PBS twice. Save for differential cell count and cell free BALF analysis (*see* **Note 2**).

4. Perfuse the pulmonary circulation with ice-cold PBS.

5. Remove the lung and place it in a sterile 50 ml falcon tube with RPMI 1640-medium.

6. Weigh the lung.

7. Working in a sterile hood P place the lung lobes on sterile gauze in a sterile petri dish and slice thinly with a scalpel blade.

8. Place the lung slices in a 50 ml Falcon tube with RPMI 1640 supplemented with 10 % FCS, collagenase (5.25 mg/ml), and DNase (3 mg/ml) and incubate in a shaking water bath at 37 °C for 90 min.

9. Filter the lung digest through a 40 μm filter and centrifuge the cell suspension at $300 \times g$ for 10 min.

10. Make a discontinuous Percoll gradient (45 and 35 %).

11. Suspend the cells in 3 ml PBS supplemented with 10 % FCS and dilute in 1 ml 90 % Percoll (density 1.03 g/ml) and layer the cells on top of the gradient and centrifuge for 30 min at $400 \times g$ without brake at 18 °C.

12. Harvest the cells in each layer with a Pasteur pipette and discard the top layer containing macrophages, dead cells, and debris.

13. Wash the cells in PBS supplemented with 0.5 % BSA.

14. Count the cells and measure viability by trypan blue test.

3.3 Magnetic Separation for Isolation and Culturing of CD34+ Cells (See Note 3)

1. Keep the cells on ice with all centrifugation performed at 4–7 °C. Centrifuge the cells and remove supernatant completely and resuspend the cell pellet in buffer in a total volume of 90 μl per 10^7 total cells.

2. Label the cells with biotinylated CD34 antibody at a concentration of 0.5 μg/μl and use 20 μl per 10^7 total cells.

3. Mix well and incubate at 4 °C for 15 min.

4. Wash carefully with 20× the labeling volume with buffer and centrifuge at $300 \times g$ for 10 min.

5. Remove supernatant completely and resuspend the pellet carefully in 90 µl buffer per 10^7 total cells.

6. To label the cells magnetically, add 10 µl MACS Streptavidin MicroBeads per 10^7 total cells. Mix well and incubate at 4 °C for 15 min.

7. Wash the cells carefully with buffer by adding 20× the labeling volume and centrifuge at $300 \times g$ for 10 min.

8. Remove supernatant completely and resuspend the cell pellet in 500 µl buffer per 10^8 total cells.

9. Place a LS column in the magnetic field of a MACS separator and prepare the column by washing with 3 ml buffer.

10. Apply the cell suspension onto the column; the unlabeled cells (i.e., negative fraction) pass through and are collected in a 15 ml Falcon tube. Rinse by adding 3 ml buffer three times.

11. Remove the column from the separator and place on a 15 ml Falcon tube. Pipette 5 ml of buffer on top of the column and flush out the labeled cells (i.e., positive fraction) using the plunger.

12. Count the positive fraction, i.e., the CD34+ cells.

13. Centrifuge at $300 \times g$ for 10 min. Remove supernatant completely and resuspend the cell pellet in complete media at a concentration of 1×10^6 cells per ml in CD34 culture medium supplemented with 10 ng/ml rmIL-5.

14. Seed the CD34+ cells in a 12-well plate at a concentration of 0.5×10^6/ml/well.

15. On day six of culture, add 100 µl RPMI-1640 supplemented with 1 % penicillin–streptomycin, 2 mM L-Glutamine supplemented with 10 ng/ml rmIL-5 (end concentration).

16. Between day 8 and 14 of culture count eosinophil colony-forming units using an inverted light microscope according to morphologic and histologic criteria (*see* **Note 4**) [12].

3.4 Immunostaining of Eosinophil-Lineage-Committed Cells

Preparation of lung tissue cells is performed as described above (Subheading 3.2). However, it is possible to obtain cells direct from **step 9**, although problems with nonspecific staining may occur (*see* **Notes 2** and **5**). Keep all cells on ice in PBS supplemented with 0.5 % BSA.

1. Prepare the specific staining protocol, all staining buffers, antibodies panel, and master mix on the day of experiment or the day before. Keep refrigerated (*see* **Note 6**).

2. Centrifuge the cells, remove supernatant completely, and suspend cells in PBS/BSA buffer in a concentration of 1×10^7/ml. Keep cells on ice.

3. Add 50 µl of the cell solution (0.5×10^6 cells) to flow tubes.

4. Add 50 µl Fc-blocking solution and incubate for 15 min at 4 °C (*see* **Note 7**).

5. Add the surface antibody mix (*see* **Note 8**).

6. Incubate for 30 min at 4 °C. From this point and until acquisition of cells in flow cytometry, samples should be protected from light.

7. Wash with 2 ml washing buffer, centrifuge at $200 \times g$ for 10 min at 4 °C, decant, and repeat washing.

8. Suspend the cells in 0.3 ml wash buffer and keep at 4 °C in dark until flow cytometry acquisition is performed. If acquisition is to be performed the next day add PFA solution at a final concentration of 2 % (*see* **Note 9**). Proceed to acquisition.

3.5 Monitoring In Situ Proliferation of Eosinophil-Lineage-Committed Cells in the Lung by Flow Cytometry

Assessment of in-situ proliferation of eosinophil-lineage-committed cells as well as other cells, i.e., CD4, in the lung can be done by in-vivo administration of a thymidine analogue such as 5-bromo-2-deoxyuridine (BrdU), a commonly used method that allow to detect the newly produced cells since they preferably incorporate BrdU into their DNA during synthesis. Thus, the cells that have incorporated BrdU can easily be evaluated by detection with an anti-BrdU fluorescence conjugated antibody. When anti-BrdU staining is combined with a DNA dye, e.g., 7-Aminoactinomycin D (7-AAD), then it is possible to detect cells that are newly produced and express a double amount of DNA, i.e., BrdU+/7-AAD^{High}. Those cells represent the cells that are currently in the S and/or G_2/M phase (*see* **Note 1**).

Here, we will describe a combined staining protocol for both surface markers for eosinophil-lineage-committed cells, i.e., CD45$^+$IL-5Ra$^+$CD34$^+$ cells, and for intracellular staining with anti-BrdU and 7-AAD. This protocol is usually divided into a two-day protocol, as the first day includes sacrificing mice and lung tissue cell sampling (Figs. 1–3). Representative plots and strategy of analysis for a sample of lung cell suspension from OVA sensitized and exposed mouse that was treated with BrdU are shown in Figs. 1–3. Cells were stained with the described protocol for surface markers and BrdU and 7-AAD for cell cycle analysis. The panel used was: CD45 FITC/IL-5Ra PE/7-AAD/ BrdU APC/ CD34 Alexa Fluor 700. Analysis was performed based on controls generated with the FMO approach.

1. Mice sensitized and exposed to allergen (OVA) are used (Chapter 25). BrdU is given at a dose of 0.8 mg in 0.2 ml of PBS by i.p. injection once a day just after allergen exposure. One mouse will serve as a control in which no BrdU will be given (*see* **Note 10**).

2. Proceed to surface staining as it is described in Subheading 3.2, until **step 8**. In the antibody panel, consider adding two more staining steps, one for anti-BrdU and one for 7-ADD.

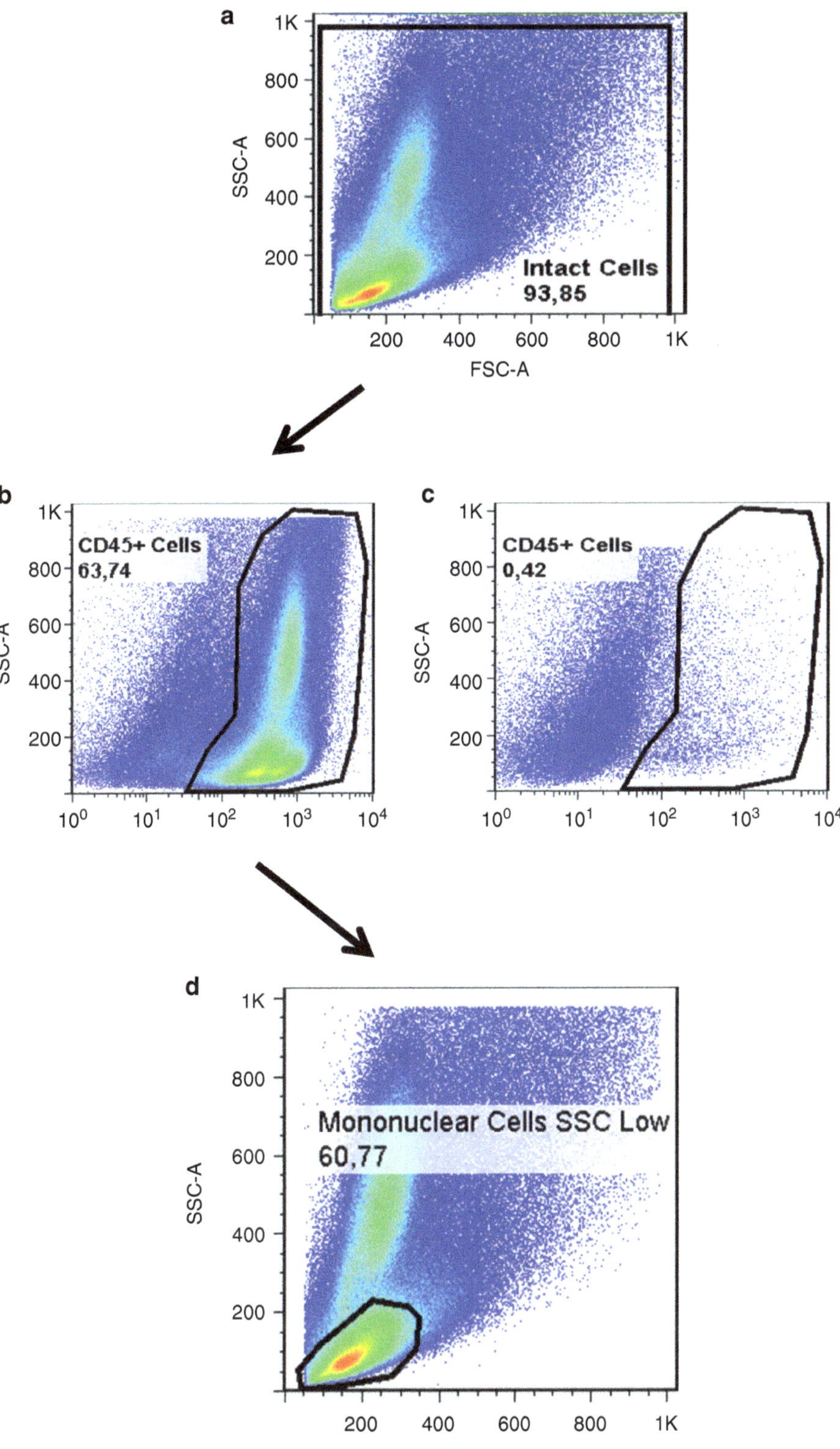

Fig. 1 Using an initial "intact cell" gate, cell debris and large aggregates were excluded (**a**) A gate for CD45 was established (**b**) based on an FMO control (**c**). Note that a small number of "false" positive cells are acceptable. Back gating revealed that these cells are distributed in the whole population, therefore not possible to exclude. (**d**) A gate on mononuclear cells (SSC^{Low}) was done (**d**). Thus, the base analysis population has been identified; mononuclear leucocytes (CD45$^+$SSC^{low})

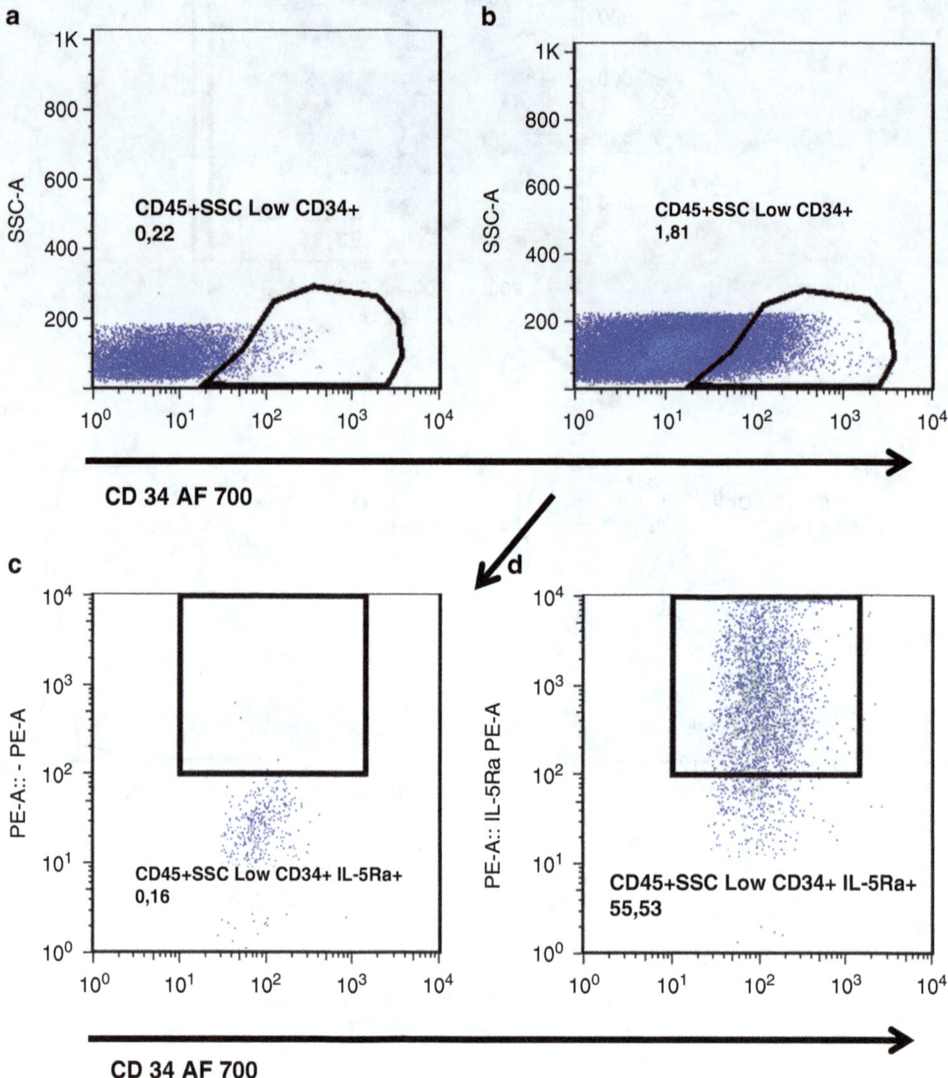

Fig. 2 Analysis continued in the population of choice CD45+SSC^{low} from Fig. 1. A gate for CD34+ cells was set (**b**) based on FMO control (**a**). Cells were then analyzed for the expression of IL-5Ra (**d**) based on FMO control (**c**). Thus, our final population is the eosinophil-lineage-committed cell: mononuclear (SSC^{low}) CD45+/CD34+/IL-5Ra+

3. Add 100 μl BD Cytofix/Cytoperm Buffer; incubate for 15 min at room temperature (RT).

4. Wash with 2 ml wash buffer, centrifuge at $200 \times g$ for 10 min at 4 °C, decant.

5. Repeat washing.

6. Suspend in 0.5 ml wash buffer and store overnight at 4 °C (*see* **Note 11**).

7. Next day centrifuge the cells and decant supernatant.

8. Add 100 μl of BD Cytoperm plus Buffer; incubate for 10 min at 4 °C.

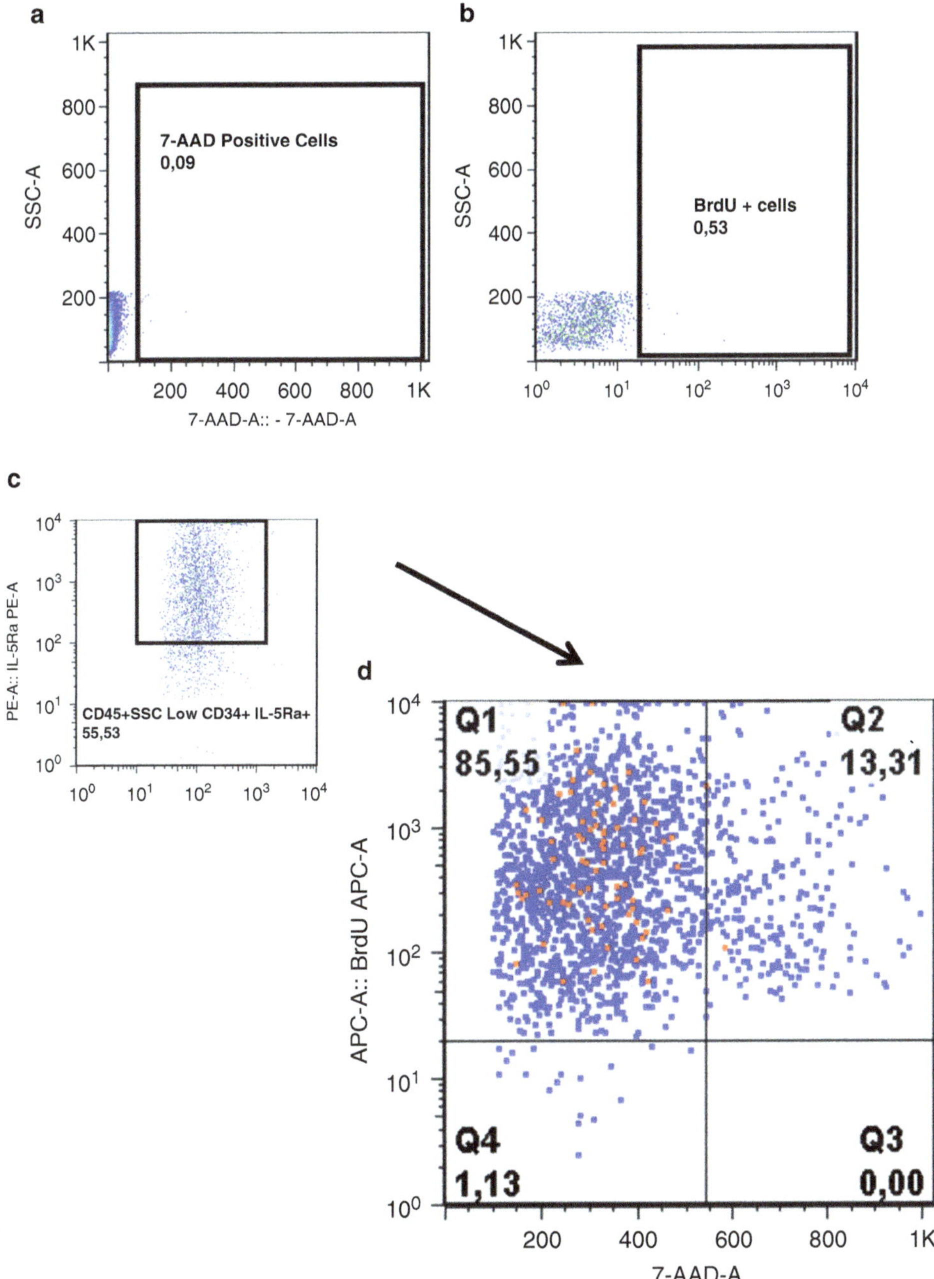

Fig. 3 Analysis for the newly produced eosinophil-lineage-committed cells (mononuclear (SSC^{low}) CD45+/CD34+/IL-5Ra+) identified in Fig. 2. (**a**) A gate for DNA analysis set on cells not stained for 7-AAD. (**b**) Gate set for the expression of BrdU on cells stained with anti-BrdU that originated from mice not treated with BrdU. (**c**) Quadrant gating of the target population based on above gates revealed three populations of interest. (**d**) Q1 cells (BrdU+/7-AAD^{low}), these are newly produced cells (i.e., during allergen exposure) that expressed normal amount of DNA, i.e., they are in the G1 phase. Q 2 cells (BrdU+/7-AAD^{high}), these are newly produced cells that express high amount of DNA, i.e., they are in the S and/or G$_2$/M phase. Q 3 cells (BrdU−/7-AAD^{low}), these are old cells that express normal amount of DNA, i.e., cells that are in the G$_0$

9. Wash with 1 ml of 1× BD Perm/Wash Buffer, centrifuge at 200×*g* for 10 min at 4 °C, decant.

10. Suspend the cells with 100 µl of BD Cytofix/Cytoperm Buffer; incubate for 5 min at RT.

11. Wash with 1 ml of 1× BD Perm/Wash Buffer, centrifuge at 200×*g* for 10 min at 4 °C, decant.

12. Suspend the cells with 100 µl DNase, incubate cells for 1 h at 37 °C.

13. Wash with 1 ml of 1× BD Perm/Wash Buffer, centrifuge at 200×*g* for 10 min at 4 °C, decant.

14. Add the anti-BrdU antibody. Incubate cells for 20 min at RT.

15. Wash with 1 ml of 1× BD Perm/Wash Buffer, centrifuge at 200×*g* for 10 min at 4 °C, decant.

16. Add 400 µl staining to each tube and resuspend cells.

17. Add the 7-AAD dye and incubate for 10 min at RT.

18. Proceed to acquisition.

3.6 Data Acquisition

1. Check the status of the flow cytometer before the experiment (*see* **Note 12**).

2. Perform the appropriate compensations. Compensation of the surface markers can be performed with either single stained populations or with the appropriate beads (*see* **Note 13**).

3. Compensation for 7-AAD as a DNA marker needs to be performed with cells fixed with BD Cytofix/Cytoperm, so the dye can pass through the cell membrane and incorporated into the DNA. Suspend 0.5×10^6 cells with 0.1 ml BD Cytofix/Cytoperm. Incubate for 15 min at RT. Wash cells as above (1 ml of 1× BD Perm/Wash Buffer, centrifuge at 200×*g* for 10 min at 4 °C, decant). Add 7-AAD dye to the cells that will serve as a positive control for the compensations. Use unstained cells as a control. Run cells in a linear mode.

4. In a "set-up" experiment evaluate the number of the cells you need to acquire in order to have sufficient numbers of cells of interest to analyze. Usually for progenitors cells, a large number of events, i.e., >250,000 events are required.

5. Consider a "doublet discrimination" strategy for your acquisition and analysis (*see* **Note 14**).

3.7 Data Analysis

1. A number of flow cytometer analysis software packages are available. It is important that you are familiar with the one that you are using for your analysis.

2. In the "set-up" experiment that is described above a full analysis should be included. If you are not familiar with flow analysis,

discuss gate-analysis strategy and results with a more experienced colleague.

3. Initially analyze your sample looking for the "dead" cells and debris. Usually cell debris is small and gathered in the lower corner of FSC vs. SSC. Often, this debris is negative for the viability dye (i.e., 7-AAD) as it is made up of disrupted membranes that lacking a nucleus required for 7-AAD staining.

4. Analysis should be performed used the "Fluorescence minus One" (FMO) approach. In this approach the "control" sample is stained with all the antibodies except the one of interest to analyze. In this way we can get the "real" background as it will increase in parallel with the number of antibodies used.

5. Several types of plots exist, i.e., "dot plots," "pseudocolours," "contour plots," and histograms. Your results should not be affected by the type of plot you choose. If it is, then you should reconsider your analysis. Choose the plot that is the most informative for your data presentation [13].

6. Use the cell population without the analyzed staining and set the gates. Remember that cells are prone to forming groups. During analysis consider twice splicing in the middle by putting a gate based on the negative population. If necessary you can perform "back gating" where the population of choice is plotted again in FSC vs. SSC. This should allow you to confirm that your population is "real" and not debris/dead cells (i.e., nonspecific binding).

7. In the gate of interest a "small" population in the control sample up to 1 % is usually accepted. However, sometimes can be larger. If so, check all your samples. Is this "high false positive" population present in all samples? Do a "back gating". Is this "false positive population" placed in a certain area of FSC vs. SSC plot that argues for dead/debris cells and nonspecific staining? Can the population be excluded? If we have a "spread population" that cannot be excluded and it will be present in all of our samples, it may be accepted. In all cases the percentage of this "false positive population" should be subtracted from the positive one. Also you should state this in the analysis and display some plots as example.

8. You may wish to evaluate the percentage of cells expressing a protein, i.e., $CD34^+$ % of $CD45^+$ cells, or the expression of the amount of the protein of interest per cells, i.e., the expression of $IL\text{-}5Ra^+$ per cell. Here two expressions are usually used; Mean Fluorescence Intensity or Median Fluorescence Intensity (MFI), or geometrical mean. A continuous discussion exists which is the most appropriate. If your population is normally distributed then you can use mean, otherwise the median is the most appropriate. State in your analysis which one is used and be consistent.

9. Initially when FACS was relatively a new technique researchers represented their "perfect" plots in their publications. Today it is acceptable to show plots that do not include perfect populations. It is important to show the populations exactly as they are and state in the paper exactly how the analysis was performed. In any case all FACS analysis is to an extent subjective.

4   Notes

1. The Fluorescence-conjugated antibodies against the antigens of choice can be sourced from various suppliers (BD Biosciences, ebioscience, R&D Systems, Abcam, etc). Several issues need to be considered when choosing antibodies.

   The first question pertains to the clone. This is an important issue as different clones attach to different epitopes and exhibit different sensitivity. A safe way to start is to choose a clone used in a referenced published paper but it will need to be tested in your hands for your experimental conditions. For example, it should be tested if the epitope of choice is destroyed by fixation and therefore the test clone is not working. In order to keep costs down, a good tip is to discuss with your in-house colleagues and borrow small amounts of the antibody of choice to test.

   A second important issue is the choice of fluorochrome that your antibody of choice will be conjugated with. Here it is important to know and understand the relative intensity of each of the fluorochromes to be used. In general, phycoerythrin (PE) and its PE-tandem fluorochromes (PE–Cy5, PE–Cy 5.5, PE–Cy7) are the brightest, followed by allophycocyanin (APC) and its tandem (APC–Alexa Fluor 700 and APC–Cy7, APC–H7). Then, the fluorescein isothiocyanate (FITC), peridinin chlorophyll-A protein (PerCP), and the Alexa Fluor series of dyes follow. New dyes such as quantum dots are developed constantly. The brightest fluorochrome should be used for the least expressed protein, i.e., CD34 or IL-5Ra, while the dimmest one for the most highly expressed, i.e., CD45. Another important issue is the emission overlap. The selected fluorochromes should have the least spectral overlap. Finally tandem dyes should be used with caution as they are sensitive to various fixation buffers, photobleaching and prone to uncoupling. Each new batch should be titrated to previous experiments [14, 15]. For proliferation studies several DNA dyes exist. The classical one is propidium iodide (PI). Although it is cheap, it excites in the PE channel that usually is kept free for other use. A good alternative is the 7-Aminoactinomycin D (7-AAD). It binds to DNA and can be used as both a viability marker as well as a cell cycle analysis marker. If it is used in live cells with an intact membrane it cannot pass though the membrane and stain the DNA. Therefore, a 7-AAD –ve population represents a viable cell population. When it is used in permeabilized cells, all the cells are positive and the difference is in the degree of the staining. Normal/low staining represents cells in the G_0/G_1 phase while, strong/bright staining represent cells that are in the S and/or G_2/M phase.

2. It may be useful to save serum and BALF if you wish to analyze cytokine and chemokine release after allergen exposure and correlate these to your assessed eosinophil-committed progenitor cells.

3. Additional protocols exist in the literature where no CD34 purification is used. Briefly, lung mononuclear cells are incubated overnight in plastic flasks at 37 °C and 5 % CO_2 to remove adherent cells and the non-adherent cells are cultured in medium containing 0.9 % methylcellulose and rmIL-5.

4. Colonies greater than 40 cells are counted by using inverse microscopy and identified by using morphologic and histologic criteria [12].

5. Lung tissue consists of many different cell types, both of hematopoietic origin and structural cells. The latter are usually damaged during the cell preparation thus, resulting in debris and dead cells. Dead cells and debris are usual stained nonspecifically with almost all antibodies during immune-staining for flow cytometry analysis. Thus, several problems during analysis may occur. Therefore, it is highly recommended that debris and dead cells should be removed before immune-staining.

6. Choice of the optimal antibodies can be demanding as described above (*see* **Note 1**). When you have chosen your antibodies, a staining-panel should be prepared. You should consider and prepare the necessary tools for your analysis. These tools include unstained cells to be used as controls for staining, and auto-fluorescence as well as isotype controls (ICs) to evaluate the nonspecific biding of your antibody. Here, it is recommended that ICs are supplied by the same supplier as the conjugated Fluorescence-conjugated antibodies. The reason for this is that different companies may have a different Fluorescence–Protein (F:P) ratio. If a F:P ratio of an antibody and its IC differ substantially it will give false results. Suspect this problem when ICs gives a very strong signal compared to unstained cells. An example of a panel designed for a five color analysis of $CD45^+CD34^+IL-5Ra^+BrdU/7-AAD$ with FMO approach is shown in Table 1.

7. Alternative staining for Fc block exists, i.e., anti-mouse CD16/CD32 (BD Bioscience). We use normal mouse serum as a more relevant method that gives very good results.

Table 1
Sample antibody-panel designed for analysis of CD34⁺ eosinophil-lineage-committed cells in the mouse lung together with cell cycle analysis

	CD45 FITC	IL-5Ra PE	7-ADD (in PercP Channel)	BrdU-APC	CD34 Alexa Fluor 700
Samples	+	+	+	+	+
FC1	–	+	+	+	+
FC2	+	–	+	+	+
FC3	+	+	–	+	+
FC4	+	+	+	–	+
FC4	+	+	+	+	–
FC5	–	–	–	–	–

The first line represents the samples followed by the controls. The Fluorescence Minus One (FMO) approach is followed. The BrdU negative control represent cells that are stained for BrdU but originate from an animal not treated with BrdU

8. Prepare a mixture of all the required Abs that will be used the day before and keep refrigerated. This will save time and help reduce incubation times.

9. When you have large amounts of samples to acquire use PFA which permeabilizes cells and keeps them in good condition. However, as some antibodies–protein interactions are affected by this treatment it will be necessary to test this before adding PFA.

10. Although an isotype control for BrdU can also be used, we have found it is more accurate to use cells from an animal that has not received BrdU and then stained with BrdU.

11. It is preferable to perform this protocol over 2 days, since during the first day animal sampling is time-consuming.

12. If the FACS is not used on a weekly basis, be sure that it is working. Open it up, do a "wash" and a setup.

13. If evaluation of large populations is required the cells of origin can be used for compensation. However, if the cells are valuable, perform compensation before the data acquisition using beads. We also use cells to set FSC and SSC.

14. Cells can aggregate and generate "doublets" and therefore give false results. This may occur in any analysis, although the most sensitive is the DNA analysis. A "doublet" of two G_1 cells will appear as a single G_2/M cell. Another sensitive area is cell sorting, as a "doublet" of a negative and a positive cell will be sorted as a positive one. In order to avoid these problems we need to have a "doublet discrimination" strategy. Such strategy includes mechanical steps, e.g., filtration of the sample and sufficient vortexing of samples as well as actions during

acquisition and analysis. During acquisition of our samples, we register both "area" and "width" of the parameter of interest (i.e., FSC, FL-2, etc.). As doublets will need more time to pass the laser beam, they can be differentiated from the single one and excluded from the analysis.

Acknowledgements

The authors would like to thank Dr. Carina Malmhäll and Dr. You Lu, Krefting Research Centre, Gothenburg University for participating in the improvement and optimization of the Flow Cytometry protocols used at Krefting Research Centre and the generation of the original data showed in the figures.

References

1. Sehmi R, Baatjes AJ, Denburg JA (2003) Hemopoietic progenitor cells and hemopoietic factors: potential targets for treatment of allergic inflammatory diseases. Curr Drug Targets Inflamm Allergy 2:271–278

2. Radinger M, Lotvall J (2009) Eosinophil progenitors in allergy and asthma—do they matter? Pharmacol Ther 121:174–184

3. Sergejeva S, Johansson AK, Malmhall C, Lotvall J (2004) Allergen exposure-induced differences in CD34+ cell phenotype: relationship to eosinophilopoietic responses in different compartments. Blood 103:1270–1277

4. Iwasaki H, Mizuno S, Mayfield R, Shigematsu H, Arinobu Y et al (2005) Identification of eosinophil lineage-committed progenitors in the murine bone marrow. J Exp Med 201: 1891–1897

5. Robinson DS, Damia R, Zeibecoglou K, Molet S, North J et al (1999) CD34(+)/interleukin-5Ralpha messenger RNA+ cells in the bronchial mucosa in asthma: potential airway eosinophil progenitors. Am J Respir Cell Mol Biol 20:9–13

6. Menzies-Gow AN, Flood-Page PT, Robinson DS, Kay AB (2007) Effect of inhaled interleukin-5 on eosinophil progenitors in the bronchi and bone marrow of asthmatic and non-asthmatic volunteers. Clin Exp Allergy 37:1023–1032

7. Dorman SC, Efthimiadis A, Babirad I, Watson RM, Denburg JA et al (2004) Sputum CD34+ IL-5Ralpha+ cells increase after allergen: evidence for in situ eosinophilopoiesis. Am J Respir Crit Care Med 169:573–577

8. Southam DS, Widmer N, Ellis R, Hirota JA, Inman MD et al (2005) Increased eosinophil-lineage committed progenitors in the lung of allergen-challenged mice. J Allergy Clin Immunol 115:95–102

9. Punia N, Smith S, Thomson JV, Irshad A, Nair P et al (2012) Interleukin-4 and interleukin-13 prime migrational responses of haemopoietic progenitor cells to stromal cell-derived factor-1alpha. Clin Exp Allergy 42:255–264

10. Radinger M, Bossios A, Sjostrand M, Lu Y, Malmhall C et al (2011) Local proliferation and mobilization of CCR3(+) CD34(+) eosinophil-lineage-committed cells in the lung. Immunology 132:144–154

11. Dyer KD, Garcia-Crespo KE, Percopo CM, Sturm EM, Rosenberg HF (2013) Protocols for identifying, enumerating, and assessing mouse eosinophils. Methods Mol Biol 1032:59–77

12. Kuo HP, Wang CH, Lin HC, Hwang KS, Liu SL et al (2001) Interleukin-5 in growth and differentiation of blood eosinophil progenitors in asthma: effect of glucocorticoids. Br J Pharmacol 134:1539–1547

13. Herzenberg LA, Tung J, Moore WA, Parks DR (2006) Interpreting flow cytometry data: a guide for the perplexed. Nat Immunol 7:681–685

14. Wood B (2006) 9-color and 10-color flow cytometry in the clinical laboratory. Arch Pathol Lab Med 130:680–690

15. Freer G, Rindi L (2013) Intracellular cytokine detection by fluorescence-activated flow cytometry: basic principles and recent advances. Methods 61:30–38

Chapter 5

Eosinophil Cell Lines

Kenji Ishihara

Abstract

Eosinophilic cell lines, HL-60 clone 15 cells and EoL-1 cells, have contributed to clarifying the mechanisms responsible for differentiation into eosinophils. These cells differentiate into eosinophils by continuous histone acetylation. Histone deacetylase inhibitors, sodium butyrate and apicidin, promote the transactivation of various genes in these cells by causing the hyperacetylation of histones, resulting in the differentiation of cells into eosinophils. In contrast, transient acetylation by histone deacetylase inhibitors such as trichostatin A does not induce eosinophilic differentiation. This chapter describes the maintenance of HL-60 clone 15 cells and EoL-1 cells and induction of the differentiation of these cell lines into eosinophils by the histone deacetylase inhibitor sodium butyrate.

Key words Eosinophils, Eosinophilic cell line, HL-60 clone 15 cells, EoL-1 cells, Sodium butyrate, Histone, Acetylation

1 Introduction

Eosinophilic cell lines, HL-60 clone 15 cells and EoL-1 cells, have been widely used to characterize eosinophils and have contributed to the understanding of the regulation and function of eosinophils [1–4]. Since the cells were established in the 1980s, sodium butyrate has been widely used for their differentiation into mature eosinophils as the most powerful chemical inducer [1–4]. However, the mechanism by which HL-60 clone 15 cells and Eol-1 cells differentiate into eosinophils on exposure to sodium butyrate remained to be elucidated. In 2004 and 2007, my colleagues and I demonstrated that sodium butyrate induces the differentiation of HL-60 clone 15 cells and EoL-1 cells into eosinophils by continuously inhibiting deacetylation using various histone deacetylase inhibitors, such as sodium butyrate, apicidin, and trichostatin A [5, 6]. Therefore, continuous acetylation of histones is necessary for the differentiation of HL-60 clone 15 cells and EoL-1 cells into eosinophils.

Garry M. Walsh (ed.), *Eosinophils: Methods and Protocols*, Methods in Molecular Biology, vol. 1178, DOI 10.1007/978-1-4939-1016-8_5, © Springer Science+Business Media New York 2014

HL-60 clone 15 cells were established in 1988 by Fischkoff, S.A. through the long-term culture of HL-60 cells under alkaline conditions (pH 7.6) [1]. Fischkoff, S.A. and colleagues indicated that the cells matured in the presence of butyric acid at 0.5 mM [2, 3]. A high percentage of cells differentiated into eosinophils when incubated in RPMI-1640 medium under alkaline conditions (pH 7.6–7.8) with butyric acid at 0.5 mM for 7 days [1].

EoL-1 cells were reported in 1985 by Saito, H. et al. [4]. This human eosinophilic leukemia cell line was established from the peripheral blood of a 33-year-old man suffering from Philadelphia chromosome-negative eosinophilic leukemia [4]. EoL-1 cells are maintained in RPMI-1640 medium supplemented with 10 % (v/v) FCS, and the cultivation of EoL-1 cells under alkaline conditions (pH 8.0) increased the eosinophilic rate to about 40 % [4]. In 2003, it was reported that peripheral cells from some patients with hypereosinophilic syndrome and EoL-1 cells have a fusion gene generated by the interstitial deletion of the fip1-like 1 (FIP1L1) gene and platelet-derived growth factor receptor (PDGFR) A gene, termed FIP1L1-PDGFRA [7–10]. The gene's product, FIP1L1-PDGFRα, is a constitutively activated tyrosine kinase and induces cell proliferation [8, 9]. Therefore, EoL-1 cells have also contributed to research as a model for chronic eosinophilic leukemia expressing FIP1L1-PDGFRα.

2   Materials

Prepare all solutions using ultrapure water (prepared by purifying deionized water to attain a sensitivity of 18 M Ω cm at 25 °C).

2.1   Preparation of RPMI-1640 Medium (pH 7.8)

RPMI-1640 medium (pH 7.8) is used for the maintenance of HL-60 clone 15 cells and for induction of the differentiation of HL-60 clone 15 cells and EoL-1 cells into eosinophils (*see* **Note 1**).

1. Add about 900 ml of water to a glass beaker. While stirring water, add the powdered RPMI-1640 medium.

2. Add sodium bicarbonate, L-glutamine, HEPES, and/or antibiotics to the medium according to the instructions accompanying the medium if necessary. The final concentration of HEPES is 25 mM (5.96 g/L). Stir until dissolved.

3. Adjust the pH to 7.8 with 1 N NaOH or 1 N HCl.

4. Adjust the final volume (1 L) with water.

5. Sterilize the medium immediately by membrane filtration with a 0.22-μm filter using a positive pressure system. Aseptically dispense the medium into a sterile container. Finally, store the medium at 4 °C.

2.2 Preparation
of RPMI-1640 Medium
(pH 7.2)

RPMI-1640 medium (pH 7.2) is used for the maintenance of EoL-1 cells. RPMI-1640 medium is generally available as liquid medium for cell culture. Alternatively, preparation from powdered RPMI-1640 medium is as follows:

1. Add about 900 ml of water to a glass beaker. While stirring the water, add the powdered RPMI-1640 medium.

2. Add sodium bicarbonate, L-glutamine, and/or antibiotics to the medium according to the instructions accompanying the medium if necessary. Stir until dissolved.

3. Adjust the pH to 7.2 with 1 N NaOH or 1 N HCl.

4. Adjust the final volume (1 L) with water.

5. Sterilize the medium immediately by membrane filtration with a 0.22-μm filter using a positive pressure system. Aseptically dispense the medium into a sterile container. Finally, store the medium at 4 °C.

2.3 Chemical
Inducer for the
Differentiation
of Eosinophils

1. Sodium butyrate: Dissolve in water. The concentration of stock solution is 0.5 M. Store at –20 °C (*see* **Note 2**).

---

3 Methods

3.1 Maintenance
of HL-60 Clone 15
Cells and EoL-1 Cells

HL-60 clone 15 cells may be obtained from the American Type Culture Collection, MD, USA (CRL-1964). EoL-1 cells may be obtained from RIKEN Cell Bank, Tsukuba, Japan (RCB0641). RPMI-1640 medium (pH 7.8 and 7.2) supplemented with 10 % FBS is used for the maintenance of HL-60 clone 15 cells and EoL-1 cells, respectively.

1. After thawing the frozen cells in a water bath at 37 °C, immediately transfer the cell suspension into a conical tube containing 5 ml of medium.

2. Centrifuge the tube for 5 min at $300 \times g$. Remove the medium completely.

3. Break the cell pellet by finger tapping. Gently resuspend the cells in 5 ml of medium and centrifuge for 5 min at $300 \times g$. Remove the medium completely.

4. Add 5 ml of medium to the conical tube, and transfer the cells to a 60-mm culture dish. Incubate at 37 °C under 5 % CO_2 for 1 day.

5. On the next day, collect the medium containing cells incubated in a 60-mm culture dish in a conical tube, and centrifuge for 5 min at $300 \times g$. Remove the culture medium completely.

6. Add an appropriate volume of medium to the cells in the conical tube. If necessary, dilute the cells with medium. Then, count the number of cells with a hemocytometer.

7. After centrifugation of the cells for 5 min at $300 \times g$, remove the medium completely.

8. Seed at a density of 1×10^5 HL-60 clone 15 cells/ml or 5×10^4 EoL-1 cells/ml in the flasks, plates, or dishes, and incubate at 37 °C under 5 % CO_2 for 3 days.

3.2 Induction of Differentiation of HL-60 Clone 15 Cells and EoL-1 Cells into Eosinophils

1. View the cultures using a microscope. Use for experiments when the cells are bright and round. If the cells are overgrown, they should be reseeded and incubated according to Subheading 3.1.

2. Collect the medium containing cells in a conical tube, and centrifuge for 5 min at $300 \times g$. Remove the culture medium completely.

3. Resuspend the cells in medium and centrifuge for 5 min at $300 \times g$. Remove the medium completely.

4. Add an appropriate volume of medium to the cells in a conical tube. If necessary, dilute the cells with medium. Then, count the number of cells with a hemocytometer.

5. After centrifugation of the cells for 5 min at $300 \times g$, remove the medium completely.

6. Add 10 % FBS-RPMI-1640 medium (pH 7.8) to the conical tube to final densities of 2×10^5 cells/ml (HL-60 clone 15 cells) and of 1×10^5 cells/ml (EoL-1 cells).

7. Dilute sodium butyrate with 10 % FBS-RPMI-1640 medium (pH 7.8) in a new conical tube to a concentration of 1 mM.

8. Add the same volume of medium containing cells (**step 6**) and the medium containing inducer (**step 7**) to the flasks, plates, or dishes labeled with the name of the cell line and date, etc. The final density of HL-60 clone 15 cells and EoL-1 cells is 1×10^5 cells/ml and 5×10^4 cells/ml, respectively. The final concentration of sodium butyrate is 500 μM.

9. Incubate at 37 °C under 5 % CO_2 for 6 days.

10. After incubation, confirm that eosinophils have differentiated from the cell lines by staining using May-Grünwald Giemsa or Luxol fast blue and the levels of expression of cell surface molecules using a flow cytometer [5, 6] (*see* **Note 3**).

---

4 Notes

1. Eosinophilic differentiation of these cell lines is induced accompanied with growth arrest. Therefore, the pH of medium on culture in the presence of inducer (sodium butyrate) is

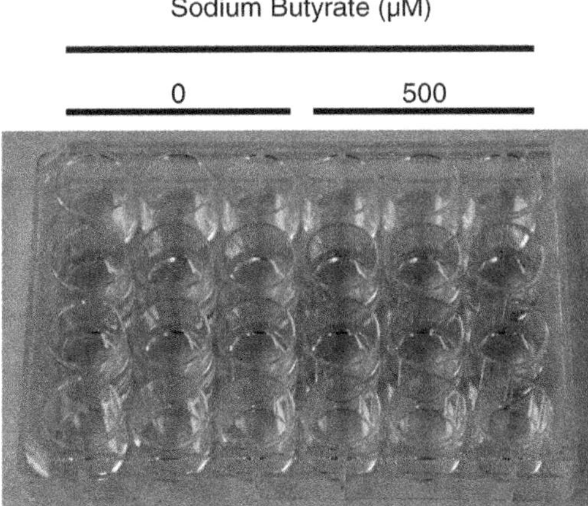

Fig. 1 Colors of medium after 6-day incubation of HL-60 clone 15 cells. HL-60 clone 15 cells (1×10^5 cells) were incubated at 37 °C for 6 days in 1 ml of RPMI-1640 medium containing 10 % FBS in the presence or the absence of 500 µM sodium butyrate

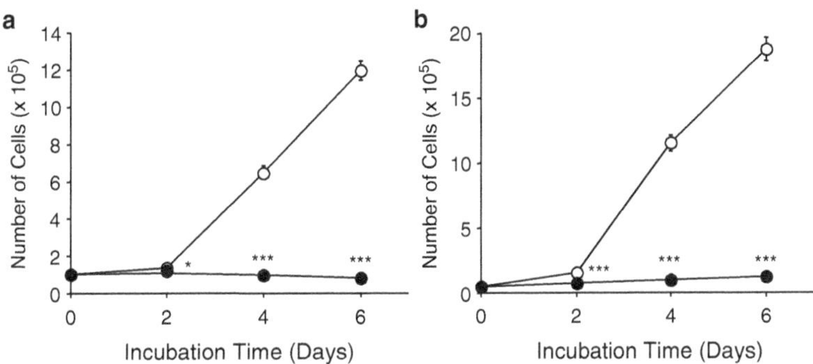

Fig. 2 Effects of sodium butyrate on the proliferation of HL-60 clone 15 cells and EoL-1 cells. (**a**) HL-60 clone 15 cells (1×10^5 cells) or (**b**) EoL-1 cells (5×10^4 cells) were incubated at 37 °C for the periods indicated in 1 ml of RPMI-1640 medium containing 10 % FBS in the presence (*closed circles*) or the absence (*open circles*) of 500 µM sodium butyrate. $*p < 0.05$, $***p < 0.001$ vs. corresponding vehicle control

higher than that of cells cultured in the absence of inducer. The progress of differentiation is clear to see if using the medium containing phenol red (Figs. 1 and 2).

2. The molecular weight of sodium butyrate (Sigma B5887-1G, Wako 193-01522) is 110.09. Dissolve 1 g of sodium butyrate in 18.2 ml of water. Sterilize this solution by membrane filtration with a 0.22-µm filter using a positive pressure system. The final concentration of this solution is 500 mM.

3. Figure 3 shows microscopic observation of HL-60 clone 15 cells and EoL-1 cells after incubation for 6 days in the medium

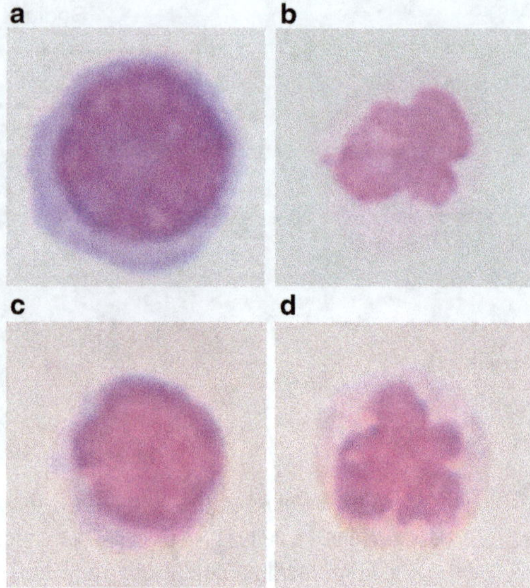

Fig. 3 Microscopic observation of HL-60 clone 15 cells and EoL-1 cells. (**a, b**) HL-60 clone 15 cells (1×10^5 cells) or (**c, d**) EoL-1 cells (5×10^4 cells) were incubated at 37 °C for the periods indicated in 1 ml of RPMI-1640 medium containing 10 % FBS in the presence (**b, d**) or the absence (**a, c**) of 500 µM sodium butyrate. After incubation, the cells were harvested, smeared on slide glasses, and stained with May-Grünwald Giemsa (×400)

with or without 500 µM sodium butyrate. Sodium butyrate changes the shape of the nucleus with increased cytoplasmic area staining with May-Grünwald Giemsa.

Acknowledgement

This work was supported by a grant-in-aid for Young Scientists (B) from the Ministry of Education, Culture, Sports, Science and Technology (MEXT) (23791098).

References

1. Fischkoff SA, Pollak A, Gleich GJ, Testa JR, Misawa S, Reber TJ (1984) Eosinophilic differentiation of the human promyelocytic leukemia cell line, HL-60. J Exp Med 160: 179–196

2. Fischkoff SA, Condon ME (1985) Switch in differentiative response to maturation inducers of human promyelocytic leukemia cells by prior exposure to alkaline conditions. Cancer Res 45: 2065–2069

3. Fischkoff SA (1988) Graded increase in probability of eosinophilic differentiation of HL-60 promyelocytic leukemia cells induced by culture under alkaline conditions. Leuk Res 12: 679–686

4. Saito H, Bourinbaiar A, Ginsburg M, Minato K, Ceresi E, Yamada K, Machover D, Bréard J, Mathé G (1985) Establishment and characterization of a new human eosinophilic leukemia cell line. Blood 66:1233–1240

5. Ishihara K, Hong J, Zee O, Ohuchi K (2004) Possible mechanism of action of the histone deacetylase inhibitors for the induction of differentiation of HL-60 clone 15 cells into eosinophils. Br J Pharmacol 142:1020–1030

6. Ishihara K, Takahashi A, Kaneko M, Sugeno H, Hirasawa N, Hong J, Zee O, Ohuchi K (2007) Differentiation of eosinophilic leukemia EoL-1 cells into eosinophils induced by histone deacetylase inhibitors. Life Sci 80:1213–1220

7. Cools J, DeAngelo DJ, Gotlib J, Stover EH, Legare RD, Cortes J, Kutok J, Clark J, Galinsky I, Griffin JD, Cross NC, Tefferi A, Malone J, Alam R, Schrier SL, Schmid J, Rose M, Vandenberghe P, Verhoef G, Boogaerts M, Wlodarska I, Kantarjian H, Marynen P, Coutre SE, Stone R, Gilliland DG (2003) A tyrosine kinase created by fusion of the PDGFRA and FIP1L1 genes as a therapeutic target of imatinib in idiopathic hypereosinophilic syndrome. N Engl J Med 348:1201–1214

8. Griffin JH, Leung J, Bruner RJ, Caligiuri MA, Briesewitz R (2003) Discovery of a fusion kinase in EOL-1 cells and idiopathic hypereosinophilic syndrome. Proc Natl Acad Sci U S A 100:7830–7835

9. Cools J, Quentmeier H, Huntly BJ, Marynen P, Griffin JD, Drexler HG, Gilliland DG (2004) The EOL-1 cell line as an in vitro model for the study of FIP1L1-PDGFRA-positive chronic eosinophilic leukemia. Blood 103:2802–2805

10. Gotlib J, Cools J (2008) Five years since the discovery of FIP1L1-PDGFRA: what we have learned about the fusion and other molecularly defined eosinophilias. Leukemia 22:1999–2010

Chapter 6

Cell Signalling During Human Eosinophil Differentiation

Miranda Buitenhuis

Abstract

Eosinophil differentiation is a complex series of events regulated by cytokines at multiple levels, including proliferation, survival, and maturation. The development of an ex vivo eosinophil differentiation model, using the current knowledge on factors involved in this process, has facilitated efforts to understand the molecular mechanisms underlying human eosinophil development. Differentiation of human hematopoietic progenitor cells, isolated by density centrifugation and immunomagnetic cell separation, towards mature eosinophils, involves a 17-day culture period in the presence of a mixture of cytokines. At early stages of differentiation, these cells can be retrovirally transduced resulting in modulation of the expression of genes of interest to examine their role in eosinophil development. Eosinophil maturation can be analyzed by combining three different methods: histochemical analysis, flow cytometric analysis, and Luxol Fast Blue staining. In addition to this ex vivo differentiation model, human hematopoietic progenitors can be transplanted into immune-deficient mice resulting in the development of all human hematopoietic lineages in the mouse bone marrow, including eosinophils. Although the ex vivo differentiation model can be used separately, combining it with the transplantation model will give insight into not only regulation of human eosinophil development but also hematopoiesis in general.

Key words Human eosinophil differentiation, Hematopoietic progenitors, CD34, Retroviral transduction, Flow cytometric analysis, β2-Microglobulin (–/–) NOD/SCID mice, Histochemical analysis

1 Introduction

The production of blood cells, or "hematopoiesis," is a complex series of events that predominantly occurs in the bone marrow of the trabecular bone and results in the formation of all blood lineages. Hematopoietic stem cells (HSCs) are defined as cells which can both self-renew and differentiate towards all hematopoietic lineages, including eosinophils. Similar to mouse HSCs, the human HSC pool can be divided into two different subpopulations based on their functionality: long-term reconstituting HSCs (LT-HSCs) and short-term reconstituting HSCs (ST-HSCs) [1]. Via a multipotent progenitor (MPP), ST-HSCs can differentiate into two distinct

Garry M. Walsh (ed.), *Eosinophils: Methods and Protocols*, Methods in Molecular Biology, vol. 1178,
DOI 10.1007/978-1-4939-1016-8_6, © Springer Science+Business Media New York 2014

committed progenitor cells, the common lymphoid progenitor [2] and common myeloid progenitor (CMP) [3], which are themselves capable of differentiating towards a subset of hematopoietic lineages. The CMP can differentiate towards the megakaryocyte/erythrocyte progenitor (MEP), granulocyte/macrophage progenitor (GMP), and committed eosinophil progenitor (Eo-P) [4], eventually resulting in the development of all myeloid lineages.

Although relatively high numbers of HSCs (0.5–3 %) can be observed in the bone marrow, HSCs can also be detected in peripheral blood (0.05–0.2 %) and umbilical cord blood (UCB) (0.1–0.5 %). In order to isolate HSCs from these sources, knowledge of the expression profiles of specific cell surface markers, including the sialomucin-like adhesion molecule CD34, is required. The human HSC population is characterized by the absence of lineage-specific markers and CD38 and the presence of CD34 and CD90 (Lin$^-$CD34$^+$CD38$^{-/lo}$CD90$^+$) [1]. Although CD34 expression is high on HSCs and is downregulated upon differentiation towards mature blood cells, hematopoietic progenitors, including CLPs [2], CMPs, GMPs, MEPs [3], and Eo-Ps [4], still express CD34 on their membrane. Antibodies directed against CD34 are generally used to isolate HSCs and those hematopoietic progenitor cells from UCB or bone marrow. These cells can be efficiently enriched to, at least, 95 % by density centrifugation over a Ficoll-Paque solution (density 1.077 g/mL) followed by immunomagnetic cell separation.

Eosinophil differentiation requires the presence of specific growth factors at different stages of development. Growth factors, such as FLT-3 L and, to a lesser extent, stem cell factor (SCF) play an important role in survival of human HSCs [5]. In addition, while the cytokines IL-3 and GM-CSF are important for regulation of proliferation and survival during differentiation of various myeloid lineages, including eosinophils, maturation of eosinophils requires the presence of IL-5 [6, 7]. An ex vivo eosinophil differentiation model has been developed utilizing this knowledge, which allows us to study the molecular mechanisms underlying eosinophil development from primary human hematopoietic progenitors. The details of this model are discussed below.

Results obtained with this differentiation model have been discussed in multiple publications [8–16]. Cytokines play an important role in directing cell fate decisions during lineage development, suggesting that the activity of cytokine-specific effectors must be regulated. Using the above-described ex vivo culture model, it has, for example, been shown that the IL-5Rα-associated protein syntenin is important for normal eosinophil development [13]. Using the same model, the roles of generally regulated molecules, such as protein kinase B (PKB/c-Akt) and p38MAPK, in regulation of eosinophil development have been successfully investigated. Although the activity of both PKB and p38MAPK is induced upon cytokine stimulation, these molecules appear to counteract each other in regulation of eosinophil development. Whereas activation of p38MAPK positively regulates eosinophil differentiation, inhibition of PKB activity appears to be required to induce final maturation of eosinophils [12]. This differential effect on eosinophil development suggests that the balance between inhibitory and activating signals induced by cytokines determines whether or not a progenitor cell becomes a mature eosinophil. Although IL-5 is essential for normal eosinophil development, our results indicate that it is not sufficient to complete eosinophil maturation [12]. It is therefore likely that additional signals, potentially provided by stromal cells in the bone marrow microenvironment, are required to induce terminal maturation of eosinophils.

This suggested that a more physiological model may be required to study eosinophil development. To determine whether the results obtained with our ex vivo culture model could be replicated under more physiological conditions, a mouse transplantation model has been developed utilizing β2-microglobulin (–/–) non-obese diabetic/severe combined immune-deficient (NOD/SCID) mice. It had been described that, in comparison to NOD/SCID mice, engraftment levels are enhanced in these mice, 6 weeks after transplantation. In addition, it had been shown that, in comparison to NOD/SCID mice, human blood cell development in the bone marrow of β2-microglobulin (–/–) NOD/SCID mice is less skewed towards lymphoid development [17, 18]. Since these two characteristics are essential to study human myelopoiesis in a mouse model, it was decided to use β2-microglobulin (–/–) NOD/SCID mice for transplantation studies. Importantly, our results revealed that human eosinophils can mature in the bone marrow of these mice [12]. Even though in our ex vivo differentiation model potentially important signals provided by the bone marrow microenvironment are absent, the in vivo transplantation studies yielded similar results [10, 12, 15]. This suggests that the ex vivo differentiation model itself provides a strong model to study human eosinophil development, especially in comparison to regularly used leukemic cell lines. The opportunity to not only examine eosinophil development but also study the effect on other hematopoietic lineages in the same experiment is of course a strong advantage of the mouse model in comparison to the ex vivo differentiation model and provides important additional information on hematopoiesis in general. To fully understand the roles of specific genes in regulation of eosinophil development, it is therefore important to combine both models.

2   Materials

All procedures, where UCB- or bone marrow-derived hematopoietic progenitors were used, were performed after protocols were approved by the local ethics committees and informed consent was provided according to the Declaration of Helsinki. Experiments with β2-microglobulin (–/–) NOD/SCID mice were performed only after protocols were approved by the local ethics committees.

2.1   Isolation of CD34⁺ Cells from Umbilical Cord Blood or Bone Marrow

1. Anticoagulant: 0.109 M Tri-sodium citrate dihydrate solution. Dissolve 32 g Tri-sodium citrate dihydrate in 1 L of H_2O. Filter the solution (0.2 μm). For 125 ml jars use 13.9 ml of anticoagulant.

2. 50 ml Tubes, 15 ml tubes, and Eppendorf tubes.

3. Phosphate-buffered saline (PBS).

4. Ficoll-Paque solution (density 1.077 g/ml).

5. Trypan blue and a counting chamber.

6. Erythrocyte lysis buffer: 155 mM NH_4Cl, 10 mM $KHCO_3$, 0.1 mM Na_2EDTA, and phenol red. Dissolve 8.3 g NH_4Cl, 1.0 g $KHCO_3$, 37.5 mg Na_2EDTA, and a few granules of phenol red in 980 ml dH_2O. Cool down the bottle overnight to 4 °C, and set the pH to 7.4. Fill up with H_2O to 1 L. Determine the osmolarity (<310 mOsm). Sterilize solution by filtration (0.2 μm) and store at 4 °C.

7. RPMI supplemented with 9 % Hyclone FetalClone I serum.

8. Isolation buffer: 2 mM EDTA and 0.5 % BSA in PBS. Sterilize the buffer by filtration (0.2 μm) and store at 4 °C.

9. MACS immunomagnetic cell separation kit (Miltenyi Biotech, Auburn, USA) containing an FcR blocking reagent and MicroBeads conjugated to monoclonal mouse anti-human CD34 antibodies and rotation wheel.

10. MACS® Cell Separation MS Columns and MiniMACS Separator.

11. Antibody incubation buffer; PBS supplemented with 5 % Hyclone FetalClone I serum.

12. CD34 antibody, 7-AAD or DAPI, flow cytometer.

2.2   Cryopreservation and Thawing of CD34⁺ Cells

1. Cryovials and a Mr. Frosty freezing container.

2. Iscove's Modified Dulbecco's Medium supplemented with 9 % Hyclone FetalClone I serum.

3. Freezing medium: Hyclone FetalClone I serum containing 10 % DMSO.

4. RPMI supplemented with 9 % Hyclone FetalClone I serum.

5. 10 mg/ml DNAseI grade II in H_2O.

6. 1 M $MgCl_2$ in H_2O.

2.3 Ex Vivo Eosinophil Differentiation

1. Culture plastics: Suspension-Culture Multiwell Plates (24-, 12-, and 6-well format) and 25 cm^2 flasks for Suspension cell culture (Greiner).

2. Hematopoietic progenitor cell culture medium: Iscove's Modified Dulbecco's Medium supplemented with 9 % Hyclone FetalClone I serum, 50 μM β-mercaptoethanol, 10 U/ml penicillin, 10 μg/ml streptomycin, and 2 mM glutamine. Filter the medium (0.2 μm).

3. Cytokines: SCF (final concentration: 50 ng/ml), FLT-3 ligand (final concentration: 50 ng/ml), GM-CSF (final concentration: 0.1 nmol/l), IL-3 (final concentration: 0.1 nmol/l), and IL-5 (final concentration: 0.1 nmol/l).

2.4 Transplantation of β2-Microglobulin (–/–) NOD/SCID Mice with Human CD34+ Cells

1. β2-Microglobulin (–/–) NOD/SCID mice.

2. Microisolator cages, Autoclaved food, Acidified water containing 111 mg/l Ciprofloxacin (Ciproxin®).

3. A ^{137}Cs source to irradiate mice and cells.

4. Culture medium (*see* Subheading 2.3).

5. Erythrocyte lysis buffer: 0.8 % NH_4Cl and 0.1 mM EDTA.

6. Antibody incubation buffer: PBS supplemented with 5 % Hyclone FetalClone I serum.

7. Blocking reagent: 5 % Hyclone FetalClone I serum and 5 % Fc block (anti-mouse CD16/32 antibodies) in PBS.

8. FACS buffer: 5 % Hyclone FetalClone I serum and a reagent to exclude nonviable cells, such as 7-AAD or DAPI, in PBS.

9. Mouse Ig,κ BD Compbead compensation particles (Becton Dickenson).

2.5 Manipulation of Eosinophil Progenitors

1. Culture plates/flasks for adherent cells: 6-Well plates, 75 cm^2 flasks.

2. Culture plates for non-adherent cells: Suspension-Culture Multiwell Plates (24 Well Format) (Greiner).

3. Phoenix-Ampho cells (available at ATCC), wild-type 293 T cells and plasmids: LZRS-EGFP or MSCV-EGFP and pCL ampho.

4. Adherent cell culture medium: DMEM supplemented with 9 % Hyclone FetalClone I serum, 10 U/ml penicillin, and 10 μg/ml streptomycin.

5. 0.25 mM $CaCl_2$ in water.

6. HBSP solution: 280 mM NaCl, 10 mM KCl, 50 mM Hepes, 1.6 mM $Na_2HPO_4 \cdot H_2O$, and 10 mM glucose. For 500 ml of

HBSP solution dissolve 8 g NaCl, 37 g KCl, 5 g Hepes, 0.0125 g $Na_2HPO_4 \cdot H_2O$, and 1 g glucose. Set the pH to 7.05 at room temperature.

7. PBS.

8. Puromycin.

9. Hematopoietic progenitor cell culture medium: Iscove's Modified Dulbecco's Medium supplemented with 9 % Hyclone FetalClone I serum, 50 μM β-mercaptoethanol, 10 U/ml penicillin, 10 μg/ml streptomycin, and 2 mM glutamine. Filter the medium (0.2 μm).

10. 0.2 μm Filter, cryovials, liquid nitrogen.

11. FuGENE-6 Transfection Reagent.

12. Retronectin : 1.25 μg/cm^2 Recombinant human fibronectin fragment CH-296 (RetroNectin; Takara, Otsu, Japan) in PBS.

2.6   Histochemical Staining of Eosinophil Progenitors

1. Microscope slides, cover slips, cytocentrifuge, disposable sample chambers (funnels).

2. PBS.

3. Methanol.

4. Buffered water: 11.7 mM NaOH and 20 mM $NaH_2PO_4 \cdot H_2O$. Dissolve 0.464 g NaOH and 2.76 g $NaH_2PO_4 \cdot H_2O$ in 1 L H_2O. Adjust pH to 7.0.

5. Eosin methylene blue solution according to May-Grunwald: 50 % May-Grunwald solution in buffered water.

6. 10 % Giemsa solution in buffered water.

7. Mounting solution: Entellan.

2.7   Luxol Fast Blue Staining

1. Microscope slides, cover slips, cytocentrifuge, disposable sample chambers (funnels).

2. PBS.

3. Fixative: Mix 3 ml of 25 % (w/w) glutaraldehyde and 97 ml MilliQ water.

4. Luxol Fast Blue staining solution: Prepare urea-saturated ethanol by adding urea to 1 L 70 % ethanol at room temperature while continuous stirring until saturation occurs (overnight mixing may be necessary). Dissolve 0.3 g Luxol Fast Blue subsequently in 200 ml urea-saturated ethanol.

5. Entellan.

2.8   Multicolor Flow Cytometric Analysis for Ex Vivo-Differentiated Cells

1. FACS tubes, antibodies, DAPI.

2. Antibody incubation buffer: PBS supplemented with 5 % Hyclone FetalClone I serum.

3. FACS buffer: 5 % Hyclone Fetal Clone I serum and a reagent to exclude nonviable cells, such as 7-AAD or DAPI, in PBS.

4. Mouse Ig,κ BD Compbead compensation particles (BD).

5. Flow-Count Fluorospheres (Beckman Coulter).

3 Methods

3.1 Isolation of CD34⁺ Cells from Umbilical Cord Blood or Bone Marrow

1. Collect umbilical cord blood or bone marrow (*see* Subheading 2.1, **item 1**) (*see* **Note 1**). Store the cells at room temperature until used.

2. Dilute UCB (or bone marrow) with sterile PBS (blood:PBS = 1:3).

3. Pipet 13 ml of Ficoll-Paque solution in 50 ml tubes. To enlarge the Ficoll-Paque surface, tilt the tube until it is almost horizontal. Carefully transfer 35 ml of the diluted blood or bone marrow onto the Ficoll-Paque solution without disturbing the Ficoll-Paque layer (*see* **Note 2**).

4. Centrifuge the tubes for 20 min at $872 \times g$ (brake low/off) to separate the mononuclear cells and hematopoietic stem and progenitor cells from the other cell types (*see* **Note 3**).

5. Remove most of the PBS-diluted plasma layer (upper layer). Collect the white interface which contains mononuclear cells and CD34⁺ cells. Dilute the collected interface with PBS (1:1) and centrifuge for 7 min at $872 \times g$.

6. When the interface appears to contain a very high number of erythrocytes, an erythrocyte lysis buffer can be used to remove most of the erythrocytes (if not necessary, continue with **step 7**). Resuspend the cells in 20 ml of ice-cold lysis buffer (*see* Subheading 2.1, **item 6**) and incubate on ice for 5 min. Subsequently centrifuge the cells for 7 min at $872 \times g$ (*see* **Note 4**) and wash once with PBS.

7. Resuspend the pellet in 14 ml RPMI supplemented with 9 % Hyclone FetalClone I serum, and determine the number of cells by trypan blue exclusion.

8. Centrifuge the cells for 7 min at 872 rpm, resuspend the pellet in 10 ml ice-cold (4 °C) isolation buffer (*see* Subheading 2.1, **item 8**), and centrifuge again for 7 min at $872 \times g$.

9. Resuspend the cells in 300 μl ice-cold isolation buffer (*see* Subheading 2.1, **item 8**). Add 100 μl blocking reagent and 100 μl CD34 antibody-coated beads to the cells (*see* Subheading 2.1, **item 9**), mix, and incubate for 30 min at 4 °C on a rotating wheel. The volumes for magnetic labelling and cell separation mentioned below are for up to 2.10^8 mononuclear cells. When working with higher cell numbers, adjust accordingly.

Table 1
Isolation of CD34⁺ cells from umbilical cord blood

Time of isolation after collection	MNC (×10⁶)/ml UCB	CD34/10⁸MNC	CD34/ml UCB	N=
0–24 h	60.3±6.2	352,657±25,234	22,166±1,428	100
24–48 h	65.9±21.6	264,990±77,969	17,469±2,114	47
48–72 h	73.0±12.9	247,586±54,321	18,076±1,668	33

10. Add 1 ml isolation buffer to the tube, and centrifuge for 7 min at $425 \times g$. Resuspend the pellet in 1 ml isolation buffer.

11. Place the MS column in the magnetic separator (*see* Subheading 2.1, **item 10**), and equilibrate the column with 500 µl isolation buffer (*see* **Note 5**).

12. Resuspend the cells in 1 ml isolation buffer, apply the cell suspension on an MS Column, and allow the cells to pass through the column.

13. Wash the column three consecutive times with 500 µl isolation buffer.

14. Remove the column from the magnetic separator, add 1 ml isolation buffer to the column, and elute the CD34⁺ cells from the column using the plunger.

15. To further improve the purity of the CD34⁺ cells, repeat **steps 12–14** once.

16. Determine the amount of viable CD34⁺ cells using trypan blue exclusion, and put the cells in culture (*see* Subheading 3.3) or freeze the cells (*see* Subheading 3.2). *See* Table 1 for expected cell numbers.

17. Determine the percentage of CD34⁺ cells after isolation using flow cytometric analysis. Incubate the cells together with a CD34 antibody (*see* **Notes 6** and 7), in antibody incubation buffer (*see* Subheading 2.1, **item 11**), on ice for 30 min. Subsequently wash the cells once, resuspend the cells in antibody incubation buffer, add a viability reagent such as 7-AAD of DAPI, and analyze by FACS. A purity of >95 % can be expected.

3.2 Cryopreservation and Thawing of CD34⁺ Cells

1. Centrifuge the CD34⁺ cells (*see* **Note 8**) for 5 min at $425 \times g$. Resuspend the cells in 500 µl of IMDM supplemented with 9 % Hyclone FetalClone I serum, transfer the cells to cryovials, and put the cells on ice.

2. Dropwise add 500 µl freezing medium (*see* Subheading 2.2, **item 3**) (*see* **Note 9**), mix, and freeze the cells using a

Mr. Frosty freezing container at −80 °C. Upon freezing, store the cells in liquid nitrogen or a −150 °C fridge.

3. Thaw the vials quickly in a 37 °C water bath until a small piece of ice is left, rinse the vials with 70 % ethanol, transfer the cells to a 50 ml tube containing 19 ml of IMDM supplemented with 9 % Hyclone FetalClone I serum, and subsequently centrifuge for 7 min at $872 \times g$.

4. Resuspend the pellet in 20 ml IMDM supplemented with 9 % Hyclone FetalClone I serum. Add 200 µl 10 mg/ml DNAse and 200 µl 1 M $MgCl_2$ to the cells (*see* **Note 10**).

5. Incubate for (at least) 30 min at 37 °C. During this period, mix the cells every 10 min. Centrifuge for 7 min at $872 \times g$.

6. Resuspend the cells in hematopoietic progenitor cell culture medium (*see* Subheading 2.3, **item 2**). Determine the quantity of viable $CD34^+$ cells using trypan blue exclusion.

3.3 Ex Vivo Eosinophil Differentiation

1. Centrifuge the cells, remove the isolation buffer, and resuspend the cells in hematopoietic progenitor cell culture medium (*see* Subheading 2.3, **item 2**) at a density of 0.25×10^6 cells/ml.

2. Add the following cytokines to the cells: SCF, FLT-3 ligand, GM-CSF, IL-3, and IL-5 (for concentrations *see* Subheading 2.3, **item 3**).

3. Culture cells at 37 °C in a humidified incubator containing 5 % CO_2 (for retroviral transduction of the cells, continue with Subheading 3.4).

4. At day 3 of culture, count the cells, and add fresh medium to a density of 0.3×10^6 cells/ml.

   Add IL-3 and IL-5 (for concentrations *see* Subheading 2.3, **item 3**) to the cells (*see* **Note 11**).

5. At days 7, 10, and 14 of culture, count the cells, and add fresh medium to a density of 0.5×10^6 cells/ml. Add IL-3 and IL-5 (for concentrations *see* Subheading 2.3, **item 3**) to the cells. A 440-fold increase in cell numbers can be expected during the 17-day culture period (Fig. 1).

6. At day 17 of culture, count the cells and analyze eosinophil differentiation.

3.4 Transplantation of β2-Microglobulin (−/−) NOD/SCID Mice with Human CD34⁺ Cells

1. To study human eosinophil development in a mouse model, use β2-microglobulin (−/−) NOD/SCID mice (*see* **Note 12**).

2. Sublethally irradiate 8–10-week-old mice with 250 cGy administered from a ^{137}Cs source.

3. Between 2 and 8 h after irradiation, transplant the mice, via tail vein injections, with 500,000 (unsorted retrovirally transduced) cord blood-derived hematopoietic progenitors along with

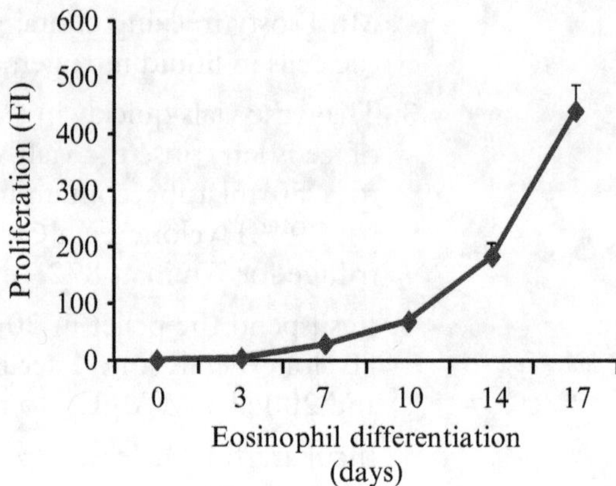

Fig. 1 Expansion of cells during ex vivo eosinophil differentiation. CD34[+] cells were cultured in the presence of IL-3 and IL-5 for 17 days to induce eosinophil differentiation. Expansion was determined by counting the trypan blue-negative cell population. *Error bars* represent SEM (*n* > 10)

1. 10^6 irradiated (6,000 cGy) CD34-depleted cord blood-derived accessory cells (if frozen, *see* Subheading 3.2, **steps 3–6**, for thawing). The volume of the cells should not exceed 0.5 ml medium.

4. Sacrifice the mice, 6 weeks after transplantation. Subsequently, flush both tibiae and femora (*see* **Notes 13** and **14**). Count the cells. Centrifuge at $425 \times g$ for 5 min. Resuspend the cells in 0.5 ml of lysis buffer (*see* Subheading 2.4, **item 5**) to remove the erythrocytes. After 1-min incubation on ice, add 1 ml antibody incubation buffer (*see* Subheading 2.4, **item 6**) to the cells. Centrifuge at $872 \times g$ for 5 min. Resuspend the pellet in blocking reagent (*see* Subheading 2.4, **item 7**) to block nonspecific binding of antibodies, incubate for 15 min on ice, divide the cells, and continue with **steps 5, 6**, and **7** (*see* **Note 15**).

5. To calculate differences in engraftment levels, determine the percentage of EGFP-positive cells within the human CD45[+] population in the mouse bone marrow by FACS and compare this to the transduction efficiency before transplantation (*see* **Note 16**). Add CD45 antibody in the optimal concentration (*see* **Note 6**), and incubate for 30 min on ice in the dark. Add 1 ml PBS, and centrifuge for 5 min at $425 \times g$. Resuspend in 300 µl of FACS buffer (*see* Subheading 2.4, **item 8**), and analyze by flow cytometer.

6. To determine lineage development in vivo, perform multicolor flow cytometric analysis using antibodies directed against CD19 (B lymphocytes), CD14 (monocytes), CD49d (lymphocytes, monocytes, and eosinophils), and Siglec-8 [19, 20] according to Subheading 3.8, **steps 1–4**. *See* Table 2 for the expected percentages of different human cells within the

Table 2
Development of human hematopoietic cells in the mouse bone marrow after transplantation

	Eosinophils		Neutrophils	Monocyte	B lymphocyte
Detection method	Luxol Fast Blue	Giemsa May-Grunwald	Giemsa May-Grunwald	CD14	CD19
Percentage	2.70±0.66	3.09±0.79	5.45±1.34	9.39±3.25	22.94±3.54

human fraction of cells in the mouse bone marrow (when cells were transduced with empty vector control virus).

7. Use the remainder of the cells to sort the EGFP-positive fraction by flow cytometer. Subsequently perform histochemical analysis (*see* Subheading 3.6) to analyze mature eosinophils, neutrophils, monocytes, and erythrocytes.

3.5 Retroviral Transduction of Eosinophil Progenitors

For virus production, different vectors can be used (*see* **Note 17**). The protocol used to generate stable transfected virus producing Phoenix-Ampho cells using the LZRS-EGFP plasmid is described below. *See* **Note 18** for transient transfection of 293T cells with MSCV-EGFP.

1. Plate Phoenix-Ampho cells (*see* **Note 19**) in 6-well plate (in adherent cell culture medium; *see* Subheading 2.5, **item 4**) in such a manner that the cells are 30–40 % confluent the next day.

2. Transfect cells the next day according to the calcium phosphate coprecipitation method (*see* **Note 20**). Add 10 µg DNA to 150 µl of 0.25 M CaCl2. Subsequently add 150 µl HBSP (*see* Subheading 2.5, **item 6**) in a dropwise manner while vortexing. Add the DNA mixture to the cells after 5–10 min of incubation. Culture cells at 37 °C in a humidified incubator containing 5 % CO_2.

3. 16 h after transfection, wash the cells with PBS and add fresh adherent cell culture medium.

4. After another 24 h, split the cells into 75 cm² flasks with 15 ml adherent cell culture medium and add puromycin (final concentration 3 µg/ml) to select transfected cells. Refresh medium and puromycin every 2–3 days. Culture the cells in the presence of puromycin for 1–2 weeks.

5. When cells are 80–90 % confluent, carefully wash the cells once with PBS and exchange the adherent cell culture medium with a minimal volume (*see* **Note 21**) of hematopoietic progenitor cell culture medium (*see* Subheading 2.5, **item 9**) without puromycin.

6. After another 24 h, carefully collect the supernatant, filter through a 0.2 μm filter, and use freshly or snap freeze aliquots in liquid nitrogen. Virus can be stored at –80 °C (*see* **Note 22**).

7. Coat the required number of dishes of a 24-well plate with retronectin (*see* Subheading 2.5, **item 12**) for 2 h at room temperature or overnight at 4 °C. Subsequently wash the dishes once with PBS, and add 0.5 ml viral supernatant to the wells.

8. Transfer 500 μl of CD34$^+$ cells, pre-cultured for 24 h (Subheading 3.3, **steps 1–3**), to the wells with viral supernatant (maximal 500,000 cells per well). Add SCF, FLT3-L, GM-CSF, IL-3, and IL-5 to the cells (for concentrations, *see* Subheading 2.3, **item 3**). As a control, use virus generated with an empty vector control.

9. 24 h after transduction, carefully remove 700 μl medium from the wells, and add 0.5 ml of viral supernatant, 0.5 ml fresh medium, and cytokines (IL-3 and IL-5) to the cells (*see* **Note 23**).

10. After another 24 h, determine the transduction efficiency by FACS. For ex vivo eosinophil differentiation, continue according to the protocol (*see* Subheading 3.3, **step 4**). For transplantation of mice with the human progenitors, continue with Subheading 3.4.

3.6 Histochemical Staining of Eosinophil Progenitors

1. Prepare cytospins from 5×10^4 differentiating granulocytes by centrifuging for 3 min at $14 \times g$. To prevent loss of cells, slides should initially be centrifuged with 50 μl PBS.

2. Fix cytospins for 3 min in methanol.

3. Place slides in an eosin methylene blue solution according to May-Grunwald (*see* Subheading 2.6, **items 4** and **5**) (*see* **Note 24**) for 15 min.

4. Rinse the slides for 10 s in buffered water (*see* Subheading 2.6, **item 4**) until excessive May-Grunwald staining has disappeared.

5. Place the slides in Giemsa solution (*see* Subheading 2.3, **item 6**) to stain the nuclei for 20 min.

6. Rinse the slices in water until excessive staining has disappeared.

7. Dry cytospin in the air.

8. Mount slides using Entellan, and analyze eosinophil development.

9. During eosinophil differentiation, cells can be characterized as differentiating from blast cells towards pro-myelocyte type I, pro-myelocyte type II, myelocyte, metamyelocyte, and finally mature eosinophils with segmented nuclei. These stages can be distinguished by the size of the cells, ratio of cytoplasm versus nucleus, presence of azurophilic granules, appearance of eosinophilic granules, and shape of the nuclei (*see* Fig. 2).

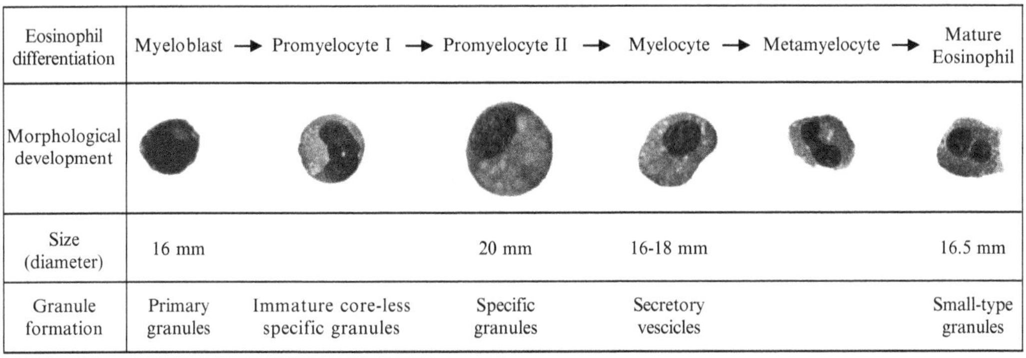

Eosinophil differentiation	Myeloblast →	Promyelocyte I →	Promyelocyte II →	Myelocyte →	Metamyelocyte →	Mature Eosinophil
Morphological development						
Size (diameter)	16 mm		20 mm	16-18 mm		16.5 mm
Granule formation	Primary granules	Immature core-less specific granules	Specific granules	Secretory vescicles		Small-type granules

Fig. 2 Eosinophil differentiation. Cells differentiating towards eosinophils undergo distinct stages: myeloblast, promyelocyte I, promyelocye II, myelocyte, metamyelocyte, and mature eosinophils. These stages are characterized by changes in morphology, size, and the development of granules

Table 3
Eosinophil differentiation after 14 and 17 days of culture

	Un-transduced		Transduced	
	Day 14	Day 17	Day 14	Day 17
Different cell types	18.3±2.7	19.5±1.8	12.8±2.5	14.9±4.5
Myeloblast/promyelocyte I	35.2±6.4	36.4±4.4	21.2±4.4	13.6±2.6
Promyelocyte II	11.8±2.4	5.8±1.4	23.6±4.5	18.8±4.5
Myelocyte	31.5±4.8	30.6±3.5	35.4±4.6	40.4±6.4
Metamyelocyte/mature	8.2±2.7	7.6±2.4	3.5±1.2	3.8±1.1
Juvenile eosinophils	51.4±7.2	44.0±3.7	62.5±6.1	63.0±6.6

See Table 3 for expected percentages of the different stages of eosinophil development after 14 and 17 days of culture in both un-manipulated and retrovirally transduced cells.

3.7 Luxol Fast Blue Staining

1. Prepare cytospins as described above (*see* Subheading 3.6, **step 1**).
2. Fix cells for 30 min at room temperature (*see* Subheading 2.7, **item 3**).
3. Wash slides with PBS.
4. Filter the freshly prepared Luxol Fast Blue staining solution (*see* Subheading 2.7, **item 4**) onto the slides and stain for 2 h at room temperature.
5. Wash slides in running tap water for 5 min.
6. Mount slides immediately using Entellan.
7. Determine the percentage of cells with Luxol Fast Blue-positive granules by microscope.

3.8 Multicolor Flow Cytometric Analysis for Ex Vivo-Differentiated Cells

Although the fast majority of the cells differentiate within the eosinophil lineage, both monocytes and neutrophils, but not basophils or mast cells, develop in low percentages during the 17-day culture period. It is therefore important to determine how many cells have differentiated towards the eosinophil lineage at different time points. To do this, the expression level of a combination of cell surface markers can be analyzed: (1) CD49 day which is expressed on both monocytes and eosinophils, but not neutrophils; (2) CD14 which is expressed on monocytes only; and (3) Siglec-8 which was found to be expressed on eosinophils. Since, to date, no eosinophil-specific markers have been identified which can determine the stage of eosinophil development in individual cells, this method should always be combined with histochemical staining (*see* Subheading 3.6).

1. Count the cells. Centrifuge at $425 \times g$ for 5 min. Resuspend the cells in 1 ml of antibody incubation buffer (*see* Subheading 2.8, **item 2**). Centrifuge again at $425 \times g$ for 5 min.

2. Resuspend the pellet in a mixture of the directly labelled antibodies (*see* **Note 6**) diluted in antibody incubation buffer. Incubate on ice for 30 min in the dark.

3. Add 1 ml antibody incubation buffer. Centrifuge for 5 min at $425 \times g$. Resuspend in 300 µl of FACS buffer (*see* Subheading 2.8, **item 3**), and analyze by FACS. To optimize fluorescence compensation settings for the multicolor flow cytometric analysis, and to preserve cells, use compensation particles (*see* **Note 25**).

4. To determine absolute cell counts on the flow cytometer, Flow-Count Fluorospheres (*see* Subheading 2.8, **item 5**) can be used. Resuspend the cells in the wells, and transfer cells to a FACS tube. Do not wash the cells. Add a fixed number of, thoroughly mixed, Flow-Count Fluorospheres and DAPI (to exclude nonviable cells) to the cells, and analyze by flow cytometer. Calculate the absolute number of viable cells in the culture.

---

4   Notes

1. UCB can be used for isolation up to 72 h after collection. However, isolating CD34[+] cells within 24 h after collection will yield higher cell numbers (*see* Table 1). On average, approximately 22,000 CD34[+] cells can be isolated from 1 ml of UCB (*see* Table 1).

2. After density gradient separation, four distinct layers can be observed: (1) The red cell pellet includes granulocytes and erythrocytes. (2) The clear (or slightly red) layer above the pellet contains the Ficoll–Paque solution. (3) The white interface contains

the mononuclear cell fraction which includes lymphocytes and hematopoietic stem and progenitor cells. The top layer, which is clear or slightly yellow, consists of plasma and platelets. Be aware that a large fraction of cells in the interface usually stick to the wall of the tube.

3. The Ficoll-Paque layer is easily disturbed. It is recommended to pipet slowly, but in a consistent pace without stopping. In addition adding the blood on top of the Ficoll-Paque layer as described above gives a much better separation of the layers in comparison to pipetting the Ficoll-Paque solution underneath the blood.

4. If necessary, the erythrocyte lysis step can be repeated once. Beware that longer incubation periods will eventually result in lysis of non-erythrocytes, including CD34$^+$ cells.

5. LS columns may be used (with the appropriate magnetic separator) when cell numbers are higher than 2.10^8.

6. Antibodies should be titrated with isotype controls to determine the most optimal concentration. This should be repeated when a new batch of antibodies is used.

7. The CD34 antibody used to determine the percentage of CD34$^+$ cells and the antibody coupled to the microbeads used during the isolation procedure should recognize different epitopes.

8. Although it is possible to freeze the mononuclear cell fraction, after thawing, both the viability and yield of the CD34$^+$ cells are reduced in comparison to cryopreservation of CD34$^+$ cells.

9. The final concentration of DMSO in this protocol is 5 %. Higher concentrations are often used (10 %). However, increasing the percentage of DMSO reduces the viability of the cells.

10. The DNAse treatment is necessary to remove the clumps of DNA that are formed after breakdown of dead cells. Although it is usually sufficient to incubate once with DNAse and $MgCl_2$, in some instances it might be necessary to repeat this step once.

11. It is important to maintain the cells in the same dish as long as possible. A stromal cell layer is formed during culture. These cells appear to positively affect eosinophil differentiation.

12. Breed and maintain the mice under sterile conditions in microisolator cages, and provide them with autoclaved food and acidified water containing 111 mg/l Ciprofloxacin (Ciproxin®).

13. To calculate absolute numbers of cells, it is preferable to crush the bones instead of flushing them.

14. Human hematopoietic cells can also be detected in the spleen of the mice, albeit in lower numbers.

15. Although it is preferred to analyze cells immediately, it is feasible to store cells on ice and analyze them within 24 h.

16. The ratio of un-transduced:empty vector-transduced cells does not decrease during the 6 weeks after transplantation.

17. For retroviral transduction of CD34$^+$ cells two different retroviral vectors can be successfully used: LZRS-EGFP and MSCV-EGFP. Both vectors have their advantages and disadvantages. Although LZRS-EGFP is very large, which makes cloning difficult, the presence of a puromycin resistance gene allows the generation of stable virus-producing cell lines resulting in higher transduction efficiencies (up to 60 % for empty vector control virus). In contrast, although MSCV-EGFP is much smaller which facilitates cloning of genes in interest, transient transfection of virus-producing cells results in lower transduction efficiencies.

18. To generate virus using the MSCV-EGFP vector the following protocol can be used. At day 1, plate 293 T cells in 6-well plate dishes (in adherent cell culture medium; *see* Subheading 2.5, **item 4**) in such a manner that the cells are 50–80 % confluent the next day. At day 2, add 97 μl of adherent cell culture medium (room temperature) to a sterile polystyrene tube. For a 3:1 FuGENE-6 Transfection Reagent:DNA ratio, add 9 μl of FuGENE Transfection Reagent to the medium and mix immediately. Add FuGENE6 Transfection Reagent directly to medium. Incubate the FuGENE6 Transfection Reagent/medium mixture for 5 min at room temperature. Add 3 μg (1 μg/μl) of plasmid DNA (1.5 μg MSCV-EGFP and 1.5 μg pCL AMPHO) to the FuGENE6 Transfection Reagent mixture, and mix immediately. Incubate the FuGENE-6 Transfection Reagent/DNA mixture for 15 min at room temperature. Subsequently, add the FuGENE-6 Transfection Reagent/DNA mixture to the cells. Culture cells at 37 °C in a humidified incubator containing 5 % CO_2. 16 h after transfection, carefully wash the cells once with PBS and exchange the adherent cell culture medium with a minimal volume (*see* **Note 21**) of hematopoietic progenitor cell culture medium (*see* Subheading 2.5, **item 9**). After another 24 h, carefully collect the supernatant, filter through a 0.2 μm filter, and use freshly or snap freeze aliquots in liquid nitrogen. Virus can be stored at −80 °C. For transduction of cells, continue with Subheading 3.5, **step 7**.

19. When virus production is not optimal, Phoenix-Ampho cells can be cultured in the presence of antibiotics for at least 1 week. In case of Phoenix-Ampho cells, hygromycin can be used to select for Gag-pol-expressing cells, while diphtheria can be used to select for cells expressing the envelope proteins.

20. If required (very low transfection efficiency), 25 μM chloroquine can be added to the cells at this stage to prevent DNA breakdown by lysosomes.

21. For 75 cm² flasks use 7.5 ml medium, and for 25 cm² flasks or 6-well plate use 2.5 ml medium.

22. Although virus can be frozen and thawed once without reducing the transduction efficiency, repeated freezing and thawing cycles are not recommended. Virus should therefore be frozen in small aliquots.

23. Although some labs perform transduction experiments by centrifuging virus and cells onto the retronectin-coated plates, this does not result in improved transduction efficiencies in CD34⁺ cells.

24. It may not always be necessary to use buffered water. However, since the composition and pH of "water" are not always the same in each institute, problems (such as weak staining) can occur when using normal water. In this case, revert back to using buffered water. To improve staining, use only freshly diluted reagents.

25. To optimize fluorescence compensation settings for the multicolor flow cytometric analysis, and to preserve cells, use compensation particles (*see* Subheading 2.4, **item 9**). Add one drop of both the beads pre-coupled to an antibody specific for mouse Ig,κ and one drop of negative control beads with no binding capacity for antibodies to 1 ml of antibody incubation buffer. Add 1 μl of antibody to 100 μl of this mixture. Separate tubes should be used for each individual antibody. Incubate for 15 min on ice (in the dark), and analyze by FACS without centrifugation.

Acknowledgements

The author thanks the current and past members of the departments of Respiratory Medicine and Immunology at the University Medical Center Utrecht (the Netherlands), the Department of Hematology at the Erasmus MC (the Netherlands), and the Hematopoietic Stem Cell Laboratory at the Lund Strategic Research Center for Stem Cell Biology and Cell Therapy in Sweden for helping develop these protocols.

References

1. Majeti R, Park CY, Weissman IL (2007) Identification of a hierarchy of multipotent hematopoietic progenitors in human cord blood. Cell Stem Cell 1(6):635–645, Pubmed: 18371405

2. Hoebeke I, De Smedt M, Stolz F, Pike-Overzet K, Staal FJ, Plum J, Leclercq G (2007) T-, B- and NK-lymphoid, but not myeloid cells arise from human CD34(+)CD38(-)CD7(+) common lymphoid progenitors expressing lymphoid-specific genes. Leukemia 21(2):311–319, Pubmed: 17170726

3. Manz MG, Miyamoto T, Akashi K, Weissman IL (2002) Prospective isolation of human

clonogenic common myeloid progenitors. Proc Natl Acad Sci U S A 99:11872–11877, Pubmed: 12193648

4. Mori Y, Iwasaki H, Kohno K, Yoshimoto G, Kikushige Y, Okeda A, Uike N, Niiro H, Takenaka K, Nagafuji K, Miyamoto T, Harada M, Takatsu K, Akashi K (2009) Identification of the human eosinophil lineage-committed progenitor: revision of phenotypic definition of the human common myeloid progenitor. J Exp Med 206(1):183–193, Pubmed: 19114669

5. Sitnicka E, Buza-Vidas N, Larsson S et al (2003) Human CD34+ hematopoietic stem cells capable of multilineage engrafting NOD/SCID mice express flt3: distinct flt3 and c-kit expression and response patterns on mouse and candidate human hematopoietic stem cells. Blood 102:881–886, Pubmed: 12676789

6. Yamaguchi Y, Suda T, Suda J et al (1988) Purified interleukin 5 supports the terminal differentiation and proliferation of murine eosinophilic precursors. J Exp Med 167:43–56, Pubmed: 3257253

7. Sanderson CJ, Warren DJ, Strath M (1985) Identification of a lymphokine that stimulates eosinophil differentiation in vitro. Its relationship to interleukin 3, and functional properties of eosinophils produced in cultures. J Exp Med 162:60–74

8. Buitenhuis M, Baltus B, Lammers JW, Coffer PJ, Koenderman L (2003) Signal transducer and activator of transcription 5a (STAT5a) is required for eosinophil differentiation of human cord blood-derived CD34+ cells. Blood 101(1):134–142, Pubmed: 12393707

9. Buitenhuis M, Verhagen LP, Cools J, Coffer PJ (2007) Molecular mechanisms underlying FIP1L1-PDGFRA-mediated myeloproliferation. Cancer Res 67(8):3759–3766, Pubmed: 17440089

10. Buitenhuis M, van Deutekom HW, Verhagen LP, Castor A, Jacobsen SE, Lammers JW, Koenderman L, Coffer PJ (2005) Differential regulation of granulopoiesis by the basic helix-loop-helix transcriptional inhibitors Id1 and Id2. Blood 105(11):4272–4281, Pubmed: 15701714

11. Ulfman LH, Kamp VM, van Aalst CW, Verhagen LP, Sanders ME, Reedquist KA, Buitenhuis M, Koenderman L (2008) Homeostatic intracellular-free Ca2+ is permissive for Rap1-mediated constitutive activation of alpha4 integrins on eosinophils. J Immunol 180(8):5512–5519, Pubmed: 18390735

12. Buitenhuis M, Verhagen LP, van Deutekom HW, Castor A, Verploegen S, Koenderman L, Jacobsen SE, Coffer PJ (2008) Protein kinase B (c-akt) regulates hematopoietic lineage choice decisions during myelopoiesis. Blood 111(1):112–121, Pubmed: 17890457

13. Beekman JM, Verhagen LP, Geijsen N, Coffer PJ (2009) Regulation of myelopoiesis through syntenin-mediated modulation of IL-5 receptor output. Blood 114(18):3917–3927, Pubmed: 19654410

14. Geest CR, Zwartkruis FJ, Vellenga E, Coffer PJ, Buitenhuis M (2009) Mammalian target of rapamycin activity is required for expansion of CD34+ hematopoietic progenitor cells. Haematologica 94(7):901–910, Pubmed: 19535348

15. Geest CR, Buitenhuis M, Laarhoven AG, Bierings MB, Bruin MC, Vellenga E, Coffer PJ (2009) p38 MAP kinase inhibits neutrophil development through phosphorylation of C/EBPalpha on serine 21. Stem Cells 27(9):2271–2282, Pubmed: 19544470

16. de Bruin AM, Buitenhuis M, van der Sluijs KF, van Gisbergen KP, Boon L, Nolte MA (2010) Eosinophil differentiation in the bone marrow is inhibited by T cell-derived IFN-gamma. Blood 116(14):2559–2569, Pubmed: 20587787

17. Kollet O, Peled A, Byk T, Ben-Hur H, Greiner D, Shultz L, Lapidot T (2000) beta2 microglobulin-deficient (B2m(null)) NOD/SCID mice are excellent recipients for studying human stem cell function. Blood 95(10):3102–3105, Pubmed: 10807775

18. Glimm H, Eisterer W, Lee K, Cashman J, Holyoake TL, Nicolini F, Shultz LD, von Kalle C, Eaves CJ (2001) Previously undetected human hematopoietic cell populations with short-term repopulating activity selectively engraft NOD/SCID-beta2 microglobulin-null mice. J Clin Invest 107(2):199–206, Pubmed: 11160136

19. Kikly KK, Bochner BS, Freeman SD, Tan KB, Gallagher KT, D'alessio KJ, Holmes SD, Abrahamson JA, Erickson-Miller CL, Murdock PR, Tachimoto H, Schleimer RP, White JR (2000) Identification of SAF-2, a novel siglec expressed on eosinophils, mast cells and basophils. J Allergy Clin Immunol 105:1093–1100, Pubmed: 10856141

20. Floyd H, Ni J, Cornish AL, Zeng Z, Liu D, Carter KC, Steel J, Crocker PR (2000) Siglec-8: a novel eosinophil-specific member of the immunoglobulin superfamily. J Biol Chem 275:861–866, Pubmed: 10625619

Chapter 7

Eosinophil Intracellular Signalling: Apoptosis

Pinja Ilmarinen, Eeva Moilanen, and Hannu Kankaanranta

Abstract

Eosinophil apoptosis is considered critical for the resolution of eosinophilic inflammation in the airways of asthmatics. Apoptosis can be mediated by an extrinsic receptor-activated pathway or alternatively by an intrinsic pathway via distortion of mitochondrial function. Both of these pathways lead to activation of the caspase cascade resulting in degradation of cellular components. We describe here two methods to explore intracellular mechanisms mediating eosinophil apoptosis. Eosinophil staining by fluorescent probe JC-1 followed by flow cytometric analysis is a reliable method for determination of the state of mitochondrial membrane potential ($\Delta\Psi_m$). Lost $\Delta\Psi_m$ indicates distorted mitochondrial function and apoptosis. We also describe a method to explore the activation of effector caspase-6 by assessing degradation of its substrate lamin A/C by immunoblotting.

Key words Eosinophils, Apoptosis, Mitochondrial membrane potential, JC-1, Caspase-6, Lamin A/C, Immunoblotting

1 Introduction

Apoptosis is an important regulator of eosinophil number in tissues, and normally eosinophils die by spontaneous apoptosis in few days. Apoptosis is inhibited by many agents such as interleukin (IL)-5, IL-3, and granulocyte macrophage-colony-stimulating factor (GM-CSF) present in the airways of asthmatics and accelerated for example by glucocorticoids and other inducers of apoptosis [1–4].

Apoptosis is characterized by cell shrinkage, chromatin condensation, DNA fragmentation, and nuclear coalescence. Apoptosis can be executed via an extrinsic receptor-mediated pathway or an intrinsic mitochondrion-centered pathway [5]. Both forms of apoptosis have been described in eosinophils [6–8]. Mitochondrial events occurring typically during intrinsic form of eosinophil apoptosis involve mitochondrial permeability transition, collapsed mitochondrial membrane potential ($\Delta\Psi_m$), mitochondrial outer membrane permeabilization, and/or release of

Garry M. Walsh (ed.), *Eosinophils: Methods and Protocols*, Methods in Molecular Biology, vol. 1178, DOI 10.1007/978-1-4939-1016-8_7, © Springer Science+Business Media New York 2014

cytochrome c [7–10]. Both extrinsic and intrinsic pathways of apoptosis may lead to activation of caspases, cysteine-dependent aspartate-specific proteases [5]. Initiator caspases (8, 9, and 10) activate effector caspases (3, 6, and 7), which in turn degrade cellular components such as lamins and poly (adenosine diphosphate-ribose) polymerase (PARP) resulting in morphological signs of apoptosis [11]. Eosinophils express at least caspases-3, -6, -7, -8, and -9, and activation of many caspases has been demonstrated during eosinophil apoptosis [9, 12–15].

Here we describe two methods for studying intracellular apoptotic signalling in eosinophils: assessment of mitochondrial membrane potential ($\Delta\Psi_m$) by JC-1 staining and activation of effector caspase-6 as determined by degradation of its substrate lamin A/C by immunoblotting.

JC-1 staining is a reliable and accurate method when the purpose is to measure whether mitochondrial membrane is roughly polarized (viable cells) or depolarized (apoptotic cells) [16, 17]. In living cells, mitochondrial inner membrane is polarized with negative charge inside and the cationic dye JC-1 accumulates into the negatively charged matrix side of the mitochondrial membrane. After a threshold concentration, JC-1 aggregates producing red fluorescence. In cells with collapsed $\Delta\Psi_m$ JC-1 remains in a monomeric form in the cytoplasm emitting green fluorescence. Cells with lost $\Delta\Psi_m$ show primarily green fluorescence and can be easily distinguished from cells with intact $\Delta\Psi_m$ showing both green and red fluorescence [16]. This method is well suitable for eosinophil work and requires no special considerations.

Immunoblotting is a standard method for studying levels of individual proteins. Proteins separated on sodium dodecyl sulphate (SDS)-polyacrylamide gel electrophoresis (PAGE) by their molecular weight are transferred to nitrocellulose or polyvinylidene difluoride membrane electrophoretically. The expression level of the desired protein is detected after staining with specific antibodies. Use of immunoblotting in eosinophils is often restrained by limited cell number available. Approximately one million eosinophils are required per sample implicating that long series with multiple time points or treatments are often impossible to conduct. We describe here the use of immunoblotting for determination of caspase-6 activity by measuring levels of the degradation product of its substrate, lamin A/C. Currently, caspase-6 is the only protease known to degrade lamin A/C [18, 19], but reversibility of this effect by caspase-6 inhibitor confirms specific activation of caspase-6. The method sums all the caspase-6 activity (deceased and current) present up to the time point studied removing the need for screening several time points to expose the ongoing caspase activity.

2   Materials

If not otherwise stated, bring all reagents to room temperature before use. Always use ultrapure water for preparation of solutions.

2.1 Mitochondrial Membrane Potential

1. rhGM-CSF and valinomycin.

2. JC-1 (5,5′,6,6′-tetrachloro-1,1′,3,3′-tetraethylbenzimidazolyl carbocyanine iodide) (Biotium Inc., Hayward, CA, USA): 1 mg/ml Stock solution in DMSO. Store at +4 °C protected from light.

3. Phosphate-buffered saline (PBS): 137 mM NaCl, 2.7 mM KCl, 1.5 mM KH_2PO_4, 7.9 mM $Na_2HPO_4 \cdot 2H_2O$, pH 7.4. To prepare 10× stock weigh 40 g NaCl, 1 g KCl, 1 g KH_2PO_4, and 7 g $Na_2HPO_4 \cdot 2H_2O$ and add water to a volume of 500 ml. To prepare 1× solution, add 800 ml water to 100 ml of PBS stock and adjust pH to 7.4. Top up to 1,000 ml with water. Store at +4 °C.

4. Pre-warmed cell culture medium: For example RPMI 1640 (Dutch modification, 1×, without L-glutamine) with additions of 10 % fetal calf serum, 50 IU/ml penicillin, 50 µg/ml streptomycin, and 2 mM L-glutamine.

5. Flow cytometer with excitation and emission wavelengths of 488 and 550 nm, respectively.

2.2 Caspase-6 Activity

1. Caspase-6 inhibitor Z-VEID-FMK (Merck, Darmstadt, Germany).

2. Ice-cold PBS: Preparation described above.

3. Protein extraction solution: Radioimmunoprecipitation assay (RIPA) buffer (65 mM Tris–HCl, pH 7.4, 150 mM NaCl, 1 % NP-40, 0.25 % sodium deoxycholate, 1 mM EDTA) (*see* **Note 2**), 10 µM *N*-octyl-β-D-glucopyranoside, 0.5 mM phenylmethylsulfonyl fluoride (PMSF), 1 mM Na_3VO_4, 42 µM leupeptin, 50 µg/ml aprotinin, 5 mM NaF, and 2 mM sodium pyrophosphate. Should be prepared on the day needed (*see* **Note 3**).

4. SDS loading buffer: 62.5 mM Tris–HCl, pH 6.8, 10 % glycerol, 2 % SDS, 0.025 % bromophenol blue, and 5 % β-mercaptoethanol (*see* **Note 4**).

5. Polyacrylamide solution for the resolving gel: 10 % Acrylamide/Bis, 375 mM Tris–HCl pH 8.8, 0.1 % SDS, 0.8 mg/ml ammonium persulfate (APS), 0.08 % TEMED (*see* **Note 5**).

6. Polyacrylamide solution for the stacking gel: 4 % Acrylamide/Bis, 100 mM Tris–HCl pH 6.8, 0.1 % SDS, 0.8 mg/ml APS, 0.08 % TEMED (*see* **Note 5**).

7. Equipment for gel casting, electrophoresis, and blotting.

8. SDS PAGE running buffer: 25 mM Tris, 250 mM glycine, and 0.1 % SDS (*see* **Note 6**).

9. Hybond ECL™ nitrocellulose membrane.

10. Transfer buffer (*see* **Note 7**).

11. Tris-buffered saline (TBS, 10×): 200 mM Tris–HCl, pH 7.6, 1.5 M NaCl.

12. TBS (1×) containing 0.05 % Tween (TBST) (*see* **Note 8**).

13. Blocking solution: 5 % Milk in TBST. Add 20 ml TBST per 1 g nonfat milk powder.

14. Lamin A/C antibody (Cell Signaling Technology Inc., Danvers, MA, USA) and secondary goat anti-rabbit IgG, horse radish peroxidase (HRP)-conjugated antibody sc-2004 (Santa Cruz Biotechnology, Santa Cruz, CA, USA).

15. HRP substrate such as Super Signal West Dura and chemiluminescence imaging system.

3   Methods

3.1 Mitochondrial Membrane Potential (See Note 1)

1. Culture cells (1×10^6/ml) in the absence and presence of the test compounds. Include eosinophils treated with 10 pM GM-CSF (negative control) and 1 μM valinomycin (positive control).

2. Transfer samples into sterile tubes. Centrifuge at $400 \times g$ for 5 min at RT. Remove the supernatant.

3. Dilute JC-1 stock 1:100 with pre-warmed medium into final concentration of 10 μg/ml just prior to use. Add 500 μl of the JC-1 solution (10 μg/ml) to each tube. Incubate the cells for 15 min at +37 °C protected from light. Centrifuge at $400 \times g$ for 5 min at RT. Remove the supernatant.

4. Resuspend the cell pellet in 2 ml of medium. Centrifuge at $400 \times g$ for 5 min at RT. Remove the supernatant.

5. Resuspend the cell pellet in 500 μl of PBS, transfer into flow cytometry tubes, and analyze immediately with flow cytometer.

6. Set up the flow cytometer. Generate a log FL1 vs. log FL2 dot plot (X vs. Y axis). Run the negative control sample (GM-CSF). Adjust PMT voltages for FL1 and FL2 so that you can see a dual-positive cell population in the dot plot (*see* **Note 9**—Fig. 1a).

7. Run the positive control sample (valinomycin). Most of the cell population should show reduced FL2 fluorescence and/or increased FL1 fluorescence as shown in Fig. 1b. This population represents the cells with lost mitochondrial membrane potential. Increase FL2-%FL1 compensation to see a clearer reduction in FL2.

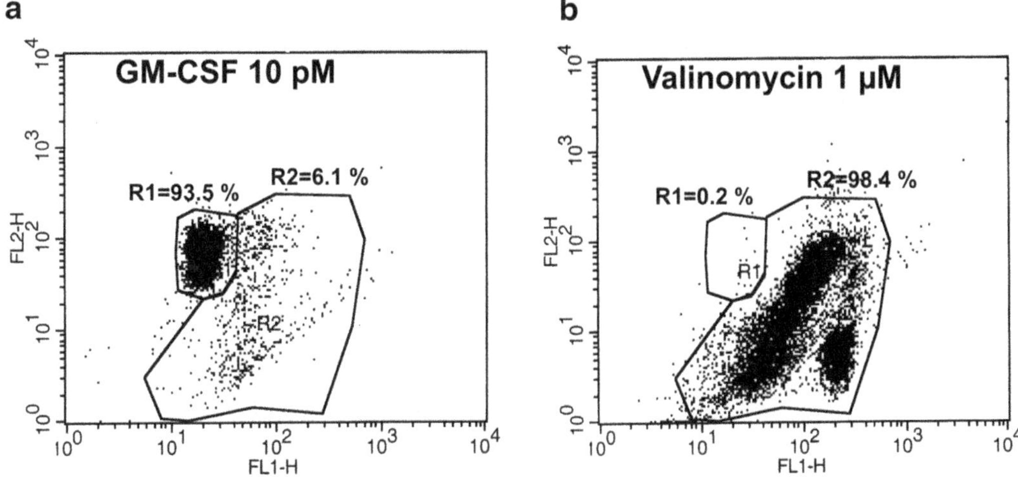

Fig. 1 Determination of mitochondrial membrane potential by JC-1 staining. (**a**) Flow cytometry plot of eosinophils treated with 10 pM GM-CSF for 40 h at +37 °C and 5 % CO_2. Mitochondrial membrane is maintained in an intact, polarized state in most eosinophils, which is shown by high fluorescence in FL2 channel. (**b**) Eosinophils treated with 1 µM valinomycin for 40 h show reduced FL2 fluorescence and/or increased FL1 fluorescence indicating lost mitochondrial membrane potential and apoptosis. Region R1 shows the percentage of healthy cells with intact mitochondrial membrane potential. Region R2 represents the percentage of cells with lost mitochondrial membrane potential

8. Run your samples by using these settings, for example 20,000 cells/sample.

9. When analyzing the samples, create region R1 that should cover approximately 90–95 % of the population of the GM-CSF-negative control sample (Fig. 1a). This region gives the percentage of healthy cells with intact mitochondrial membrane potential. Create region R2 that should cover approximately 95–99 % of the population of the positive control (valinomycin) sample (Fig. 1b). R2 represents the percentage of cells with lost mitochondrial membrane potential (*see* **Note 10**).

3.2 Caspase-6 Activity

Immunoblotting experiments should be planned with particular care because of the limited cell number available. Unless otherwise specified, carry out all procedures at room temperature.

1. *Cell culture experiment.* In experiments where high degree of apoptosis is expected it is preferred to use at least 1.5 million eosinophils per sample to obtain sufficient protein for immunoblotting. Otherwise, one million eosinophils/sample should be sufficient. For example eosinophils treated with 10 pM GM-CSF in the absence and presence of 1 mM SNAP for 40 h are good choices as negative and positive controls, respectively. We recommend including samples containing the test compound in the

absence and presence of caspase-6 inhibitor such as Z-VEID-FMK (200 μM). Incubations should be carried out at +37 °C with 5 % CO_2.

2. *Cell lysis and protein extraction.* After incubation for the desired time in the presence and absence of the inducers of apoptosis, centrifuge cells and remove the supernatant. Add 1 ml of ice-cold PBS, centrifuge cells, remove the supernatant, and add ice-cold protein extraction solution (for example 25 μl/1.5 million cells). Incubate the cells for 20–30 min at +4 °C and centrifuge at 12,000 × *g* for 10 min at +4 °C. Proteins are in the supernatant. Take a sample of 2 μl for protein quantification, and prepare a dilution of 1:10 in water (*see* **Note 11**). Carefully transfer the remaining protein supernatant to another Eppendorf tube, and add one part of SDS loading buffer per three parts of protein supernatant (1:4). Store at –20 °C.

3. *SDS-PAGE.* Mix compounds of 10 % resolving gel (*see* **Note 6**) and cast within a gel apparatus (mini/large gel apparatus). Leave space for the stacking gel, and add ultrapure water to the gel surface. Allow the resolving gel to polymerize at RT for 45–60 min. Absorb the water from the gel surface using a filter paper. Mix ingredients of 4 % stacking gel, and add the mixture onto the resolving gel with the well-comb. Let stand at RT for 15 min. Boil protein samples for 10 min, and centrifuge the condensate. Depending on whether you use mini-gels or large gels, load 2–5 μl of pre-stained molecule weight marker onto the first gel well and equal protein quantities (*see* **Note 11**) onto the following wells. Conduct electrophoresis in SDS-PAGE running buffer. Running time varies according to the gel size, machinery, and voltage used. Continue until the 70 and 28 kDa proteins are well separated according to the molecule weight markers. Stop electrophoresis when the dye front is at the bottom of the gel.

4. *Blotting.* Following electrophoresis, pry the gel plates open and cut the gel into a size that comprises at least 20–80 kDa proteins. Transfer the gel carefully to a container with transfer buffer. Cut nitrocellulose membrane to the size of the gel and immerse in transfer buffer. Many different systems exist for the transfer of proteins from the gel to the membrane (blotting). The blot sandwich is prepared and transfer conducted according to the manufacturer of your transfer apparatus.

5. *Membrane blocking.* After successful transfer of the proteins to the nitrocellulose membrane, place the membrane protein side up in a container containing approximately 20 ml of blocking solution. Incubate for 1 h at RT on a shaker.

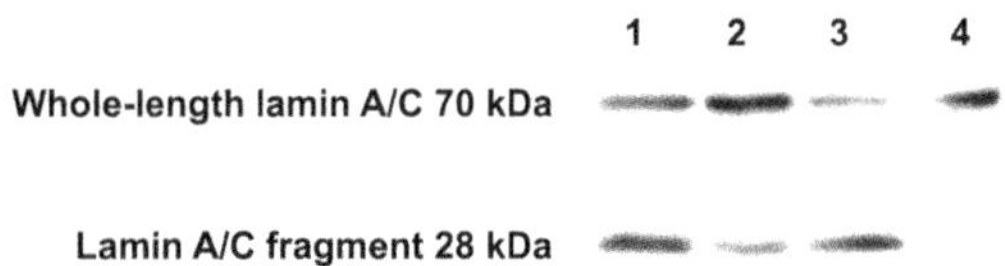

Fig. 2 Caspase-6 activation in eosinophils as determined by degradation of full-length lamin A/C (70 kDa) into a 28 kDa fragment by immunoblotting. Eosinophils were treated with (1) solvent, (2) GM-CSF 10 pM, (3) GM-CSF 10 pM + SNAP 1 mM, and (4) GM-CSF 10 pM + SNAP 1 mM + caspase-6 inhibitor Z-VEID-FMK 200 µM for 40 h at +37 °C and 5 % CO_2. Z-VEID-FMK was added 20 min before other substances. Cell lysis, protein extraction, and immunoblotting were carried out as explained in the text. 25 µg of protein was added onto each well. Decreased levels of full-length lamin (70 kDa) and increased levels of the 28 kDa fragment (as shown in wells 1 and 3) indicate caspase-6 activation and apoptosis. Reproduced from Pulmonary Pharmacology & Therapeutics 2010 [13] with permission from Elsevier Ltd

6. *Incubation with the primary antibody.* Pour off the blocking solution, and add lamin A/C antibody solution (e.g., 20 ml 1:1,000 dilution in 5 % milk in TBST). Incubate overnight at +4 °C on a shaker. Pour the antibody solution in a tube and store at –20 °C. You can reuse the antibody solution 3–5 times.

7. *Washing.* Wash the membrane three times in TBST, 5 min each, by using a shaker.

8. *Incubation with the secondary antibody.* Add secondary goat anti-rabbit, HRP-conjugated antibody (e.g., 20 ml 1:2,000 dilution in 5 % milk in TBST). Incubate for 30 min at RT using a shaker. Pour the antibody solution in a tube and store at –20 °C. You can reuse the antibody solution 4–10 times.

9. *Washing.* Repeat **step 7**.

10. *Detection.* Remove the excess TBST off by holding the membrane against a paper towel for a few seconds. Transfer the membrane on a plastic sheet, protein side up. Add chemiluminescent substrate such as Super Signal West Dura according to the instructions of the manufacturer, incubate for 5 min, cover the membrane with another plastic sheet, and detect proteins by using a chemiluminescence imaging system.

11. *Analysis.* Protein bands of approximately 28 kDa (lamin A/C, fragment) and 70 kDa (lamin A/C, full length) should be visible (Fig. 2). Define band intensities. Decreased level of full-length lamin A/C and increased level of fragmented lamin A/C that are reversible by inhibitor of caspase-6 indicate activation of caspase-6 and apoptosis. We recommend presenting the results as the ratio of 28 kDa fragment to the full-length lamin A/C (70 kDa) (*see* **Note 12**).

4   Notes

1. We recommend the use of 500,000 eosinophils per sample to ensure adequacy of the sample when adjusting flow cytometric settings. However, when the settings are adjusted, this assay can be performed with 250,000 eosinophils/sample. With this lower number of cells, use only half the volume of JC-1 solution and PBS. If sufficient number of cells are obtained, prepare each sample as duplicates. Use sterile tubes and pipette tips at least until JC-1 staining has been conducted.

2. For protein extraction solution you can use 2× RIPA stock prepared as follows: Weigh 1.58 g Tris base and 1.8 g NaCl and dissolve into approximately 50 ml of water. Adjust pH to 7.4 with HCl. Add 2 ml of 100 % NP-40, 5 ml of 10 % sodium deoxycholate, and 2 ml of 100 mM EDTA. Make up to 100 ml with water. Store in a dark bottle at +4 °C. Prepare 10 % sodium deoxycholate by weighting 0.5 g sodium deoxycholate and dissolving it into 5 ml of water. Sodium deoxycholate solution is best to prepare fresh because it strongly crystallizes when stored at +4 °C. To prepare 100 mM EDTA, weight 3.722 g $Na_2EDTA{\cdot}2H_2O$ and add 40 ml water. The compound dissolves slowly by increasing pH to 7.4 by NaOH. Make up to 100 ml with water. Store the EDTA solution at +4 °C.

3. Prepare 5 ml protein extraction solution by mixing 2.5 ml 2× RIPA stock with 1.8 ml water and 100 µl 0.5 mM N-octyl-β-D-glucopyranoside. Add the following inhibitors of proteases and phosphatases: 25 µl of 0.1 M PMSF stock in 2-propanol, 25 µl of 0.2 M Na_3VO_4 stock in water, 25 µl of 8.4 mM stock leupeptin in water, 25 µl of 10 mg/ml aprotinin stock in water, 250 µl of 0.1 M NaF stock in water, and 250 µl of 40 mM sodium pyrophosphate stock in water.

4. For SDS loading buffer, mix 45.6 ml of water, 12 ml of 0.5 M Tris–HCl, pH 6.8, 9.6 ml of glycerol, 19.2 ml of 10 % SDS, 4.8 ml of 0.5 % bromophenol blue, and 4.8 ml of β-mercaptoethanol. Store at +4 °C. Prepare 0.5 M Tris–HCl by weighting 12.12 g Tris base and dissolving it into 100 ml of water. Adjust pH to 6.8 by using strong HCl. Make up to 200 ml with water, and store at +4 °C. 10 % SDS solution is prepared by weighing 10 g SDS and dissolving it into 100 ml of water (foaming). Store at RT. Prepare 0.5 % bromophenol blue solution by weighting 0.25 g bromophenol blue and dissolving it into 50 ml of water. Store at +4 °C.

5. Prepare gels by using 40 % acrylamide/Bis solution (37.5:1), water, 1.5 M Tris–HCl pH 8.8 (for resolving gel) and 0.5 M Tris–HCl pH 6.8 (for stacking gel), 10 % SDS, 100 mg/ml APS, and TEMED. APS and TEMED should be added last because their addition initiates polymerization. Unpolymerized

acrylamide is a neurotoxin; prepare gels in a fume hood and wear gloves. You can prepare the gels in advance; they can be stored at +4 °C folded in wet paper towels.

6. Prepare 10× stock of running buffer by weighting 30.2 g Tris base, 188 g glycine, and 10 g SDS, and fill up to 1 l with water. Dissolve slowly overnight. Store at RT. For 1× running buffer, add 100 ml 10× stock to 900 ml water and mix.

7. Composition of transfer buffer depends on the use of blotting method (semidry or wet). In wet transfer use transfer buffer with 24 mM Tris, 193 mM glycine, 0.5 % SDS, and 20 % methanol. Store at +4 °C.

8. TBST is made by mixing 100 ml of 10× TBS with 900 ml of water. Add 1 ml Tween last to prevent foaming. Mix, and store at +4 °C.

9. Typical flow cytometry settings for JC-1 staining in FACScan (Becton Dickinson, San Jose, CA) are as follows: FL1 PMT voltage 390, FL2 PMT voltage 320, and compensations FL1-4 % FL2 and FL2-17 % FL1.

10. Several distinct populations with different levels of decreased mitochondrial membrane potential may be distinguished in cells treated with valinomycin or other inducers of apoptosis. This is normal, and all the populations can be counted under region R2.

11. You can determine protein content of each sample beforehand by Bradford method based on binding of Coomassie blue to protein [20]. Use of 25 µg protein/well typically gives good bands.

12. Alternatively, you can normalize the level of lamin A/C 28 kDa fragment against the level of β-actin at each sample. In that event, strip off the previous antibodies (stripping solution 62.5 mM Tris–HCl, pH 6.8, 2 % SDS, 0.68 % β-mercaptoethanol), block the membrane, and carry out incubations with the primary and secondary antibodies to detect β-actin (use for example primary β-actin (C-11) rabbit IgG antibody and secondary goat anti-rabbit IgG, HRP-conjugated antibody sc-2004 (Santa Cruz Biotechnology, Santa Cruz, CA, USA)).

References

1. Ilmarinen P, Hasala H, Sareila O et al (2009) Bacterial DNA delays human eosinophil apoptosis. Pulm Pharmacol Ther 22:167–176

2. Zhang X, Moilanen E, Kankaanranta H (2000) Enhancement of human eosinophil apoptosis by fluticasone propionate, budesonide, and beclomethasone. Eur J Pharmacol 406:325–332

3. Zhang X, Moilanen E, Adcock IM et al (2002) Divergent effect of mometasone on human eosinophil and neutrophil apoptosis. Life Sci 71:1523–1534

4. Kankaanranta H, Moilanen E, Zhang X (2005) Pharmacological regulation of human eosinophil apoptosis. Curr Drug Targets Inflamm Allergy 4:433–445

5. Galluzzi L, Vitale I, Abrams JM et al (2012) Molecular definitions of cell death subroutines: recommendations of the Nomenclature

Committee on Cell Death 2012. Cell Death Differ 19:107–120

6. Letuve S, Druilhe A, Grandsaigne M et al (2001) Involvement of caspases and of mitochondria in Fas ligation-induced eosinophil apoptosis: modulation by interleukin-5 and interferon-gamma. J Leukoc Biol 70:767–775

7. Gardai SJ, Hoontrakoon R, Goddard CD et al (2003) Oxidant-mediated mitochondrial injury in eosinophil apoptosis: enhancement by glucocorticoids and inhibition by granulocyte-macrophage colony-stimulating factor. J Immunol 170:556–566

8. Ilmarinen-Salo P, Moilanen E, Kinnula VL et al (2012) Nitric oxide-induced eosinophil apoptosis is dependent on mitochondrial permeability transition (mPT), JNK and oxidative stress: apoptosis is preceded but not mediated by early mPT-dependent JNK activation. Respir Res 13:73. doi:10.1186/1465-9921-13-73

9. Dewson G, Cohen GM, Wardlaw AJ (2001) Interleukin-5 inhibits translocation of Bax to the mitochondria, cytochrome c release, and activation of caspases in human eosinophils. Blood 98:2239–2247

10. Tait SW, Green DR (2010) Mitochondria and cell death: outer membrane permeabilization and beyond. Nat Rev Mol Cell Biol 11:621–632

11. Pop C, Salvesen GS (2009) Human caspases: activation, specificity, and regulation. J Biol Chem 284:21777–21781

12. Zangrilli J, Robertson N, Shetty A et al (2000) Effect of IL-5, glucocorticoid, and Fas ligation on Bcl-2 homologue expression and caspase activation in circulating human eosinophils. Clin Exp Immunol 120:12–21

13. Ilmarinen-Salo P, Moilanen E, Kankaanranta H (2010) Nitric oxide induces apoptosis in GM-CSF-treated eosinophils via caspase-6-dependent lamin and DNA fragmentation. Pulm Pharmacol Ther 23:365–371

14. Kankaanranta H, Ilmarinen P, Zhang X et al (2006) Antieosinophilic activity of orazipone. Mol Pharmacol 69:1861–1870

15. Hasala H, Giembycz MA, Janka-Junttila M et al (2008) Histamine reverses IL-5-afforded human eosinophil survival by inducing apoptosis: pharmacological evidence for a novel mechanism of action of histamine. Pulm Pharmacol Ther 21:222–233

16. Salvioli S, Ardizzoni A, Franceschi C et al (1997) JC-1, but not DiOC6(3) or rhodamine 123, is a reliable fluorescent probe to assess delta psi changes in intact cells: implications for studies on mitochondrial functionality during apoptosis. FEBS Lett 411:77–82

17. Perry SW, Norman JP, Barbieri J et al (2011) Mitochondrial membrane potential probes and the proton gradient: a practical usage guide. Biotechniques 50:98–115

18. Orth K, Chinnaiyan AM, Garg M et al (1996) The CED-3/ICE-like protease Mch2 is activated during apoptosis and cleaves the death substrate lamin A. J Biol Chem 271:16443–16446

19. Takahashi A, Alnemri ES, Lazebnik YA et al (1996) Cleavage of lamin A by Mch2 alpha but not CPP32: multiple interleukin 1 beta-converting enzyme-related proteases with distinct substrate recognition properties are active in apoptosis. Proc Natl Acad Sci U S A 93:8395–8400

20. Bradford MM (1976) A rapid and sensitive method for the quantitation of microgram quantities of protein utilizing the principle of protein-dye binding. Anal Biochem 72:248–254

Chapter 8

Identification of Human Eosinophils in Whole Blood by Flow Cytometry

Caroline Ethier, Paige Lacy, and Francis Davoine

Abstract

Identification of eosinophils in whole blood samples by flow cytometry is often problematic. There are usually only a low number and percentage of cells that may be detected, and it may be difficult to discriminate eosinophils from other granulocytes. Here, we propose a simple approach using the eosinophil's intrinsic autofluorescence properties, combined with detection of CCR3 expression, to reliably identify eosinophils in a mixed leukocyte population.

Key words Flow cytometry, Eosinophils, Granulocytes, White blood cell differential, CCR3, CD193

1 Introduction

The identification of eosinophil granulocytes in whole blood samples represents a challenge. These cells are part of a rare population and are usually difficult to discriminate from other granulocytes simply by the measurement of light scattering properties. Isolation of circulating eosinophils requires large quantities of blood (50–100 ml) as well as lengthy manipulation procedures. Moreover, many of the techniques used for eosinophil isolation may activate granulocytes and/or deplete important subpopulations, such as hypodense or CD16-positive subpopulations. For example, CD16 expression on eosinophils can vary in pathological conditions such as asthma or by cytokine stimulation [1–6]. This can be circumvented through whole blood staining of eosinophils in combination with standard flow cytometry equipment using simple gating strategies and specific eosinophil markers. The use of intrinsic physical and optical characteristics of eosinophils in order to identify these cells in whole blood has been elegantly demonstrated by Lavigne et al. [7]. They reported the use of depolarized orthogonal light scattering to allow better discrimination of neutrophils from eosinophils. Unfortunately, it may not be possible or

Garry M. Walsh (ed.), *Eosinophils: Methods and Protocols*, Methods in Molecular Biology, vol. 1178,
DOI 10.1007/978-1-4939-1016-8_8, © Springer Science+Business Media New York 2014

81

practical to modify side scatter settings in most flow cytometry facilities with a depolarized light filter, which poses a major technical limitation. Here, we describe the use of simple physical-optical attributes of light scattering, autofluorescence, and specific receptor expression of CCR3 to reliably identify human eosinophils in a mixed leukocyte population from whole venous blood samples.

2 Materials

Sterile distilled water must be used to prepare all solutions. No sodium azide should be added to any reagents.

1. Lysis buffer: Ammonium chloride–potassium bicarbonate lysing solution. Add 800 ml of water to a glass beaker. Weigh 8.29 g of NH_4Cl, 1 g of $KHCO_3$, and 0.0372 g of Na_2EDTA and transfer to the beaker. Mix, and adjust the pH to 7.35 with HCl. Transfer to a 1 L graduated glass cylinder, and make up to 1 L with distilled water. Store at room temperature, and use within 4 weeks.

2. Phosphate-buffered saline (PBS): Add 800 ml of distilled water to a glass beaker. Weigh 8 g of NaCl, 1.15 g of Na_2HPO_4, 0.2 g KH_2PO_4, and 0.2 g of KCl, transfer to the beaker, and dissolve thoroughly with stirring. Adjust pH to 7.35 with HCl. Transfer to a graduated glass cylinder, and make up to 1 L. Keep at room temperature (*see* **Note 1**).

3. 10× PBS: Add ~70 ml of water to a glass beaker. Weigh 8 g of NaCl, 1.15 g of Na_2HPO_4, 0.2 g KH_2PO_4, and 0.2 g of KCl, transfer to the beaker, and dissolve thoroughly with stirring. Transfer to a graduated glass cylinder, and make up to 100 ml. Keep at room temperature (*see* **Note 1**).

4. Blocking buffer: 5 % Goat serum in PBS. Add 0.5 ml of goat serum in 10 ml of PBS. Mix well, and keep at 4 °C.

5. Flow buffer: 5 % Bovine serum albumin in PBS. Weigh 50 g of bovine serum albumin and add to 1 L PBS in a beaker. Mix well, and keep at 4 °C. Prepare fresh on the day of use, preferentially, and discard within a week of preparation as this is easily contaminated by microbial growth.

6. Paraformaldehyde (4 %): Warm 80 ml of PBS to 65 °C in a beaker using a microwave (i.e., not boiling!) (*see* **Note 2**). Weigh 4 g of paraformaldehyde and add to the warm water under the fume hood. Add a magnetic stirrer, and mix for 10 min until the solution is fully suspended and cloudy. Then add one drop of NaOH (4 M) to the solution. The solution will turn almost instantly clear. If not, add another drop of NaOH and repeat until the solution is absolutely clear (*see* **Note 3**). Cool down the solution for 30 min in an ice

bucket under the fume hood. When the solution is ice cold adjust pH to 7.3 with HCl. Then using a graduated glass cylinder, add PBS to make up to 100 ml. Aliquot the solutions in 15 ml tubes and keep at -20 °C (*see* **Note 4**).

---

3 Methods

3.1 Staining of Whole Blood Leukocytes

1. Venous blood is usually collected in Vacutainer™ collection tubes containing anticoagulant (*see* **Note 5**).

2. To 5 ml of blood, add 10 ml of lysis solution in a 50 ml Falcon conical tube (*see* **Note 6**).

3. Incubate for 10 min at room temperature on a rocking plate (gentle mixing at 30 rpm). Add PBS (room temperature) to 50 ml to stop the reaction, and centrifuge at $200 \times g$ for 7 min.

4. Remove the supernatant by aspiration. Recap the tube, and resuspend the pellet of cells by flicking the bottom of the tube with your fingers (*see* **Note 7**). Then add 5 ml blocking buffer, and count cells using a hemocytometer. If there are still some red blood cells, this will not cause a problem for staining and flow cytometry acquisition.

5. Adjust the cell concentration to 10^7 cells/ml with blocking buffer. Mix gently by manually flicking the cell suspension without using a pipette or vortexing. This is important for maintaining cell integrity.

6. Add 100 µl of cell suspension to a flow cytometry tube (5 ml snap cap tubes) for each sample (*see* **Note 8**). Typically, you will need one tube for an isotype control (e.g., IgG_1 if the test antibody is an IgG_1 antibody) and a second tube for the test control (i.e., the antibody of interest which is IgG_1 in this example) where you wish to carry out single staining. If performing multiple marker labeling with antibodies conjugated to different fluorescent dyes, you will need to generate a multiple isotype control for each antibody used by combining isotype control antibodies in one tube. It is also recommended to include an additional tube as an unstained autofluorescence control that lacks antibodies.

7. For a demonstration experiment, we used conjugated antibodies against human CD4-FITC, CD45-FITC, CD8-PE, CD3-PERCP, CCR3-APC, and CD25-APC. *See* Table 1 for the staining protocol.

8. Add antibodies according to your staining plan (e.g., Table 1). Since monoclonal antibodies may come from different sources and production batches, refer to the manufacturer's instructions for optimal concentrations required. Add the antibodies directly in the cell suspension at the bottom of respective tubes. Mix gently without vortexing.

Table 1
Spreadsheet of fluorescent antibody combinations

Tube numbers	Purpose	Antibodies (mix)	Comments
1	Autofluorescence	None	Process the cells as the other tubes for washing, centrifugation, and fixation
2	Isotype control APC	Matched isotypes for FITC, PE, PERCP, and APC	Use same isotype concentration than the respective test antibodies
3	Compensation control	CD4-FITC	Individual staining to control overlapping of fluorescence
4	Compensation control	CD8-PE	
5	Compensation control	CD3-PERCP	
6	Compensation control	CCR3-APC	
7	TEST CCR3	CD4-FITC+CD8-PE+CD3-PERCP+CCR3-APC	
8	Compensation control	CD25-APC	
9	TEST CD25	CD4-FITC+CD8-PE+CD3-PERCP+CD25-APC	
10	TEST CD45	CD45-FITC+CCR3-APC	

The concentration of antibodies should be adjusted to manufacturer technical data sheet. The optimal concentration should be determined for individual application and cell concentration. We stained cells with a concentration of antibody proteins of 1 μg/million cells or 10 μg/ml

9. Incubate antibodies with cell suspensions. Ideally, incubate on ice for 20 min protected from light.

10. After incubation, add 4 ml flow buffer to each tube and centrifuge at $200 \times g$ for 5 min at 4 °C (*see* **Note 9**).

11. Remove supernatants, and discard liquid directly into a beaker containing a small volume of bleach for biohazard control. The last remaining drop of liquid at the tube collar should be wiped using absorbent tissue paper (*see* **Note 10**).

12. Resuspend each pellet by gentle tube flicking.

13. Add 100 μl of paraformaldehyde (4 %) solution, mix each tube by gentle agitation, and keep on ice for 10 min.

14. After fixation, add 300 μl of flow buffer (*see* **Note 11**).

15. Keep in the dark at 0–4 °C until ready for flow cytometry acquisition.

3.2 Distinguishing Eosinophils from Other Blood Leukocytes by Flow Cytometry

Since there are a wide variety of flow cytometers available, we will not discuss specific instrument settings here, but instead will provide strategies to obtain the desired results. Results shown as an example in this section were obtained using a BD FACSCanto™ II Flow Cytometer.

1. To begin acquisition, we recommend performing a baseline setting of the instrument's photomultipliers using Tube #1 (autofluorescence, Table 1). Using forward scattering (FS) and side scattering (SSC), adjust the voltage settings of the photomultipliers to visualize the entire cell population. In our example, we used a log scale for SSC to spread the scale and allow better grouping of different populations depicted on flow cytometry density plots. Increase the voltage and gain as much as necessary for FS and SS properties of your cell population to ensure that you visualize the entire population. Too low a voltage setting will result in grouping all cells in the lower left corner of the density plot and render it impossible to discriminate intact cells from debris and erythrocytes. In Fig. 1, a representative flow cytometry density plot of side scatter (SSC-log) and forward scatter (FS-linear) is shown in a whole blood sample. Granulocytes, monocytes, and lymphocytes are easily discriminated based on their light scattering properties using the argon 488 nm laser. However, it is usually difficult to clearly distinguish eosinophils from neutrophils in the granulocyte population using only forward and side scattering characteristics.

2. Next, examine the FITC-related fluorescence in the cell population by acquisition of data using the argon 488 laser.

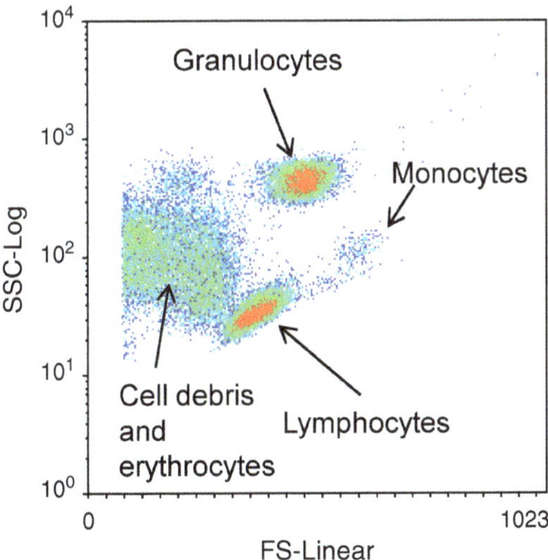

Fig. 1 A typical 488 nm light scattering density plot of whole blood after lysis of erythrocytes with ammonium chloride solution

Neutrophils are less autofluorescent than eosinophils when excited by the argon laser, allowing discrimination of these two cell types. Figure 2a shows a typical FITC isotype control result. This density plot reveals a small population of cells (eosinophils) exhibiting high SSC-log along with higher autofluorescence. Using different antibodies against CD4, CD3, CD8, CD45, and CD25 receptors conjugated to common fluorophores (FITC, PE, PERCP, APC), it is possible to distinguish a population of CD4$^+$ cells (Fig. 2b). CD45 is present on all leukocytes, to varying intensities, as depicted in Fig. 2c. This density plot depicts CD45$^+$ cells shifted to the right side of the graph, while CD45$^-$ erythrocytes and debris remain in their original position on the left side of the density plot. In Fig. 2a–c, autofluorescent eosinophils are clearly discernible from neutrophils.

3. Eosinophil autofluorescence may also be detected with other commonly used photomultipliers for PE (585 nm) and PERCP (670 nm) when excited with 488 nm argon laser. Figure 3a, c shows eosinophil autofluorescence observed with isotype controls for PE and PERCP, respectively. Staining for CD8-PE and CD3-PERCP (Fig. 3b, d) as well as CD4-FITC (Fig. 2b) did not affect the autofluorescence of eosinophils.

4. To confirm the identity of eosinophils, a specific marker is required. Good surface markers for flow cytometry identification of human eosinophils include VLA-4 (CD49) [8], CRTH2 (CD294) [9], and CCR3 (CD193) [10]. In our example, we confirmed eosinophil identification by autofluorescence using a far-red wavelength HeNe (633 nm) laser. In contrast to the use of the 488 nm argon laser to detect eosinophil autofluorescence, eosinophils fail to autofluoresce distinctly from neutrophils when excited with the 633 nm laser, as seen in Fig. 4a using the isotype control for APC (660 nm). This allows a clear identification of eosinophils using anti-CCR3-APC in Fig. 4b. The CCR3$^+$ population of cells with high SSC-log (eosinophils) was back-gated on autofluorescent cells in Figs. 2a and 3a, c to confirm their identification as eosinophils, shown in Fig. 5 for PE autofluorescence. Figure 4c shows an additional control (staining with anti-CD25-APC, the IL-2 receptor) indicating the absence of autofluorescent high SSC-log cells as well as confirming the absence of nonspecific binding in the isotype control in Fig. 4a and CCR3-APC (Fig. 4b).

5. Using autofluorescence-based identification strategies for eosinophils, it is possible to collect highly purified eosinophils by sorting using flow cytometry. Sorting should be carried out only on unlabeled cells to ensure that they are not activated for additional measurements.

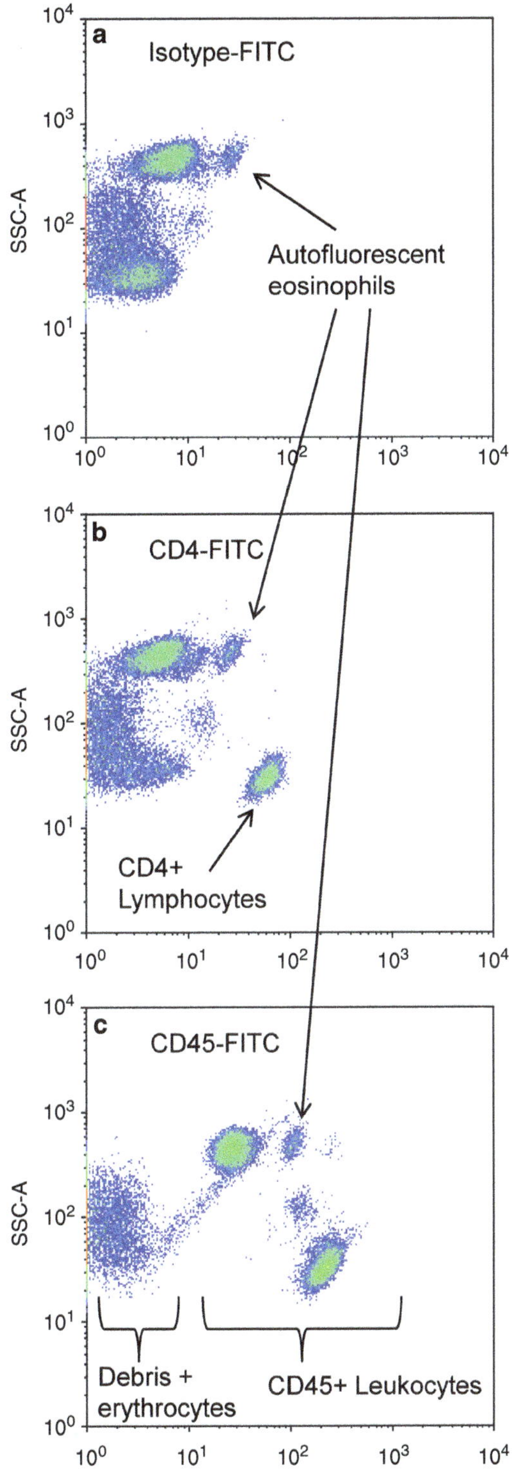

Fig. 2 Density plots of 488 nm argon laser excitation and green (530 nm) emission of whole blood leukocytes. (**a**) Emission from isotype control (mouse IgG) coupled with FITC (nonspecific staining control). (**b**) Staining of CD4$^+$ T cells with anti-CD4-FITC. (**c**) Staining of total leukocytes with anti-CD45-FITC

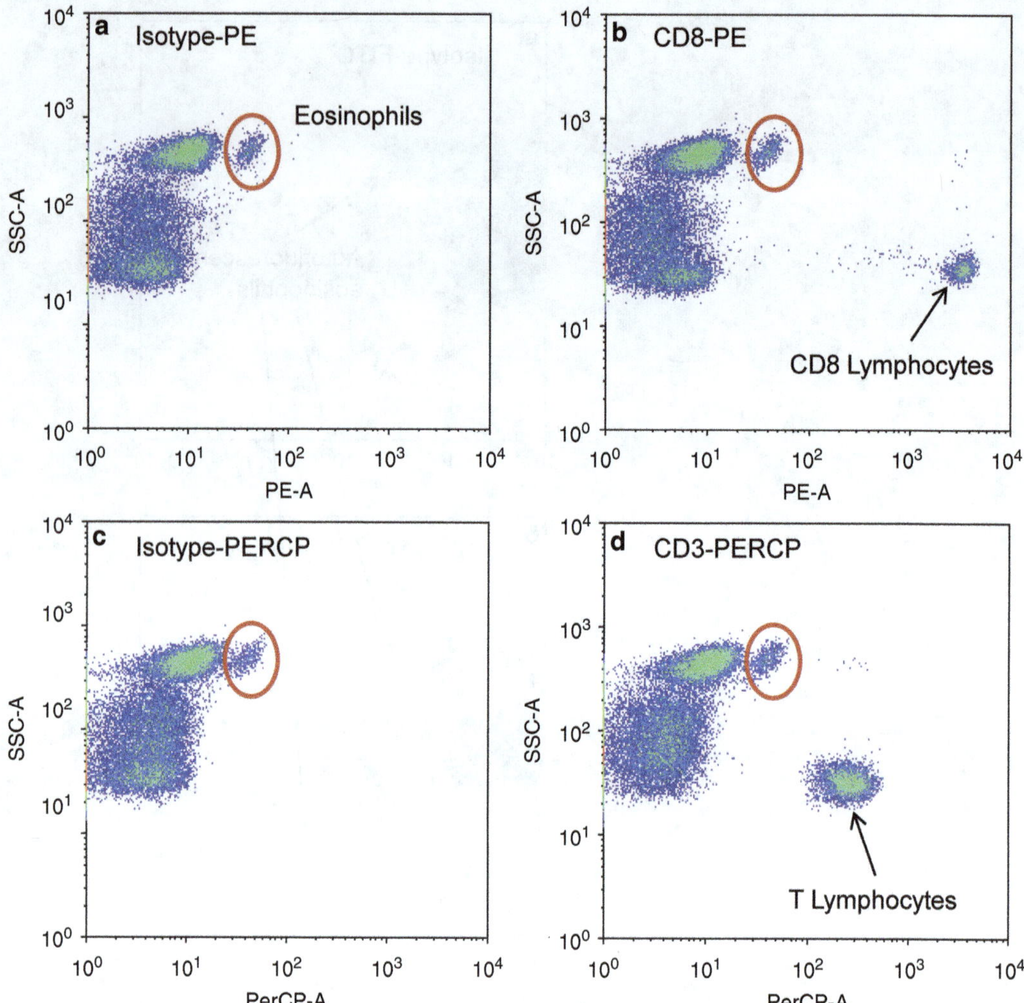

Fig. 3 Density plots of 488 nm argon laser excitation and *orange* (585 nm) and *red* (670 nm) emission of whole blood leukocytes. (**a** and **c**) Isotype controls for PE and PERCP, respectively. (**b** and **d**) Specific staining for CD8+ T cells (CD8-PE) and all T cells (CD3-PERCP). Autofluorescent eosinophil cell populations are *circled* in each density plot

4 Notes

1. You can also use ready-made PBS and 10× PBS from laboratory suppliers. To prevent clumping of leukocytes, use PBS without Mg^{2+} and Ca^{2+}; these cations contribute to coagulation. PBS must be prepared fresh on the day of use and must be discarded if unused as it is prone to microbial contamination.

2. Wear a mask and gloves when weighing paraformaldehyde. Cover the weigh boat with another weigh boat of similar size to avoid dispersion of paraformaldehyde powder when transporting to the fume hood. Keep the solution under the fume

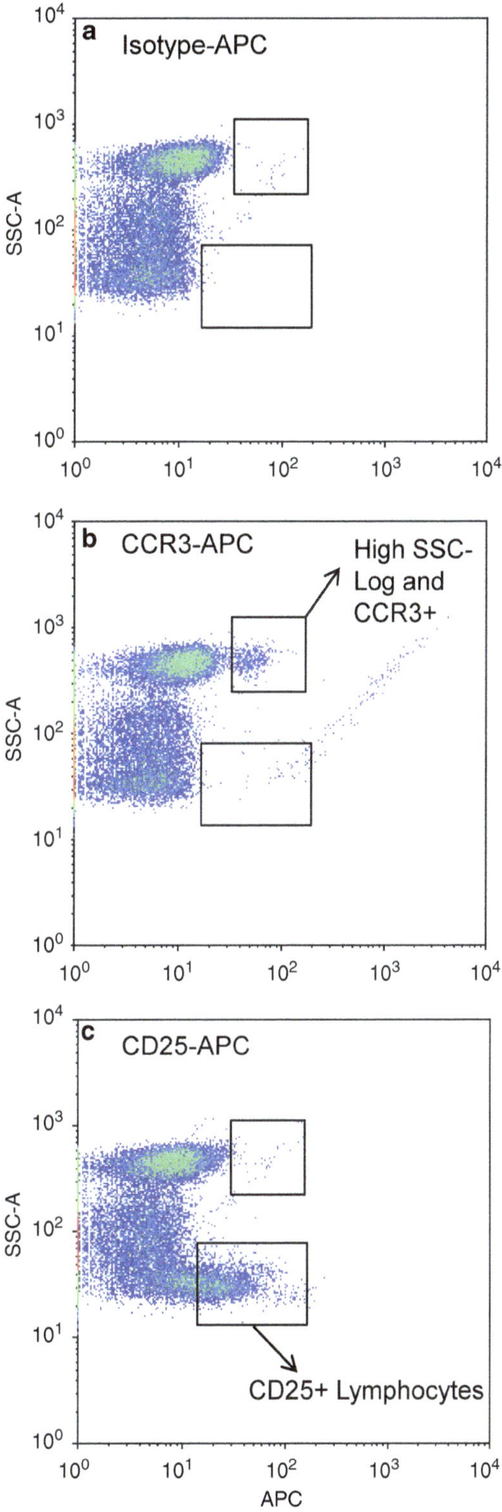

Fig. 4 Density plots of 633 nm HeNe laser excitation and *red* (660 nm) emission of whole blood leukocytes. (**a**) Isotype control emission (mouse IgG coupled with APC). (**b**) Leukocytes stained with anti-CCR3-APC to confirm eosinophils. (**c**) Staining for anti-CD25-APC to detect cells expressing IL-2 receptor. Rectangles in density plots show positive staining of high SSC-log (SSC-A) for CCR3 in (**b**) and CD25[+] T cells in (**c**)

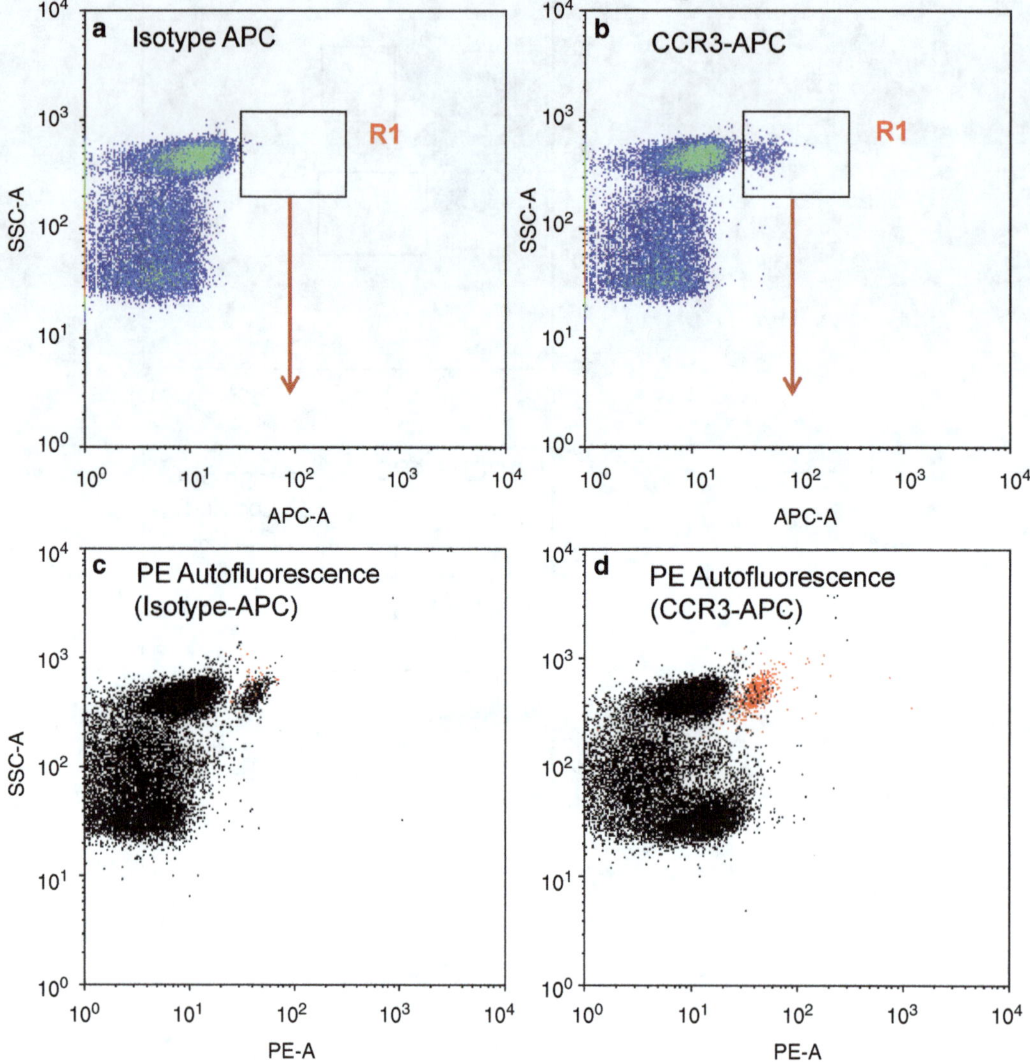

Fig. 5 Confirmation of specific eosinophil granulocyte autofluorescence. The *red* events in panels (**c** and **d**) are coming from the sort rectangle gate in (**a** and **b**), respectively. CCR3[+] cells in (**b**) are shown in *red* in panel (**d**) confirming that high SS/CCR3[+] cells are also high SS/high autofluorescent cells

hood until it is ice cold. We highly recommend adding PBS at this stage, because buffered paraformaldehyde is superior to paraformaldehyde prepared in water. The reason for this is that paraformaldehyde becomes formaldehyde in solution, which then breaks down into formic acid very readily if the solution is not buffered. Even if it is frozen at −20 °C, thawing paraformaldehyde in water increases formic acid development. Formic acid degrades cells and does not fix them appropriately.

3. Paraformaldehyde is very difficult to solubilize unless you warm and increase the pH of the solution. Usually one or two drops of NaOH (4 M) is sufficient to dissolve paraformaldehyde powder.

4. Paraformaldehyde solution will stay stable for at least 1 year when stored at −20 °C. It is highly recommended to use PBS to dissolve paraformaldehyde, because buffered paraformaldehyde is superior to paraformaldehyde prepared in water. The reason for this is that when paraformaldehyde becomes formaldehyde in solution, it rapidly produces formic acid if the solution is not buffered. Even if frozen at −20 °C, thawing paraformaldehyde in water will result in formic acid generation. Formic acid does not fix cells and instead degrades them. Once paraformaldehyde is prepared in this manner, aliquot the solution in 15 ml conical tubes, and thaw the minimum amount necessary for daily use. If after thawing the solution is slightly cloudy, place the hermetically closed tube in lukewarm water (50–60 °C) for 10 min until clear again. Then place tube in an ice bucket to cool it down.

5. Vacutainer™ blood collection tubes may contain EDTA (purple cap) or heparin (green cap) to prevent coagulation. EDTA is the preferred anticoagulant to use when working with granulocytes.

6. All these manipulations should be done in a biosafety laminar flow cabinet in a level 2 laboratory and in compliance with your institution's biosafety regulations regarding handling of human samples.

7. Flicking the tubes: Hold one well-closed tube by the cap, and tap the bottom side with one finger to cause the cell pellet to gently break down. If this flicking does not work you can carefully use a 2 ml pipette and, by gentle up–down aspiration, break up the pellet.

8. Carefully pipette 100 μl cell suspensions without up and down aspirations, since shear stress through the pipette tip may cause cells to disintegrate. Slowly dispense cell suspensions directly to the bottom of the tube. The resulting number of cells per tube should be $10^6/100$ μl. Keep tubes in an open tube rack and place over crushed ice in a large ice box.

9. This is a washing step to remove unbound antibodies. You should be able to see a similar small pellet of cells at the bottom of each tube. Some remaining red blood cells may give the pellet a pink color.

10. Our experience suggests that pouring out supernatants (direct dispensation) is less likely to cause loss of cells and may be less time consuming than aspiration of supernatants directly from tubes. With top-to-bottom aspiration of supernatant liquid,

there is more of a risk of turbulence and inadvertent loss of cells. Perform this step in one gentle motion without shaking the tube. There is usually about 50 μl of liquid remaining in the tube after direct dispensation. This also prevents exposure of cells to air, which causes degradation of cell integrity.

11. Fixation of labeled cells with paraformaldehyde will stabilize antibodies on cell surfaces and prevent further degradation of cells. The final concentration of paraformaldehyde will be a little less than 17 % which is sufficient to preserve cell integrity and staining for at least 72 h.

Acknowledgements

This work was supported by funding from Agriculture Life and Environmental Science (ALES) and Campus Saint-Jean research funds from University of Alberta to FD.

References

1. Hartnell A, Moqbel R, Walsh GM, Bradley B, Kay AB (1990) Fc gamma and CD11/CD18 receptor expression on normal density and low density human eosinophils. Immunology 69:264–270

2. Davoine F, Labonte I, Ferland C, Mazer B, Chakir J, Laviolette M (2004) Role and modulation of CD16 expression on eosinophils by cytokines and immune complexes. Int Arch Allergy Immunol 134:165–172

3. Davoine F, Lavigne S, Chakir J, Ferland C, Boulay ME, Laviolette M (2002) Expression of FcgammaRIII (CD16) on human peripheral blood eosinophils increases in allergic conditions. J Allergy Clin Immunol 109:463–469

4. Valerius T, Repp R, Kalden JR, Platzer E (1990) Effects of IFN on human eosinophils in comparison with other cytokines. A novel class of eosinophil activators with delayed onset of action. J Immunol 145:2950–2958

5. Zhu X, Hamann KJ, Munoz NM, Rubio N, Mayer D, Hernrreiter A, Leff AR (1998) Intracellular expression of Fc gamma RIII (CD16) and its mobilization by chemoattractants in human eosinophils. J Immunol 161:2574–2579

6. Hartnell A, Kay AB, Wardlaw AJ (1992) IFN-gamma induces expression of Fc gamma RIII (CD16) on human eosinophils. J Immunol 148:1471–1478

7. Lavigne S, Bosse M, Boulet LP, Laviolette M (1997) Identification and analysis of eosinophils by flow cytometry using the depolarized side scatter-saponin method. Cytometry 29:197–203

8. Thurau AM, Schylz U, Wolf V, Krug N, Schauer U (1996) Identification of eosinophils by flow cytometry. Cytometry 23:150–158

9. Faucher JL, Lacronique-Gazaille C, Frebet E, Trimoreau F, Donnard M, Bordessoule D, Lacombe F, Feuillard J (2007) "6 markers/5 colors" extended white blood cell differential by flow cytometry. Cytometry A 71:934–944

10. Ponath PD, Qin S, Post TW, Wang J, Wu L, Gerard NP, Newman W, Gerard C, Mackay CR (1996) Molecular cloning and characterization of a human eotaxin receptor expressed selectively on eosinophils. J Exp Med 183:2437–2448

Chapter 9

Isolation and Functional Assessment of Eosinophil Crystalloid Granules

Renata Baptista-dos-Reis, Valdirene S. Muniz, and Josiane S. Neves

Abstract

Cell-free granules, upon extrusion from human eosinophils, remain fully competent to secrete granule-derived proteins in receptor-mediated processes in response to different stimuli. However, in order to avoid the shrinkage and damage of granules, as well as preserve their structure, properties, and functionality, the use of an optimized process of subcellular fractionation using an isoosmotic density gradient is needed. Here, we describe a detailed protocol of subcellular fractionation of nitrogen-cavitated eosinophils on an isoosmotic iodinated density gradient (iodixanol) and the isolation of well-preserved and functional membrane-bound specific granules.

Key words Granules, Iodixanol, Subcellular fractionation, Isoosmotic gradient, Eosinophils

1 Introduction

Eosinophils are leukocytes notably associated with allergic conditions, anti-helminthic host defense, and immunoregulatory responses. Mature eosinophils have a single population of secondary (or specific or crystalloid) granules ultrastructurally characterized as membrane-bound organelles that contain a crystalloid core surrounded by a matrix. These granules store a variety of preformed proteins including cationic proteins such as eosinophil cationic protein (ECP), major basic protein (MBP), eosinophil peroxidase (EPO), eosinophil-derived neurotoxin (EDN), enzymes, and over 36 cytokines, chemokines, and growth factors [1, 2]. The intriguing presence of membrane-bound cell-free granules extruded from eosinophils has been long recognized in tissues associated with eosinophilia, including allergic diseases and responses to helminths [3, 4]. However, over the years, the presence and relevance of these eosinophil granules in tissue sites have been underestimated and at times attributed to "crush artifacts." Recently, we presented evidence for the functional capability of intact extracellular cell-free granules [5, 6]. Eosinophil granules express receptors on their

Garry M. Walsh (ed.), *Eosinophils: Methods and Protocols*, Methods in Molecular Biology, vol. 1178,
DOI 10.1007/978-1-4939-1016-8_9, © Springer Science+Business Media New York 2014

membranes that recognize eotaxin-1 (CCL11), interferon-γ, and cysteinyl leukotrienes [5–7]. In response to these ligands, cell-free granules selectively secrete cationic proteins and cytokines by signal-transducing, kinase pathway-dependent processes. Cell-free granules, upon extrusion from human eosinophils, remain fully competent to secrete granule-derived proteins in receptor-mediated processes in response to select chemokines, cytokines, and cysteinyl leukotrienes [5–7]. However, in order to isolate functional well-preserved membrane-bound eosinophil crystalloid granules, the use of an optimized process of subcellular fractionation using an isoosmotic density gradient is needed. Here we describe a detailed protocol of subcellular fractionation of nitrogen-cavitated eosinophils on an isoosmotic iodinated density gradient and the isolation of functional membrane-bound specific granules.

2   Materials

Prepare all solutions using ultrapure water (deionized water) and analytical grade reagents.

2.1 Eosinophil Disruption and Gradient Components

1. Disruption buffer: 0.25 M Sucrose, 10 mM Hepes, 1 mM EGTA—pH 7.4. Add about 50 mL to a 100 mL graduated cylinder or a glass beaker. Weight 8.55 g of sucrose, 260 mg of Hepes, and 38 mg of EGTA and transfer to the cylinder. Add water to a volume of 90 mL. Mix, and adjust pH with HCl. Make up to 100 mL with water. Store 6 mL aliquots of disruption buffer at −20 °C until use.

2. Diluent: 0.25 M Sucrose, 60 mM Hepes, 6 mM EGTA, pH = 7.4. Add about 50 mL to a 100 mL graduated cylinder or a glass beaker. Weight 8.55 g of sucrose, 1.43 g of Hepes, and 228 mg of EGTA and transfer to the cylinder. Add water to a volume of 90 mL. Mix, and adjust pH with HCl. Make up to 100 mL with water. Store 6 mL aliquots of diluent at −20 °C until use.

3. Iodixanol solution 45 %: Iodixanol solution 45 % is prepared from a ready-made mixture of iodixanol/water 60 % (w/v) commercially available under the name of OptiPrep (OptiPrep, Axis-Shield, Oslo, Sweden, density 1.32 ± 0.001 g/mL; osmolality 170 ± 15 mOsm). It was prepared after two subsequent dilution steps as follows. First, prepare a 50 % (w/v) solution: mix 250 mL of iodixanol 60 % with 50 mL of diluent. To reach a 45 % (w/v) gradient solution, mix 300 mL of iodixanol 50 % with 33.33 mL of the disruption buffer. According to the OptiPrep manufacturer, the density of the iodixanol 45 % (w/v) gradient solution prepared as described above is between

1.243 and 1.252 g/mL. The density of iodixanol 45 % (w/v) in our conditions was 1.248 g/mL. Store 6 mL aliquots of iodixanol 45 % (w/v) at –20 °C until use.

4. Ultracentrifugation tubes for gradient preparation and subcellular fractionation—open top polyclear centrifuge tubes—14 × 89 mm.

5. Cell disruption bomb (Parr Instrument, Moline, IL, USA).

6. Phenylmethylsulfonyl fluoride (PMSF), $MgCl_2$, ATP, pepstatin, N-alpha-p-tosyl-L-arginine methyl ester hydrochloride (TAME), aprotinin, 1,4-dithio-DL-threitol (DTT), and leupeptin.

2.2 Granule-Enriched Fraction Identification Components

1. Substrate solution for EPO: 100 mM Tris–HCl, 3 mM H_2O_2, 16 mM O-phenylenediamine dihydrochloride (OPD), and 0.1 % Triton X-100, pH = 8. Add about 45 mL of water to a 50 mL clean tube. Weight 788 mg of Tris–HCl and transfer to the tube. Mix, and adjust the pH to 8. Weight 144.8 mg of OPD, transfer to the tube, and mix. Add 50 μL of Triton X-100. Mix gently. Make up to 50 mL with water. Just right before starting the substrate addition add 17 μL of a 30 % H_2O_2 commercial solution. Prepare the solution on the day of the experiment. Keep the tube in the dark during all steps.

2. Stop solution for EPO activity measurement (H_2SO_4 4 M): Caution: H_2SO_4 is a strong acid. Add 21.39 mL of H_2SO_4 (MW = 98.08 and density = 1.84 kg/L) to a 50 mL graduated cylinder. Add small volumes of H_2SO_4 to a 100 mL cylinder or a glass beaker containing 78.61 mL of water. This is an exothermic reaction and the acid must be added very slowly.

3. Digital densitometer.

3 Methods

Carry out all procedures in the laminar flow hood and at room temperature unless otherwise specified.

3.1 Isolation of Human Eosinophils from Peripheral Blood

1. Isolate eosinophils from the blood of healthy donors by previously described methods [8] and as described in Chapter 2.

3.2 Continuous Iodixanol Gradient Preparation

1. For gradient preparation use a standard two-chamber gradient maker connected to a peristaltic pump set to ~180 μL/min (Fig. 1) (*see* **Notes 1** and **2**).

2. Thaw one 6 mL aliquot of disruption buffer, one 6 mL aliquot of diluent, and one 6 mL aliquot of iodixanol 45 % (w/v).

3. Lay a cushion of 0.5 mL iodixanol 45 % (w/v) on the bottom of the ultracentrifugation tube.

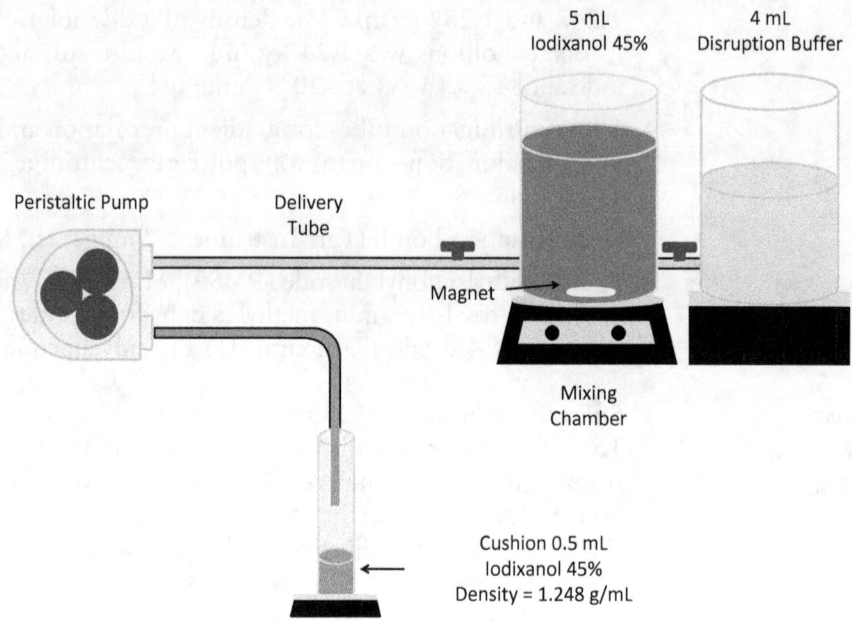

Fig. 1 Continuous gradient-forming device showing the reservoir containing the lower density solution (4 mL disruption buffer) connected to the mixing chamber containing the higher density solution (5 mL iodixanol 45 %) via a channel with a stopcock. A delivery tube leads from the mixing chamber to a peristaltic pump and then to the top wall of the centrifuge tube containing a cushion of 0.5 mL iodixanol 45 %

4. Place 5 mL of iodixanol 45 % in the mixing chamber of the gradient maker (the one connected to the delivery tube) (*see* **Note 3**) and 4 mL of the disruption buffer in the other chamber. The tip of the delivery tube needs to be placed against the wall of the ultracentrifuge tube close to its top (Fig. 1).

5. Open the stopcocks, and turn on the peristaltic pump. The incoming gradient is allowed to flow in a steady stream down the wall of the tube (Fig. 1).

6. Under these described conditions, the gradient takes around 1 h to be formed.

7. Keep the gradient at 4 °C until use.

3.3 Disruption of Eosinophils for Subcellular Fractionation

1. Start this step when the eosinophil purification is ready.

2. For subcellular fractionation, use a number of eosinophils not less than 10×10^6 and not more than 35×10^6 in order to obtain a reasonable amount of eosinophil-specific granules and to prevent overloading the gradient, respectively.

3. Using a plastic Pasteur pipette, resuspend the isolated eosinophils ($10–35 \times 10^6$) in 1 mL of disruption buffer (0.25 M sucrose, 1 mM EGTA, 10 mM Hepes—pH 7.4) previously supplemented with 100 µg/mL PMSF, 2 mM $MgCl_2$, 1 mM ATP, and 5 µg/mL each of pepstatin, TAME, aprotinin, DTT, and leupeptin, all of them added just before use (*see* **Note 4**).

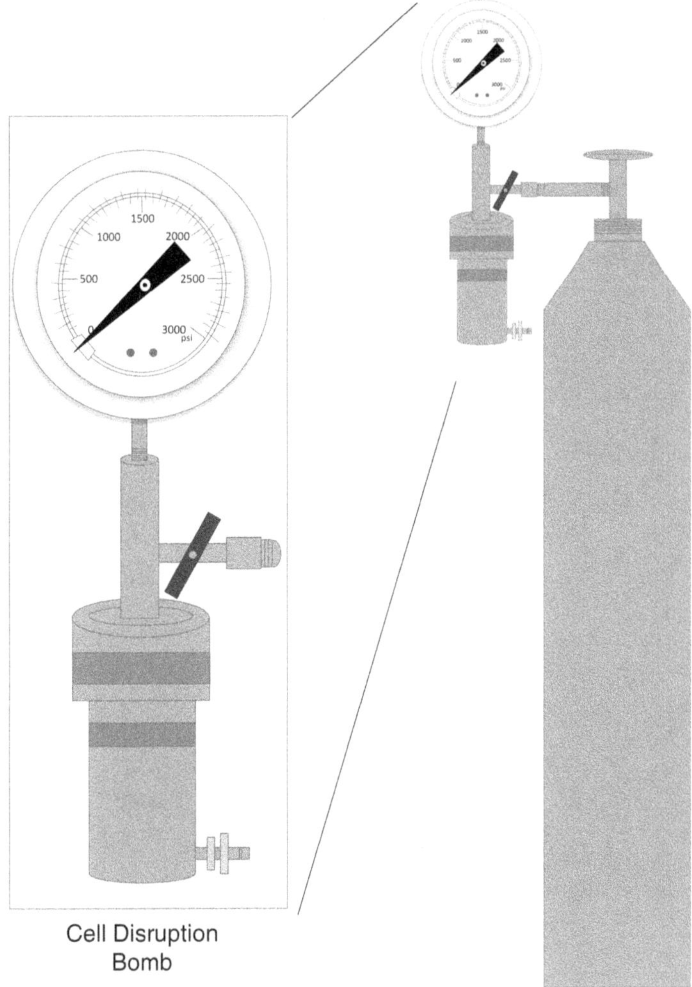

Fig. 2 Nitrogen cavitation. Cell disruption bomb connected to a nitrogen tank. Eosinophils were pressurized under nitrogen for 10 min at 600 psi

4. Place the eosinophil suspension in a cell disruption bomb connected to a nitrogen tank, and pressurize the cells under nitrogen atmosphere for 10 min at 600 psi (4 °C) (Fig. 2) (*see* **Note 5**).

5. Collect the cavitate drop by drop very slowly and gently.

6. Centrifuge the cavitate at $200 \times g$ at 4 °C for 10 min to pellet nuclei and intact cells.

7. Carefully decant the post-nuclear supernatant (S1), and keep it at 4 °C.

8. Resuspend the pellet in another 1 mL of disruption buffer supplemented with protease inhibitors, and submit the suspension to a second nitrogen cavitation (*see* **Note 6**).

9. Centrifuge the second cavitate ($200 \times g$, 4 °C, 10 min), and decant the second post-nuclear supernatant (S2).

10. Join S1 and S2, centrifuge again (200×*g*, 4 °C, 10 min), decant, and save the supernatant (S3).

11. Analyze the supernatant (S3) content by light microscopy to ensure the absence of intact cells or nuclei.

3.4 Gradient Loading and Subcellular Fractionation

1. Apply the 2 mL post-nuclear supernatant (S3) slowly through a plastic Pasteur pipette on the top of the precooled gradient.

2. Ultracentrifuge the loaded gradient at 100,000×*g* for 1 h at 4 °C. After ultracentrifugation, the eosinophil-specific granule band can be visualized at denser gradient fractions as indicated in Fig. 3.

3. Collect fractions at 4 °C in 1.5 mL centrifuge tubes by aspiration from the bottom through a capillary tube attached to a polyethylene tube connected to a peristaltic pump and a fraction collector (total of 20 fractions—~500 µL each, ~12 drops). The granule-enriched fractions are normally fractions number 5 and 6 (from the bottom to the top—*see* **Note** 7).

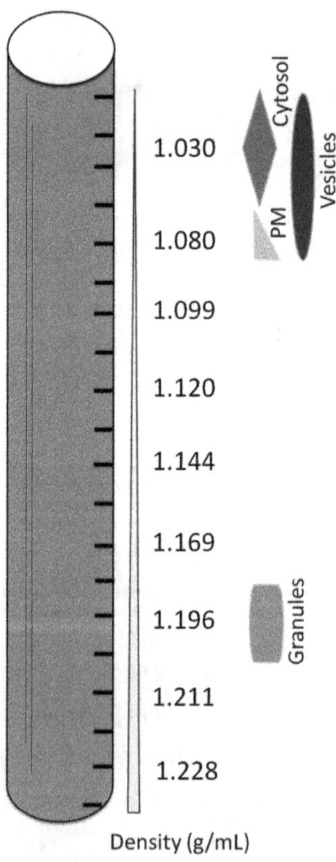

Fig. 3 After centrifugation at 100,000 × *g* for 1 h, the gradient shows an eosinophil granule band as indicated. The less dense vesicle-, plasma membrane- (PM), and cytoplasm-containing fractions are also indicated. Eosinophil subcellular fractions were separated on the basis of their density range (1.228–1.030 g/mL) on iodixanol gradient

4. It is recommended to verify the density of the gradient fractions by the use of a digital densitometer. The gradient fraction densities are reported in Fig. 3 (*see* **Note 8**).

3.5 Granule Fraction Identification

After collecting the fractions, the next step is to identify the granule-enriched fractions. From the bottom to the top, granule-enriched fractions are usually fractions 5 and 6. However, the measurement of EPO activity can be used as a marker for granule-enriched fractions. EPO activity can be measured by a colorimetric assay as described below.

1. Add 20 μL of each fraction to a 96-well plate.

2. Add 100 μL of EPO substrate solution (100 mM Tris–HCl, 3 mM H_2O_2, 16 mM OPD, and 0.1 % Triton X-100, pH = 8).

3. Stop the reaction after 2 min by the addition of 100 μL 4 M H_2SO_4.

4. Read the plate at 492 nm.

3.6 Granule Isolation and Stimulation

After granule-enriched fraction identification:

1. Pool and split granule-enriched fractions into aliquots depending on experimental groups (*see* **Note 9**) using 1.5 mL centrifuge tubes.

2. Add 1 mL of calcium–magnesium-free HBSS to each sample to help wash away the gradient component residues (sucrose, etc.).

3. Pellet the granules by centrifugation using a swinging-bucket rotor (to ensure that the granule pellet will be located on the bottom of the tube) at $2,500 \times g$ for 10 min.

4. Resuspend the granule pellets in proper medium. For granule stimulation and measurement of their secretory proteins in the supernatants, granules can be resuspended in RPMI plus 0.1 % ovalbumin (acceptable volumes 200–250 μL). After appropriate stimulation, pellet the granules at 2,500 g for 10 min using a swinging-bucket rotor and freeze the supernatants at –20 °C for further evaluations.

---

4   Notes

1. Prepare the gradient freshly on the day of the experiment. The gradient must be cold at the time of loading. The best approach is to start preparing the gradient right after the eosinophil purification initiation.

2. The gradient maker system must be cleaned exhaustedly with deionized water each time it is used to avoid deposition of sucrose residues.

3. The mixing chamber contains a small magnet that gently mixes the medium before it reaches the delivery tube.

4. Prepare concentrated stock solutions of the supplements in order to add small volumes (range 1–10 μL) to the 1 mL disruption buffer.

5. This procedure can be performed in a cold room. We recommend performing all the cell and granule manipulation very gently with plastic Pasteur pipettes at 4 °C in order to minimize cell damage or activation.

6. The second nitrogen cavitation is performed to optimize the eosinophil disruption and increase the granule yield.

7. Collection from the top to the bottom should be avoided in order to prevent possible contamination with secretory vesicles and plasma membrane fragments.

8. According to iodixanol (OptiPrep) specification sheet, the osmolarity of the iodixanol solutions in the referred fraction densities is in the range of 295–310 mOsm.

9. To check if granules secrete their preformed proteins in response to a new stimuli, for instance, in three different concentrations, split the 1 mL pooled fractions in four (250 μL each): not stimulated, stimulated in concentration 1, stimulated in concentration 2, and stimulated in concentration 3.

Acknowledgment

The authors thank Conselho Nacional de Pesquisas (CNPq—Brazil), Comissão de Aperfeiçoamento de Nível Superior (Capes—Brazil), and Fundação de Amparo à Pesquisa do Estado do Rio de Janeiro (FAPERJ—Brazil) for the financial support.

References

1. Gleich GJ (2000) Mechanisms of eosinophil-associated inflammation. J Allergy Clin Immunol 105:651–663

2. Rothenberg ME, Hogan SP (2006) The eosinophil. Annu Rev Immunol 24:147–174

3. Muniz VS, Weller PF, Neves JS (2012) Eosinophil crystalloid granules: structure, function, and beyond. J Leukoc Biol 92:281–288

4. Neves JS, Weller PF (2009) Functional extracellular eosinophil granules: novel implications in eosinophil immunobiology. Curr Opin Immunol 21:694–699

5. Neves JS, Perez SA, Spencer LA, Melo RC, Reynolds L, Ghiran I et al (2008) Eosinophil granules function extracellularly as receptor-mediated secretory organelles. Proc Natl Acad Sci U S A 105:18478–18483

6. Neves JS, Radke AL, Weller PF (2010) Cysteinyl leukotrienes acting via granule membrane-expressed receptors elicit secretion from within cell-free human eosinophil granules. J Allergy Clin Immunol 125:477–482

7. Neves JS, Perez SA, Spencer LA, Melo RC, Weller PF (2009) Subcellular fractionation of human eosinophils: isolation of functional specific granules on isoosmotic density gradients. J Immunol Methods 344:64–72

8. Akuthota P, Shamri R, Weller PF (2012) Isolation of human eosinophils. In: Wiley, J. & Sons (ed) Curr Protocols Immunol 7: 31

Chapter 10

Eosinophil Chemotaxis

Gordon Dent

Abstract

Chemotaxis assays have a number of applications in the study of leukocyte biology and immune/inflammatory pathology. Multiwell "blind chamber"-type assays allow a large number of parallel measurements within a single assay. The development of fluorescence assays using microplate-based chemotaxis chambers has permitted a degree of automation to be applied to these assays. Here, a method is described for the quantitative measurement of eosinophil migration using a 96-well assay with numbers of cells that may realistically be obtained from blood samples.

Key words Cell-based assays, Chemotaxis, Eosinophils, Fluorescence, Leukocytes, Migration

1 Introduction

Measurement of cell leukocyte migration has a number of applications in biomedical research. Migration assays using specific cell types may be used to identify, quantify, and characterize chemotactic activity for those cells in biological samples such as body fluids [1] or cell/tissue culture supernatants [2]. They may also be used to determine alterations to cellular migratory responses associated with disease [3] or to determine the roles of specific receptors and/or signalling pathways in migratory responses [4].

A number of approaches have been applied to the measurement of leukocyte migration. Some, such as the under-agarose method [5], permit sensitive analysis of directional cell movement under a variety of complex conditions. Such assays are, however, time consuming and are not appropriate for simultaneous measurements of migratory responses under a large number of different conditions within the same assay. Where multiple rapid measurements of cell migration are required, the "blind chamber" chemotaxis approach is more convenient and cost effective. Based on the original Boyden chamber technique [6], this type of assay measures the movement of leukocytes through bare or endothelial cell-coated porous membranes. The membranes are arranged to

Garry M. Walsh (ed.), *Eosinophils: Methods and Protocols*, Methods in Molecular Biology, vol. 1178,
DOI 10.1007/978-1-4939-1016-8_10, © Springer Science+Business Media New York 2014

separate two chambers: one containing the chemoattractant and the other containing the cells under investigation. Diffusion of soluble chemoattractant across the membrane creates a chemotactic gradient, along which leukocytes migrate so that they move from the upper cell-containing chamber (low concentration) to the lower chemoattractant-containing chamber (high concentration). The use of chequer-board designs, in which chemoattractant is present in the lower chamber, upper chamber, both chambers, or neither chamber, allows distinction between chemokinetic responses (increased random cell movement) and genuine chemotaxis (directed movement along a chemotactic gradient).

Traditionally, chemotaxis assays used uncoated polycarbonate or nitrocellulose filter membranes, with cell migration assessed as the number of cells adhering to the lower surface of the filter; cells were visualized using visual stains and counted using a light microscope [7]. This process is time consuming, inaccurate, and prone to bias in the selection of visual fields for counting. The use of fluorescent dyes to label cells allows automated, and more reliable, quantification of the magnitude of migratory responses [1]. However, the measurement of fluorescence in/on the filters has two obvious drawbacks. First, it is impractical to derive an actual number of migrated cells from the fluorescence signal. Secondly, if the cells do not adhere firmly to the lower surface of the filter, or if the number of cells migrating is too large to allow them all to come into contact with the lower surface, there may be separate compartments of migrated cells on the filter and in the fluid in the lower chamber, necessitating the combining of two separate fluorescence measurements made by different methods [8].

The use of filter membranes treated with the wetting agent, polyvinylpyrrolidone (PVP), allows migrated cells to drop off the lower side of the filter. Consequently, all migrated cell-associated fluorescence may be measured in the fluid in the lower chambers. This, combined with the development of 96-well microplate-based assay chambers, has allowed a relatively straightforward approach to the measurement of chemotaxis in the blind chamber-type assay.

2   Materials

Basic solutions (PBS, HBSS, HEPES, EDTA) should either be purchased as ready-made sterile solutions or prepared from tablets/sachets using sterile deionized water. Throughout this chapter, PBS refers to simple phosphate-buffered saline containing Na^+, K^+, H^+, Cl^-, and PO_4^{3-} only: do not use formulations containing Ca^{2+}, Mg^{2+}, or glucose. Solutions prepared in the laboratory should be sterilized immediately after preparation, either by filtration through 0.2 μM pore-size sterile filters (for protein-containing solutions) or by autoclaving.

2.1 Component Solutions: Incubation and Washing Buffers

1. BSA stock solution: Bovine serum albumin (BSA) 25 % w/v in PBS. Add 25 g lyophilized, fatty acid-free, low-endotoxin BSA (cell culture grade) to 100 mL PBS. Allow to dissolve fully before stirring (*see* **Note 1**). Sterilize by filtration. May be stored at 4–10 °C for up to 2 weeks if kept sterile.

2. Chemotaxis buffer: Hanks's balanced salts solution (HBSS) supplemented with 10 mM HEPES and 0.25 % BSA. To 490 mL of HBSS (containing Ca^{2+} and Mg^{2+}), add 5 mL of 1 M HEPES solution (pH range 7.2–7.5) and 5 mL of BSA stock solution. Use on the day of preparation.

3. Washing buffer: PBS containing 2 mM EDTA and 0.25 % BSA. To 246.5 mL of PBS, add 1 mL of 0.5 M sterile EDTA solution and 2.5 mL of BSA stock solution. Keep on ice until required. May be stored at 4–10 °C for up to 3 days if kept sterile.

2.2 Reagent Solutions

1. Calcein AM stock solution: Calcein 1 mM in dimethyl sulfoxide (DMSO). To 1 mg calcein acetoxymethyl ester (calcein AM), add 1 mL anhydrous DMSO. Divide into 50 μL aliquots, and store at –20 °C until required.

2. PAF stock solution: Platelet-activating factor 1 mM. To 1 mg lyophilized (water-soluble) PAF, add 2 mL sterile deionized water. Allow to dissolve fully before mixing by gentle stirring with a sterile pipette tip (*see* **Note 2**). Retains significant biological activity if stored at –80 °C for up to a week. However, it cannot be guaranteed that the activity will not decline to some extent during that time.

3. PAF working solution: Platelet-activating factor 1 μM. Perform three serial 1:10 dilutions of PAF stock solution in chemotaxis buffer to produce a 1 μM solution. Use immediately.

3 Methods

Once solutions and cells have been prepared, all procedures should be performed at room temperature as quickly as possible, except where stated. Avoid rapid changes in temperature of cell suspensions.

Chemotaxis may be measured in blood-derived eosinophils, or the Eol-1 cell line following differentiation with dibutyryl cyclic AMP [9]. The AML14.3D10 cell line, which is otherwise useful as a model of eosinophils [10], is not motile and will not function in assays of chemotaxis.

3.1 Fluorescent Labelling of Eosinophils

The method is based upon the loading of cells with a fluorescent dye that is retained by the cells throughout the assay. Calcein AM is highly cell permeant but non-fluorescent. Within cells it is cleaved by esterase enzymes to form calcein, which is fluorescent but only slightly cell permeant. Therefore, once cleaved, the fluorescent dye will predominantly remain within the cells. A small amount of dye will leak out of cells over time. This procedure would not, therefore, be appropriate for assays involving very long incubation periods.

Calcein has been demonstrated to have no significant effect on migratory responses [11], indicating that it may be used with confidence to label cells for migration assays.

1. After purification of eosinophils or harvesting of growth-arrested eosinophilic cell lines, count cells and then centrifuge ($400 \times g$ for 10 min) and discard supernatant. Resuspend cells in chemotaxis buffer at a density of 1×10^7/mL.

2. Add 1 μL of calcein AM stock per mL of cell suspension. Mix gently, and incubate at 37 °C for 45 min. For optimal maintenance of pH, perform this step in a cell culture incubator with an atmosphere of 5 % CO_2 and leave the cap of the culture tube unscrewed. Agitate the tube gently at 15-min intervals.

3. Wash cells three times with PBS to remove any unabsorbed calcein AM and any calcein that has leaked from the cells. Resuspend cells in chemotaxis buffer at a density of 4×10^6/mL (*see* **Note 3**).

3.2 Measurement of Chemotaxis

The method utilizes specialized apparatus in which two discrete fluid-filled chambers are separated by a filter membrane. Chemoattractant is added to the lower chamber, and cells are added to the upper chamber. The filter is coated with a wetting agent, which prevents cells from adhering to the filter. Consequently, cells that have migrated through the filter may be collected in the lower chamber and their fluorescence measured. A number of lower chambers are preloaded with fixed numbers of calcein-labelled cells (without chemoattractant) to allow quantification of migrated cell numbers from fluorescence measurements.

Fluorescence-based assays of chemotaxis were developed using neutrophils [12], while the method described here was applied to the study of Jurkat T-cell lines [13]. In the author's laboratory it has been used routinely for measurement of chemotaxis in differentiated promyelocytes and eosinophil cell lines as well as blood-derived neutrophils and eosinophils.

The recommended apparatus is supplied by Neuroprobe Inc., Gaithersburg, MD, USA (www.neuroprobe.com). To allow automated measurement of cell-associated fluorescence, it is most convenient to use the 96-well format chambers (Fig. 1), which allow reading of lower chamber plates in standard fluorescence microplate readers. The following instructions refer to the MBC96 chamber (50 μL upper chamber volume) using MP30 lower chamber

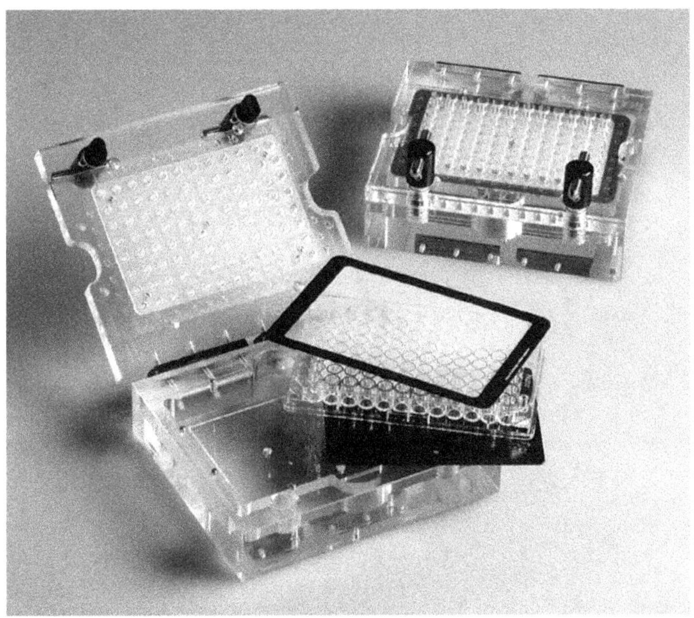

Fig. 1 The Neuroprobe® MB series 96-well chemotaxis system. The assembled system is shown in the upper right-hand corner; the components are shown in the foreground. Image reproduced with permission from http://www.neuroprobe. com/products/mbseries.html

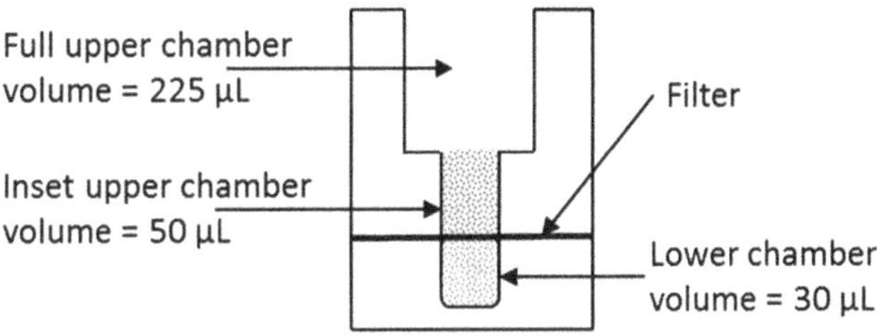

Fig. 2 Cross-sectional diagram of the components of a single chamber. The Neuroprobe® MBC chamber with low-volume microplate is illustrated

plates (30 µL well capacity, Fig. 2) and PRD-series self-adhesive framed filters. Different components may be used if larger volumes of chemoattractant or cell suspension are required.

1. Pipette 30 µL chemotaxis buffer into wells A1, A2, A3, H1, H2, and H3 of the lower chamber microplate. To triplicate wells in columns 1–3, add 30 µL volumes of eosinophil

suspension containing a known numbers of cells. The following numbers are recommended if 2×10^5 cells will be added to the upper chambers:

Row B—1×10^4

Row C—2×10^4

Row D—5×10^4

Row E—1×10^5

Row F—2×10^5

2. Pipette 30 µL of PAF working solution into wells G1, G2, and G3. This will serve as a positive control for the experiment: if no measureable chemotactic response to 1 µM PAF can be observed, it is likely that a step in the cell preparation or the chemotaxis experiment has been performed incorrectly or the cells are, for some reason, unresponsive.

3. Working quickly (*see* **Note 4**), pipette 30 µL volumes of all assay samples or chemoattractant solutions into appropriate wells. It is recommended that all samples/solutions are assayed in triplicate. If insufficient cells are available, duplicate assays may be performed. It is not recommended to rely on a single measurement for any sample or chemoattractant solution. Pipette 30 µL chemotaxis buffer into all the remaining wells.

4. For eosinophil chemotaxis measurements, it is recommended that PVP-coated polycarbonate track-etch (PCTE) filters with a pore size of 5 µm are used (*see* **Note 5**). Remove the backing strip from the self-adhesive framed filter membrane. Hold the frame at an angle of approximately 10° to the horizontal, with the fingers of the right hand against the upper long edge and the thumb against the lower long edge. Place the left-hand edge against the left-hand edge of the microplate, and use the fingers of the left hand to press these edges firmly together while gently lowering the rest of the filter onto the surface of the microplate. Press all edges to ensure a firm adhesion of the filter frame to the microplate. (Left-handed people may wish to attach the right-hand edges first.)

5. Place the assembled microplate/filter unit into the MBC che-motaxis chamber using any spacers that may be required for the specific microplate. Place the appropriate silicone rubber gasket against the underside of the upper chamber section. Close the chamber, and hold the upper chamber section down firmly while tightening the thumb screws.

6. Pipette 50 µL of cell suspension into the upper chamber wells for which samples/solutions have been added to the corre-sponding lower chamber wells, ensuring that (a) the pipette tip does not puncture the filter membrane and (b) no air is trapped between the cell suspension and the filter (*see* **Note 6**).

Swirl the cell suspension in its tube frequently to prevent sedimentation of cells.

7. Place the chamber in a non-sterile incubator or oven at 37 °C (*see* **Note 7**). Incubate for the required time. A minimum of 1 h is likely to be required for reproducibly measurable responses.

8. At the end of the incubation, remove the bulk of the liquid from the upper chamber wells using a multichannel pipette, being careful to avoid puncturing the filter membranes. Pipette 50 μL washing buffer into each well, and place the chamber in a refrigerator for 20 min. During this time, cells will detach from both sides of the filter owing to the presence of EDTA.

9. Remove the bulk of the liquid from the upper chamber wells using a multichannel pipette. Loosen the thumb screws, and open the chamber. Remove the microplate/filter unit, and scrape the upper surface of the filter membrane with a rubber scraper, moving from center to edges. Dip the scraper in clean washing buffer, and scrape the upper surface of the filter again.

10. Place the microplate/filter unit in a centrifuge microplate adapter. Centrifuge at low speed (maximum $100 \times g$) for 5 min to ensure that all migrated cells remain in the wells when the filter is removed.

11. Starting at one corner, detach the filter frame from the edge of the microplate and gently lift the filter off the plate.

12. Place the microplate in a fluorescence microplate reader with excitation wavelength $(\lambda_{ex}) = 485$ nm and emission wavelength $(\lambda_{em}) = 535$ nm (*see* **Note 8**), and read the fluorescence of all wells. The reader should be blanked on well A1 or, if possible, on the average of wells A1, A2, and A3. If there is no significant fluorescence in the positive control wells (G1, G2, G3), or if there is fluorescence in wells that did not have cells added to the upper chambers, it is inadvisable to use the results from this plate.

13. Construct a standard curve for fluorescence of known numbers of cells (Fig. 3), and use this to calculate numbers of migrated cells in other wells.

4 Notes

1. Do not vortex-mix, shake, stir, or otherwise agitate solutions to which BSA powder has been added. Sprinkle the protein powder onto the surface of the solution, and allow it to dissolve fully before mixing. Shaking or stirring will cause the powder to form clumps which cannot readily be broken up.

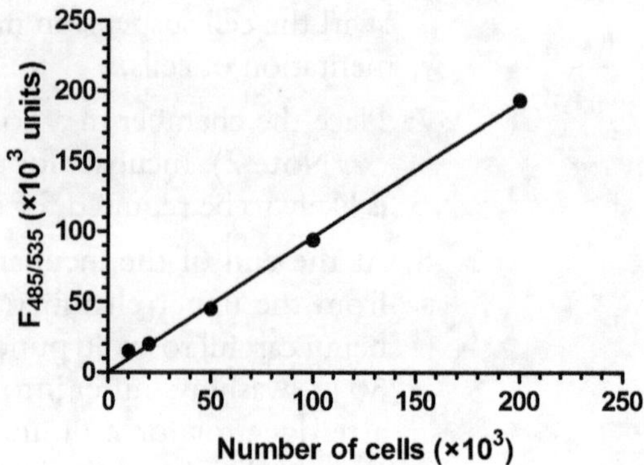

Fig. 3 Typical standard curve for calcein-labelled human blood eosinophils. The linear regression line is constrained to pass through the origin, as the fluorimeter is "blanked" on a well containing no cells (*see* **Note 9**). Therefore, the number of migrated cells (C) in a chamber may be calculated from the measured fluorescence (F) and the gradient (G) of the line by the formula C = F/G. Data taken from Hasan 2009 [14]

2. Do not use vigorous mixing (e.g. vortex-mixing) for PAF solutions. PAF is a phospholipid and is hydrophobic. A proportion of the PAF in a solution will adhere to the walls of polystyrene or polycarbonate test tubes. Vortex-mixing greatly increases the area of the plastic tube that the solution comes into contact with. Consequently, more of the lipid will be lost from solution. When performing serial dilutions, draw a small volume of the diluted solution into the pipette tip and eject it back into the tube to mix the solution.

3. A cell density of 4×10^6/mL corresponds to 2×10^5 cells in 50 µL. This number of cells gives a strong signal in assays of blood-derived eosinophil chemotaxis in response to chemoattractants such as PAF and CCL11 (eotaxin 1). For experiments to assess chemotactic activity in biological specimens (e.g. culture supernatants), or using less efficacious chemoattractants, the number of cells might need to be increased.

4. Rapid and accurate pipetting is *essential*. The liquid pipetted into the lower chamber wells should form a slight positive meniscus above the wells: this will allow the filter membrane to be placed on top of the lower chamber microplate without trapping air bubbles. If samples/solutions are pipetted too slowly, evaporation will lead to the earlier wells containing a smaller volume than the later wells. If pipetting is inaccurate, the wells will also contain unequal volumes. It is recommended that reverse pipetting be used [15].

5. Eosinophils will not readily migrate through smaller pores (e.g. 2 or 3 µm). Using filters with larger pore sizes (e.g. 8 µm) results in higher spontaneous movement of cells between

chambers and may lead to high levels of background cell-associated fluorescence.

6. Migration of cells across the filter requires a contiguous column of liquid in contact with each surface. It is, therefore, vital that no air bubbles are trapped above or below the filter: no cells will migrate across areas of the filter that are in contact with air rather than liquid. Reverse pipetting is necessary. The pipette tip should be wetted with chemotaxis buffer several times before use with cell suspension, and the same tip should be used throughout. When ejecting cell suspension into the upper chamber well, place the pipette tip against the internal wall of the well 1–2 mm above the filter and exert a firm but even pressure on the operating button. Excessively rapid operation of the pipette is likely to result in trapping of air bubbles; excessively gentle operation will result in the dispensing of unequal volumes of cell suspension.

7. Chemotaxis chambers are made of acrylic and must *not* be exposed to organic solvents, including ethanol. It is, therefore, not possible to sterilize them before placing them in an incubator. If it is essential that incubations be conducted under sterile conditions, it will be necessary to use disposable chemotaxis chambers, such as the Neuroprobe® Chemo Tx® system. After use, reusable chambers should be soaked in enzymatic detergent (e.g. Terg-a-zyme®) for at least 4 h, rinsed several times in distilled water, finally rinsed in deionized water, and then left to air-dry. They may be sterilized periodically by soaking in weak chlorine solution or 1 M NaOH (followed by extensive rinsing in sterile water), or by gas sterilization with ethylene oxide.

8. Technical data sheets give the excitation (λ_{ex}) and emission (λ_{em}) maxima for calcein as 495 nm and 515 nm, respectively [16]. The publication by Taylor et al. [13] used wavelengths of 485 nm and 535 nm, respectively, which are well within the peaks shown in the technical data [16]. For devices with filter slides/wheels rather than monochromators, wavelengths should be selected within the range of 480–505 nm and 500–535 nm for excitation and emission, respectively. To minimize interference from scattered incident light, it is preferable to use $\lambda_{ex} < 500$ and $\lambda_{em} > 510$ nm.

9. Most microplate readers will allow a single well to be defined as a blank. The value returned for this well is subtracted from all other measurements. Some readers will allow multiple wells to be defined as blank. The average of the readings from these wells will be subtracted from all other measurements. If these arrangements are not available, simply measure the absolute fluorescence signal and subtract the value for the "blank" wells from each other measurement.

References

1. Dent G, Hadjicharalambous C, Yoshikawa T et al (2004) Contribution of eotaxin-1 to eosinophil chemotactic activity of moderate and severe asthmatic sputum. Am J Respir Crit Care Med 169:1110–1117

2. Furukawa E, Ohrui T, Yamaya M et al (2004) Human airway submucosal glands augment eosinophil chemotaxis during rhinovirus infection. Clin Exp Allergy 34:704–711

3. Fujishima H, Fukagawa K, Okada N et al (2013) Chemotactic responses of peripheral blood eosinophils to prostaglandin D_2 in atopic keratoconjunctivitis. Ann Allergy Asthma Immunol 111:126–131

4. Hasan AM, Mourtada-Maarabouni M, Hameed MS, Williams GT, Dent G (2010) Phosphoinositide 3-kinase γ mediates chemotactic responses of human eosinophils to platelet-activating factor. Int Immunopharmacol 10:1017–1021

5. Heit B, Liu L, Colarusso P, Puri KD, Kubes P (2008) PI3K accelerates, but is not required for, neutrophil chemotaxis to fMLP. J Cell Sci 121:205–214

6. Boyden S (1962) The chemotactic effect of mixtures of antibody and antigen on polymorphonuclear leucocytes. J Exp Med 115:453–466

7. Dent G, Hosking LA, Lordan JL et al (2002) Differential roles of IL-16 and CD28/B7 costimulation in the generation of T-lymphocyte chemotactic activity in the bronchial mucosa of mild and moderate asthmatic individuals. J Allergy Clin Immunol 110:906–914

8. Hadjicharalambous C, Dent G, May RD et al (2004) Measurement of eotaxin (CCL11) in induced sputum supernatants: validation and detection in asthma. J Allergy Clin Immunol 113:657–662

9. Al-Rabia MW, Blaylock MG, Sexton DW, Walsh GM (2004) Membrane receptor-mediated apoptosis and caspase activation in the differentiated Eol-1 eosinophilic cell line. J Leukoc Biol 75:1045–1055

10. Baumann MA, Paul CC (1998) The AML14 and AML14.3D10 cell lines: long overdue model for the study of eosinophils and more. Stem Cells 16:16–24

11. Denholm EM, Stankus GP (1995) Differential effects of two fluorescent probes on macrophage migration as assessed by manual and automated methods. Cytometry 19:366–369

12. Sunder-Plassmann G, Hofbauer R, Sengoelge G, Hörl WH (1996) Quantification of leukocyte migration: improvement of a method. Immunol Invest 25:49–63

13. Taylor ML, Dastych J, Sehgal D et al (2001) The Kit-activating mutation $D^{816}V$ enhances stem cell factor-dependent chemotaxis. Blood 98:1195–1199

14. Hasan AM (1999) Intracellular signalling in eosinophils: differential roles for phosphoinositide 3-kinase and p38 MAP kinase in cellular responses to chemoattractants. PhD thesis, Keele University

15. Suominen I (2009) Application note AN-HP-REVPIPET-0909: dispense liquids containing proteins more reliably with reverse pipetting. http://www.thermoscientific.com/content/dam/tfs/LPG/LCD/LCD%20Documents/Application%20&%20Technical%20Notes/Manual%20and%20Automated%20Liquid%20Handling/Pipet%20Tips/Standard%20Pipet%20Tips/D00177~.pdf. Accessed 2 Dec 2013

16. Life Technologies Corp (2013) Calcein, AM, cell-permeant dye. http://www.lifetechnologies.com/order/catalog/product/C3100MP. Accessed 2 Dec 2013

Chapter 11

Eosinophil Shape Change and Secretion

Lian Willetts, Sergei I. Ochkur, Elizabeth A. Jacobsen, James J. Lee, and Paige Lacy

Abstract

The analysis of eosinophil shape change and mediator secretion is a useful tool in understanding how eosinophils respond to immunological stimuli and chemotactic factors. Eosinophils undergo dramatic shape changes, along with secretion of the granule-derived enzyme eosinophil peroxidase (EPX) in response to chemotactic stimuli including platelet-activating factor and CCL11 (eotaxin-1). Here, we describe the analysis of eosinophil shape change by confocal microscopy analysis and provide an experimental approach for comparing unstimulated cells with those that have been stimulated to undergo chemotaxis. In addition, we illustrate two different degranulation assays for EPX using OPD and an enzyme-linked immunosorbent assay technique and show how eosinophil degranulation may be assessed from in vitro as well as ex vivo stimulation.

Key words Chemotaxis, Platelet-activating factor, Eotaxin, Chemokine, Confocal microscopy, Secretion, Degranulation, Eosinophil peroxidase

---

1 Introduction

Eosinophil shape change is an important cellular event that precedes the movement and transmigration of cells from the blood to tissue compartments in response to chemotactic stimuli [1–3]. Shape change occurs following chemokine receptor stimulation, which activates actin cytoskeleton remodeling through a plethora of actin-binding proteins [4]. Dynamic actin reorganization is a fundamental process in cell motility and involves the reversible transformation of soluble G-actin to filamentous F-actin [4]. The movement of actin throughout cells allows eosinophils to form leading edges, pseudopods, filopodia, lamellipodia, and uropods, and provides directionality and force to cellular migration. Many chemokines are capable of inducing migration in eosinophils, among which platelet-activating factor (PAF) and CCL11 (eotaxin-1) are among the most potent [5, 6]. Concurrently with

Garry M. Walsh (ed.), *Eosinophils: Methods and Protocols*, Methods in Molecular Biology, vol. 1178,
DOI 10.1007/978-1-4939-1016-8_11, © Springer Science+Business Media New York 2014

chemokine-stimulated shape changes, and depending on the stimulus used, eosinophils can also undergo secretion of granule-derived mediators. PAF is additionally capable of inducing eosinophil degranulation in parallel with increased shape change [7]. Actin remodeling and degranulation in eosinophils have been shown to be regulated by Rho guanine triphosphatases (GTPases), which are monomeric intracellular signaling molecules that are evolutionarily conserved from yeast to mammalian cells [8]. Specifically, the Rho GTPase Rac2 has an active role in eosinophil F-actin formation and shape change and contributes to degranulation and superoxide release [9]. The importance of these events in asthmatic patients is underscored by the recent finding that eosinophil shape change and granule release correlate strongly with acute exacerbations of asthma in children [10]. Eosinophils in peripheral blood samples obtained from asthmatic children undergoing exacerbations were found to have increased cell spreading, formation of pseudopods, and released clusters of free granules suggestive of degranulation and/or cytolysis [10].

Cellular F-actin may be visualized by the addition of the F-actin-binding phallotoxin, phalloidin, which is conjugated to a fluorescent dye such as rhodamine or Alexa Fluor molecules. Phalloidin is a member of a group of toxins produced by the death cap mushroom (*Amanita phalloides*), which binds F-actin much more tightly than G-actin monomers and prevents F-actin depolymerization. When conjugated to fluorescent dyes, phalloidin displays intensely detailed staining of the F-actin cytoskeleton in adherent cells that have been fixed and permeabilized. Using confocal laser scanning microscopy on rhodamine-phalloidin-stained eosinophils, we have examined the effects of PAF and CCL11 on eosinophil shape change in mouse eosinophils obtained from wild-type controls and Rac2 gene knockout mice [9].

We have also assayed for the release of eosinophil peroxidase (EPX) into supernatants of PAF and calcium ionophore-stimulated cells using a cell-impermeable assay with *o*-phenylenediamine (OPD) as the substrate for extracellular peroxidase activity [11]. This will be compared with using an enzyme-linked immunosorbent assay (ELISA) for EPX which has ten times greater sensitivity for EPX than the OPD assay. In addition, we describe an ex vivo degranulation assay in which purified mouse eosinophils have been intratracheally administered into triple-transgenic mice overexpressing interleukin-5 (*IL-5*) and human eotaxin-2 (*hE2*) and lacking EPX expression (*IL-5/hE2/EPX^{-/-}* mice). These animals have potent eosinophil-stimulating conditions in their airways and are useful for determining EPX release from exogenously introduced eosinophils. The ex vivo degranulation assay is superior to in vitro degranulation assays for mouse eosinophils for inducing maximal degranulation responses, as these cells are difficult to degranulate in vitro [12].

2 Materials

Where appropriate, prepare solutions with ultrapure water that has been generated by purified deionized, endotoxin-free water to attain a sensitivity of 18 MΩ-cm at 25 °C and using cell culture-grade reagents. All reagents should be prepared and used at room temperature unless otherwise indicated. Use the proper waste disposal protocols appropriate for each reagent.

2.1 Actin Staining in Adherent Eosinophils

1. Human or mouse eosinophils, approximately 10–100×10^6 cells, in RPMI 1640 cell culture media: Cells may be kept on ice or at room temperature until used. Cells should be purified according to appropriate protocols detailed elsewhere [13, 14] and Chapter 2.

2. Hanks' balanced salt solution (HBSS), 10× stock solution: Dilute 1:10 using ultrapure water to 1× stock solution on the day of use. Always use 1× HBSS, and never use 10× stock HBSS with cells under any circumstances, as 10× solutions will lyse cells.

3. Phosphate-buffered saline (PBS), 10× stock solution (pH 7.4): Dilute 1:10 using ultrapure water to 1× stock solution on the day of use. Always use 1× PBS, and never use 10× stock PBS with cells under any circumstances, as 10× solutions will lyse cells.

4. Cell culture-grade dimethylsulfoxide (DMSO).

5. Platelet-activating factor (PAF, C18, β-acetyl-O-octadecyl-L-α-phosphatidylcholine in DMSO, Sigma-Aldrich, St. Louis, MO, P6537): PAF is lipid soluble and must be dissolved in organic solvents. Prepare a stock solution of 1 mM PAF in cell culture-grade DMSO by adding 1.812 ml DMSO to 1 mg PAF, dissolve thoroughly, then aliquot in 20 μl, and freeze at −20 °C. PAF degrades readily and must be used fresh on the day of preparation. To prepare a working stock of PAF (and achieve a final concentration of 10 nM), thaw one aliquot of 1 mM PAF and dilute as follows.

    (a) First prepare 10 μM PAF by diluting the freezer stock 1:1,000 in HBSS (add 1 μl freezer stock to 999 μl HBSS).

    (b) Then dilute 4.75 μl of working stock PAF in 995.3 μl HBSS to generate 47.5 nM solution.

    (c) Finally, add 100 μl of this to 375 μl cell suspension to achieve the desired concentration of 10 nM. Scale up or down the volume of PAF to accommodate the number of samples that will be analyzed.

6. Recombinant mouse CCL11: Prepare a stock solution of 5 μg/ml in PBS, and prepare 20 μl aliquots for storage at −80 °C. To use in experiments, thaw one aliquot of 5 μg/ml

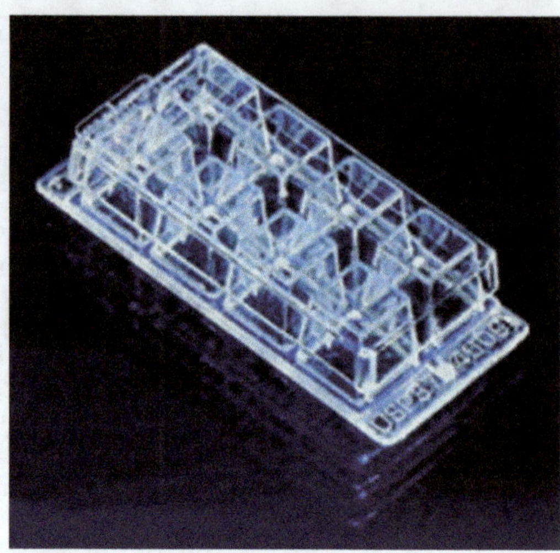

Fig. 1 LabTek 8 Chambered Coverglass. Working volume is 0.5 ml, and chambers are made of polystyrene material attached to a glass cover slip of 1.5 borosilicate glass, suitable for high-definition immunofluorescence imaging by confocal microscopy or similar systems. Modified from the Sigma-Aldrich website for this product

CCL11 and dilute as follows. Add 9.5 μl of stock CCL11 to 990.5 μl HBSS to generate 47.5 ng/ml, and then add 100 μl of this to 375 cell suspension to achieve the final concentration of 10 ng/ml. CCL11 is also easily degraded and must be used fresh on the day of preparation. Scale up or down the volume of CCL11 to accommodate the number of samples that will be analyzed.

7. Incubation slides (Lab-Tek Chambered #1.0 Borosilicate Coverglass System, 8 Chamber, Fig. 1).

8. 4 % Paraformaldehyde: Prepare using analytical grade paraformaldehyde powder. To prepare 100 ml, weigh 4 g paraformaldehyde and add to 50–75 ml water in a clean 150 ml glass beaker. Heat while stirring with a stirrer bar on a heated stirring platform to 55 °C, and add 1, 5, or 10 M NaOH gradually until the solution clears. Ensure that the temperature of the solution does not exceed 60–65 °C (*see* **Note 1**). Cool the solution to room temperature, and vacuum filter through a 0.45 μm filter to remove large particles. Add 10 ml 10× PBS, and then bring up to the final volume of 100 ml. Adjust pH of solution to 7.4 or slightly higher (*see* **Note 2**), and prepare aliquots of 5 or 10 ml. Freeze at –20 °C. Thaw at room temperature or at 37 °C, but never at 50 °C or higher. This can be refrozen and thawed up to three times.

9. 0.1 % Triton X-100 in PBS: First prepare a stock solution of 10 % Triton X-100 in water which can be stored at 4 °C for up

to 1 year. Weigh 2 g Triton X-100 in a 50 ml conical centrifuge tube, and add up to 20 ml ultrapure water. Dilute 1:100 to obtain 0.1 % for permeabilization of cells by adding 100 μl 10 % Triton X-100 to 9.9 ml PBS.

10. 2 % Bovine serum albumin (BSA) in PBS: Weigh 0.2 g BSA and make up to 10 ml in PBS.

11. Rhodamine-phalloidin (Molecular Probes, Invitrogen): This comes as a solution which can be diluted on the day of use. Dilute 1:200 by adding 5–995 μl PBS. Scale up or down the volume to accommodate the number of samples that will be analyzed.

12. ProLong Gold DAPI-containing mounting media: This should be a ready-made solution which is used directly from a small bottle.

2.2 In Vitro Degranulation Assay	1. 96-Well flat-welled microtitre plates.

2. Microcentrifuge tubes (1.5 ml).

3. Human or mouse eosinophils, approximately $10–100 \times 10^6$ cells, in RPMI 1640 cell culture media: Cells may be kept on ice or at room temperature until used. Cells should be purified according to appropriate protocols detailed elsewhere [13, 14] and Chapter 2.

4. Phenol red-free RPMI 1640 medium: For convenience, purchase the ready-made media and ensure that this is used prior to the expiry date. It does not have to contain HEPES, bicarbonate, or glutamine as this medium is not required for incubation of cells for long periods.

5. Cell culture-grade DMSO.

6. PAF (C18, β-acetyl-*O*-octadecyl-L-α-phosphatidylcholine in DMSO, Sigma-Aldrich, P6537). *See* #5 above for preparation of stock PAFIonomycin. Prepare as a stock solution of 5 μg/ml in DMSO, aliquot in 20 μl, and freeze at –20 °C until needed.

2.3   Ex Vivo Degranulation Assay

1. Microcentrifuge tubes (1.5 ml).

2. Human or mouse eosinophils, approximately $10–100 \times 10^6$ cells, in RPMI 1640 cell culture media: Cells may be kept on ice or at room temperature until used. Cells should be purified according to appropriate protocols detailed elsewhere [13, 14] and Chapter 2.

3. PBS, 10×: Dilute 1:10 to use 1× PBS for all experiments.

4. Recipient mice (*IL-5/hE2/EPX$^{-/-}$*, Lee Labs, Mayo Clinic, AZ).

5. Isoflurane, USP liquid for inhalation (Novaplus; *see* **Note 3**): Isoflurane inhalation is carried out using a precision vaporizer instrument.

6. 2 % Fetal bovine serum (FBS) in PBS: Aliquot 1 ml FBS to 49 ml PBS in a conical centrifuge tube.

7. 18 G Blue tip catheter (30 mm).

8. 1 ml Sterile syringes.

9. 75 % Ethanol with water.

10. Nembutal sodium solution (pentobarbital sodium, 50 mg/ml).

2.4 o-Phenylene-diamine (OPD) Assay

1. 96-Well flat-welled microtitre plates.

2. 1 M Tris buffer, pH 8.0: Prepare 100 ml by adding 12.1 g Tris base to 80 ml ultrapure water, and then adjust pH to 8.0 using concentrated hydrochloric acid. Make up to 100 ml with water, filter through 0.45 μm, and store for up to 1 year at 4 °C.

3. 30 % H_2O_2: This is a ready-made solution that should be stored at 4 °C.

4. OPD HCl substrate solution: OPD should be prepared fresh immediately before use as it degrades rapidly. Add 9 mg OPD to 1 ml ultrapure water. In a separate tube, mix 4 ml 1 M Tris (pH 8.0), 6 ml ultrapure water, and 1.25 μl H_2O_2 (30 %). Keep these separate, and then add 800 μl OPD to this mixture just before use in the assay (*see* **Note 4**).

5. Optional: If an ultrasound probe is not available, prepare 10 % 3-[(3-cholamidopropyl)dimethylammonio]-1-propanesulfonate (CHAPS) detergent, which is used to lyse cells. Weigh out 1 g CHAPS and make up to a final volume of 10 ml with ultrapure water. This may be stored at room temperature for up to 1 year. Always dilute to 0.1 % for lysing cells.

6. 4 M Sulfuric acid.

2.5 EPX Enzyme-Linked Immunosor-bent Assay

1. 96-Well flat-welled microtitre plate (Nunc-Immuno Plate MaxiSorp, Thermo Fisher Scientific, Waltham, MA): These must be MaxiSorp plates, and not standard 96-well plates used in other assays, for optimal antibody coating.

2. Hexadecyltrimethylammonium bromide (CTAB) in 0.3 M sucrose.

3. EPX Standards: These may be prepared by isolating peripheral blood eosinophils from NJ.1638 mice [13] or human blood [14]. Prepare standards starting with a purified eosinophil suspension (>98 % purity) at 14.6×10^6 cells/ml in PBS with 2 % FBS. To prepare stock lysate for standards, spin 250 μl of eosinophil suspension at $950 \times g$ for 10 min at 4 °C. Remove 200 μl supernatant, add 250 μl of 0.22 % CTAB in 0.3 M sucrose to the cells, and lyse the cell pellet with repeated pipetting. Vortex the lysate for 1 min and flash-freeze in liquid nitrogen for storage in 25 μl aliquots at −80 °C. On the day of use, lysates should be thawed at 37 °C until just melted, then

Table 1
Serial dilution of eosinophils to generate standards for EPX ELISA

Standard #	Eosinophil equivalents/50 µl	PBS (µl)	Extract (µl)	Total (µl)	Serial dilution with PBS
1	22531	650	25	675	Take 25 µl of neat extract, put in tube 1 with 650 µl PBS, mix well
2	7510	450	225	675	Take 225 µl from tube 1, put in tube 2 with 450 µl of PBS, mix well
3	2503	450	225	675	Take 225 µl from tube 2, put in tube 3 with 450 µl of PBS, mix well
4	834	450	225	675	Take 225 µl from tube 3, put in tube 4 with 450 µl of PBS, mix well
5	278	450	225	675	Take 225 µl from tube 4, put in tube 5 with 450 µl of PBS, mix well
6	93	450	225	675	Take 225 µl from tube 5, put in tube 6 with 450 µl of PBS, mix well
7	31	450	225	675	Take 225 µl from tube 6, put in tube 7 with 450 µl of PBS, mix well
8	0	450	0	450	Transfer 450 µl of PBS in tube 8

Prepare standards starting with an eosinophil suspension of 14.6×10^6 cells/ml

pulse-spun at $10,000 \times g$ at 4 °C, and placed on ice. Use one 25 µl aliquot to carry out a sequential dilution of lysates to generate a standard curve (*see* Table 1). Once dilution series is completed, use 50 µl of each standard in the EPX ELISA. This technique is described in detail by Ochkur et al. [15]. Alternatively, EPX standards may be prepared using commercially available human EPX from several suppliers.

4. Coating Solution, 10× (KPL Inc., Gaithersburg, MD): Dilute 1:10 before use by mixing 1 ml of concentrate with 9 ml ultrapure water.

5. 10 % BSA diluent/blocking solution kit:

    (a) For use as a diluent, use 1:15 dilution for samples/standards and antibodies.

    (b) For blocking, use 1:10 dilution to block plastic surfaces after coating with capture antibody.

6. Wash solution concentrate, 20× (KPL Inc.): Dilute 1:20 by adding 60 ml concentrate to 1.14 L ultrapure water to give 1.2 L of wash buffer.

7. Capture Antibody (mouse anti-mouse EPX, 1 mg/ml, clone MM25-429.1.1, Lee Labs, Mayo Clinic, AZ): Dilute by adding 20 μl of 1 mg/ml stock antibody to 10 ml of coating solution to make a 2 μg/ml final concentration.

8. Detection Antibody (biotinylated rat anti-EPX monoclonal antibody, clone MM25-82.2.1, Lee Labs, Mayo Clinic, AZ): Prepare 0.8 μg/ml from 1.4 mg/ml stock solution by diluting 1:1,750. For one 96-well plate, add 5.7 μl antibody to 10 ml PBS and use 100 μl per well.

9. Streptavidin–alkaline phosphatase: Dilute 1:500 to 1:1,000 in 1 % BSA, 0.05 % Tween 20, 0.025 M Tris (pH 7.4), and 0.5 M NaCl. For a 1:500 dilution to use for a 96-well microtitre plate, add 22 μl streptavidin–alkaline phosphatase to 11 ml diluent, and use 100 μl per well.

10. Trizma hydrochloride buffer solution, pH 7.5: This solution is ready-made for use in this assay.

11. BluPhos Microwell Phosphatase Substrate System, 600 ml (KPL Inc.): Prepare 26 ml of substrate solution no earlier than 15 min before the reaction. Mix 13 ml of solution A with 13 ml of solution B, and add 100 μl per well.

12. EDTA (2.5 %) stop solution: Prepare a 0.5 M EDTA stock solution by adding 14 g EDTA (acid form) to 100 ml and autoclaving to dissolve salt with a final concentration of 14 % EDTA. Alternatively, 10 M NaOH may be added with continuous stirring to keep pH of the solution neutral and allow dissolving of EDTA. Take care not to exceed a neutral pH range of 7.0–7.5. Before use, dilute this by adding 2.5 ml 14 % EDTA to 11.5 ml ultrapure water to make 2.5 % EDTA.

3 Methods

3.1 Actin and Nuclear Staining in Adherent Eosinophils to Detect Eosinophil Shape Change

1. Prepare eosinophils as described in Chapter 2. Resuspend eosinophils to 5–6×10^6 cells/ml in HBSS (no serum). If any serum or protein is present in media, cells will not adhere to glass surfaces, which is essential for imaging.

2. Plate 375 μl of cell suspension (containing 2–2.5×10^6 cells in HBSS) in each well of a LabTek chamber slide (Fig. 1). Incubate for 15 min at 37 °C in tissue culture incubator to adhere cells to glass surfaces. Each slide should have alternating control and test samples for direct comparison.

3. Prewarm agonists for 15 min at the same time in separate tubes (PAF, recombinant mouse CCL11).

4. Set up a timer to record a time of 10 s per well.

5. Before adding agonist, load two micropipettes: one with 100 µl agonist and the other with 200 µl paraformaldehyde.

6. To start stimulation, add the following reagents with the incubator door open and the LabTek slide on the incubator shelf:

    (a) Control (100 µl HBSS + 0.0001 % DMSO).

    (b) PAF (100 µl, final concentration 10 nM).

    (c) Recombinant mouse CCL11 (100 µl, final concentration 10 ng/ml).

7. Incubate for 10 s. Stagger the timing of stimulation of plates if more than one plate is used.

8. At the end of the incubation, immediately aspirate media with micropipette without dislodging cells, and add 200 µl 4 % paraformaldehyde, again without disturbing cells. A useful method is to place the micropipette tip at an angle in the corner of the well so that liquid forces do not impact cells excessively and detach them.

9. Fix cells at room temperature for 20 min. Do not let slides incubate in fixative for longer than 30 min.

10. Wash wells twice with PBS. Fill each well to the top with PBS each time to ensure that they are adequately washed. Aspirate washings using a vacuum trap for this and all subsequent steps. Prior to the next step, aspirate all PBS out of wells and quickly add the next reagent to avoid dehydrating cells.

11. Permeabilize cells with 200 µl 0.1 % Triton X-100 for 3 min.

12. Wash wells twice with PBS. After the last wash, aspirate all PBS and quickly add the next reagent.

13. Block with 200 µl of 2 % BSA in PBS for 20 min at room temperature.

14. Wash cells twice with PBS. After the last wash, aspirate all PBS and quickly add the next reagent.

15. Stain cells with 200 µl rhodamine-phalloidin (diluted 1:200) for 1 h at room temperature. Keep slides in the dark from this point onwards to avoid bleaching of fluorescence.

16. Wash cells three times for 5 min each with PBS. After the last wash, aspirate all PBS and quickly add the next reagent.

17. Add several drops per well of ProLong Gold DAPI-containing mounting media. Make sure that the cells are fully covered with mounting media to prevent cells from drying out.

18. Place slides in a petri dish and wrap in foil for transport to a confocal microscope for immediate analysis, or store slides at 4 °C in a dark container until analysis by confocal microscopy (Fig. 2).

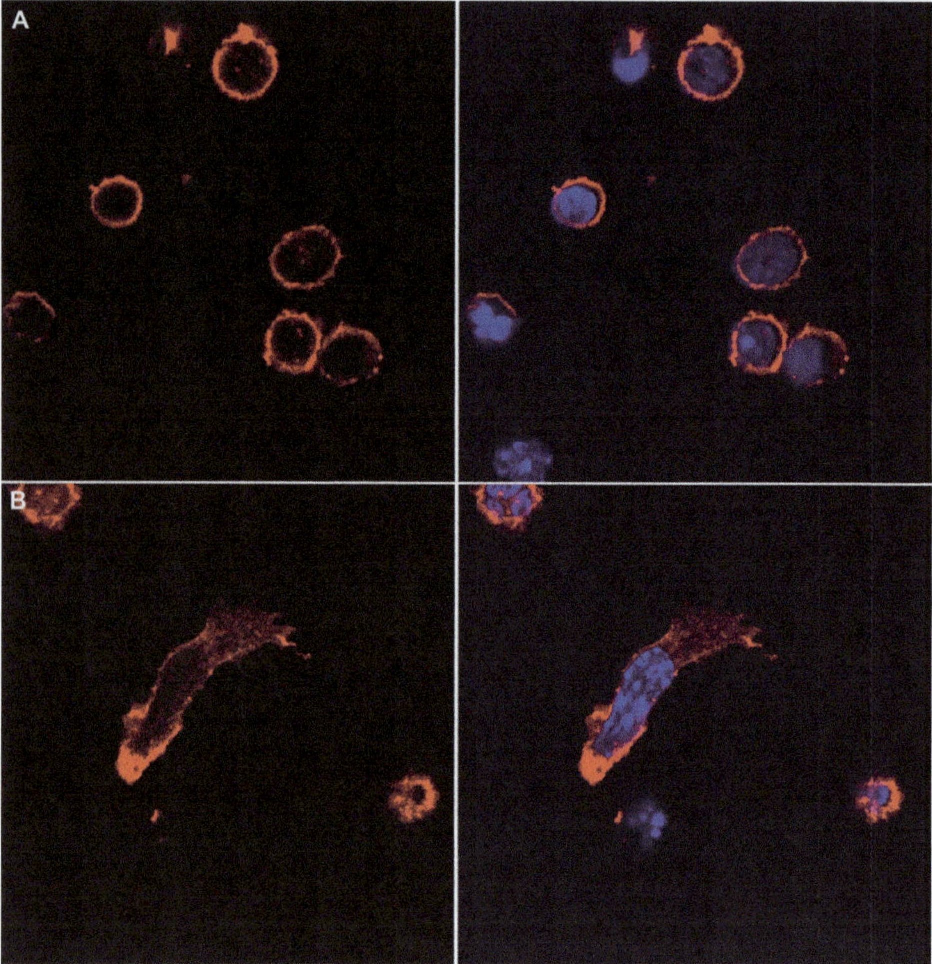

Fig. 2 Confocal microscopy images of (**a**) adherent unstimulated normal mouse eosinophils stained for visualization of nuclei (*blue*, using DAPI) and actin cytoskeleton (*red*, using rhodamine-phalloidin). The *left panel* shows actin staining alone, and the *right panel* shows merged images. Eosinophils undergo striking shape changes upon stimulation within 10 s following addition of 10 ng/ml CCL11/eotaxin (**b**), as evident from a stretched cellular morphology. Original magnification, 60×

19. For confocal microscopy analysis, use 405 nm diode lasers to visualize DAPI and 543 nm helium–neon laser to visualize rhodamine. Use the appropriate settings for the confocal microscope, preferably a 60× oil immersion Plan Apo objective (at least 1.4 N.A.). Images should be collected and arranged using Adobe Photoshop CS (see Fig. 2 for examples of microscopy).

20. A statistical test to compare "round" vs. "stretched" morphology can be applied using frequency plots to compare different shapes of cells together with Fisher's exact test, 2-sided (GraphPad Prism, v. 6) [9].

3.2 In Vitro Degranulation Assay

1. Isolate mouse or human peripheral blood eosinophils as described previously [13, 14], Chapter 2.

2. Centrifuge ($300 \times g$ at 4 °C for 5 min) and resuspend purified eosinophils in phenol red-free RPMI 1640 at 2.5×10^6 cells/ml. Use phenol red-free RPMI for all steps to prevent interference with absorbance in later assays.

3. Prepare lysed unstimulated cells for obtaining total EPX activity or concentration. Sonicate separate tubes of cells for lysate values using a sonication probe (Ultrasonic), set at power level 3, for 5 s, in a microcentrifuge tube on ice containing 2.5×10^5 cells in 100 μl RPMI. Alternatively, use a detergent such as CHAPS and add this to a final concentration of 0.1 % to cells. Place on ice during incubation of cells in the following steps.

4. Add 100 μl cell suspension (containing 2.5×10^5 cells) to each well in a 96-well microtitre plate. In separate wells, add agonists (150 μl each of PAF, 400 ng/ml, and/or ionomycin, 100 ng/ml, in RPMI). Carry out all stimulation in triplicate for more accurate average values.

5. Prepare DMSO vehicle controls for additional cells in separate wells using the percentage of DMSO used after dilution of the original stock solutions for PAF and ionomycin.

6. Prewarm the whole plate for at least 15 min at 37 °C (*see* **Note 5**).

7. Add 100 μl of PAF (for a final concentration of 200 ng/ml) and/or ionomycin (for a final concentration of 50 ng/ml) or DMSO in RPMI.

8. Incubate plate for 30 min.

9. Spin down microtitre plate at $300 \times g$ for 5 min at 4 °C using an appropriate microtitre plate rotor. Collect 200 μl from each supernatant without disturbing cell pellets.

10. Add cells to a separate series of wells to check their viability later using trypan blue or an equivalent viability assay.

11. Centrifuge the collected supernatants again at $500 \times g$ (or higher speeds) for 5 min at 4 °C to remove cells, organelles, and debris. These supernatants can be analyzed for EPX using the OPD assay (Subheading 3.4) to determine EPX activity and/or the EPX ELISA technique (Subheading 3.5) to determine total EPX concentration.

12. Store supernatants and lysates at −80 °C for further analysis.

3.3 Ex Vivo Degranulation Assay

This procedure involves intratracheal instillation of peripheral blood eosinophils into *IL-5/hE2/EPX⁻ᐟ⁻* recipient mice (Fig. 3).

1. Isolate mouse eosinophils as described previously [13].

2. Resuspend purified mouse eosinophils in PBS at 1×10^7 cells in 25 μl and keep on ice until needed.

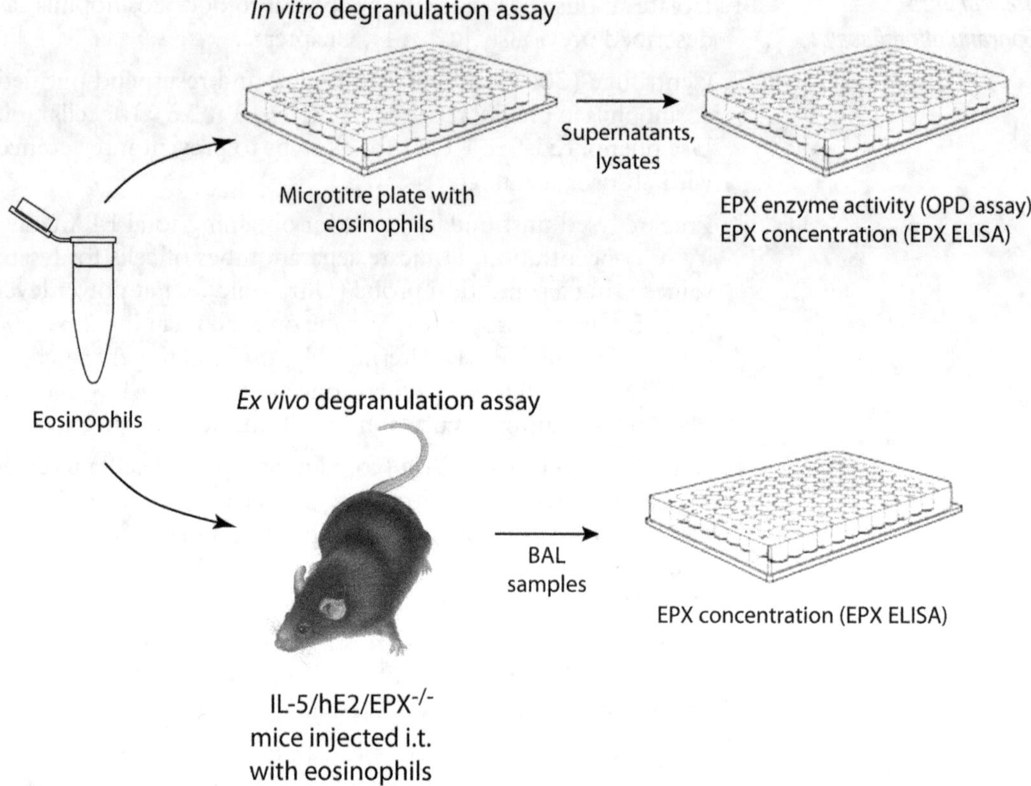

Fig. 3 In vitro and ex vivo degranulation assays. For the in vitro degranulation assay, either mouse or human eosinophils may be subjected to stimulation by various secretagogues using a microtitre plate (or microcentrifuge tubes, if more appropriate). Cell samples may then be assessed by OPD assay for EPX activity and/or EPX ELISA for the concentration of EPX. In the case of the ex vivo degranulation assay, only mouse eosinophils may be used. Resulting BAL samples can then be assayed, preferably by using the EPX ELISA approach

3. Anesthetize recipient mice (IL-$5/hE2/EPX^{-/-}$) with isoflurane as appropriate (*see* **Note 3**).

4. Suspend mice by their front teeth using an intratracheal instillation apparatus (*see* **Note 6**) to expose the trachea through the oral cavity.

5. Instill a volume of 25 μl of eosinophil suspension using a micropipette or a vehicle control (PBS) into the trachea of the mice.

6. Allow the recipient mice to recover from anesthesia posttransfer with appropriate care.

7. After 24 h, euthanize the mouse with an intraperitoneal injection of sodium pentobarbital (100 μl/mouse).

8. Carry out surgical incision in the upper thoracic area of the mouse to expose the trachea. Ensure that blood vessels are not compromised and limit bleeding in the tracheal area.

9. Cut a horizontal incision in the trachea with fine scissors.

10. Slowly introduce 1 ml PBS using a 1 ml syringe via the tracheal incision into the lungs, and then gently retrieve the solution into the same syringe. This generates the bronchoalveolar lavage (BAL) sample.

11. Eject BAL from the syringe into a labeled microcentrifuge tube, place on ice, and repeat for each mouse.

12. Centrifuge BAL samples at $500 \times g$ for 5 min at 4 °C to remove cells and debris.

13. Centrifuge the supernatants again at $10,000 \times g$ for 10 min at 4 °C to remove cellular debris and clarify supernatants.

14. Store supernatants at −80 °C for later analysis by OPD assay or EPX ELISA.

3.4 OPD Assay for EPX Activity

There are two ways to carry out the OPD assay for EPX activity. The simplest approach is to measure EPX activity in supernatants of stimulated eosinophils (after centrifugation) with OPD substrate solution. The way to carry out the OPD assay on supernatants is as follows:

1. Prepare OPD substrate solution as detailed in the Materials (Section 2.4). Store solution in the dark until needed, and keep OPD separate from the rest of the mixture until just before use.

2. Thaw or prepare supernatants and lysates from in vitro or ex vivo degranulation assays. If thawing previously frozen supernatants, place tubes in 37 °C until just thawed, and then place on ice until use.

3. Add 50 μl supernatants to each well of a 96-well microtitre plate. Include a series of wells with RPMI alone ("blanks") for background subtraction, and include a series of lysed cells to give total EPX activity.

4. Add 50 μl OPD substrate solution.

5. Incubate the plate at room temperature for up to 30 min depending on the color development. Place the plate in the dark during incubation as OPD is light sensitive. Color reaction should show a rapid development to a light orange/brown. Do not allow the reaction to proceed to too dark a color, as this will generate off-scale readings on the plate reader (>2.0 absorbance units).

6. Terminate the reaction by the addition of 100 μl 4 M H_2SO_4. Subtract background from each well using the absorbance

value obtained with the blanks. Divide the supernatant values into the lysed values to get a percentage of total EPX release.

However, EPX is highly adhesive due to its cationic nature and precipitates readily out of solution, making its recovery from supernatants very difficult if not impossible. In addition, some EPX activity from supernatants is lost upon freeze–thaw. A more appropriate technique is to incubate OPD substrate solution directly with live, viable eosinophils following their activation [11]. OPD is soluble in aqueous media and does not require organic solvents to dissolve it. This has the added advantage of preventing damage to eosinophils when OPD substrate solution is added to live cells or leading to inadvertent detection of intracellular EPX. The following technique describes how to incubate OPD substrate solution with live eosinophils for detection of EPX activity immediately after its release.

7. Prepare OPD substrate solution as detailed in the Materials (Section 2.4). Store solution in the dark until needed, and keep OPD separate from the rest of the mixture until just before use (*see* **Note 7**).

8. Resuspend eosinophils in phenol red-free RPMI to a concentration of 2.5×10^6 cells/ml. All steps in this assay require phenol red-free RPMI to avoid interference with the colored product generated by OPD substrate.

9. Prepare lysed unstimulated cells for obtaining total EPX activity or concentration. Sonicate separate tubes of cells for lysate values using a sonication probe (Ultrasonic), set at power level 3, for 5 s, in a microcentrifuge tube on ice containing 2.5×10^5 cells in 100 μl RPMI. Alternatively, use a detergent such as CHAPS and add this to a final concentration of 0.1 % to cells. Place on ice during incubation of cells in the following steps.

10. Add 100 μl cell suspension (containing 2.5×10^5 cells) to each well in a 96-well microtitre plate. In separate wells, add agonists (150 μl each of PAF, 400 ng/ml, and/or ionomycin, 100 ng/ml, in RPMI). Carry out all stimulation in triplicate for more accurate average values.

11. Prepare DMSO vehicle controls for additional cells in separate wells using the percentage of DMSO used after dilution of the original stock solutions for PAF and ionomycin.

12. Prewarm the whole plate for at least 15 min at 37 °C (*see* **Note 5**).

13. Add 100 μl of PAF (for a final concentration of 200 ng/ml) and/or ionomycin (for a final concentration of 50 ng/ml) or DMSO in RPMI.

14. Incubate plate for 30 min. While incubating cells, prepare fresh OPD solution.

15. At the end of the incubation period, add 200 µl of OPD solution into each well of cells, blanks, and lysates and wait for 2 min. Color reaction should show rapid development to light orange/brown. Do not allow the reaction to proceed to too dark a color as this will be off-scale (absorbance value > 1.0) in the plate reader.

16. Add 100 µl of 4 M H_2SO_4 into each well to stop the reaction using a multichannel pipette.

17. Read plate on spectrophotometric plate reader at wavelength 490 nm. Subtract the background absorbance using the blank wells (containing RPMI only) from all sample wells. Divide the value obtained for stimulated cells into the lysed cell absorbance average to obtain the percentage of EPX release.

3.5 EPX ELISA

This technique measures the concentration of EPX in mouse or human eosinophil samples, as opposed to the OPD assay which measures EPX activity. The EPX ELISA can be used to measure human [16] or mouse [17] samples.

1. Add 100 µl capture antibody diluted in coating solution to appropriate wells in a 96-well microtitre MaxiSorp plate, and incubate for 1 h at room temperature or overnight at 4 °C.

2. Discard solution, and tap out residual liquid on paper towels.

3. Wash plate by filling each well to the top with wash solution. Discard solution into sink, and tap out residual liquid onto clean paper towels (*see* **Note 8**). Repeat three times. The same paper towels can be used throughout the wash procedure.

4. Add 300 µl blocking solution to each well.

5. Incubate for 15 min.

6. Discard solution into sink, and tap out residual liquid onto clean paper towels.

7. Add 50 µl sample, standard, or blank solution (RPMI) into each well. Be sure to include the standards shown in Table 1 and carry out all samples, standards, and blanks in triplicate for more accurate averages.

8. Incubate for 1 h at room temperature or overnight at 4 °C.

9. Remove samples with a multichannel pipette and discard to prevent cross-contamination of neighboring wells.

10. Tap out residual liquid onto clean paper towels.

11. Wash plate by filling each well to the top with wash solution. Discard solution into sink, and tap out residual liquid onto clean paper towels. Repeat three times.

12. Add 100 µl detection antibody to each well.

13. Incubate for 1 h at room temperature.

14. Discard solution into sink, and tap out residual liquid onto clean paper towels.

15. Wash plate by filling each well to the top with wash solution. Discard solution into sink, and tap out residual liquid onto clean paper towels. Repeat three times. Leave the final wash solution for 5 min to fully wash wells before discarding and tapping plate out.

16. Add 100 μl streptavidin–alkaline phosphatase solution to each well.

17. Incubate for 20 min at room temperature.

18. Discard solution into sink, and tap out residual liquid onto clean paper towels.

19. Wash plate by filling each well to the top with wash solution. Discard solution into sink, and tap out residual liquid onto clean paper towels. Repeat three times.

20. Dispense 100 μl BluePhos Microwell Phosphatase Substrate into each well.

21. Incubate for up to 1 h.

22. If desired, after sufficient color development, and add 100 μl of stop solution to each well.

23. Take care to remove all bubbles from the well surfaces as these interfere with absorbance readings. In addition, clean the bottom of the plate if there is any material there to prevent interference.

24. Read the absorbance of wells at 595–650 nm. Subtract the background absorbance obtained in blank wells from all samples and standards.

---

4   Notes

1. Ensure that this procedure is done in a suitable fume hood with functional extraction fans to avoid inhaling toxic fumes. Handle this solution with great care, and avoid breathing fumes during the heating step, as formaldehyde is a known carcinogen. If the paraformaldehyde solution exceeds 60–65 °C, discard the solution through suitable chemical waste disposal and start again with a new preparation using clean glassware.

2. Paraformaldehyde forms formaldehyde when in solution and must be buffered to prevent degradation into inactive products. Adjusting the pH to higher values than 7.4 (e.g., 7.6–7.8) is advantageous as formaldehyde fixes better at higher pH values. It is critical that the pH range of the formaldehyde solution is kept in this range as this maintains its ability to fix specimens for detailed high-magnification microscopy.

Formaldehyde in water readily breaks down into formic acid, leading to poor fixation and specimen degradation. Avoid using commercially prepared buffered formalin as this is less effective at fixation of fine intracellular structures than freshly prepared buffered and filtered paraformaldehyde solution.

3. Isoflurane produces rapid induction and recovery from anesthesia, and the depth of anesthesia can be altered easily. There are minimal adverse effects, toxicity, or interference with drug metabolism when using isoflurane. Start with 0.5 % isoflurane, and increase by 0.5 % increments every few breaths. If the animal becomes agitated or excited, then quickly deliver a higher percentage of anesthetic to no more than 5 %. Maintain the animal on isoflurane (0.5–3.0 %) and oxygen mixture during the procedure. Once intratracheal injection is completed, remove the animal from isoflurane, allow it to breathe oxygen until fully recovered, and then place it in recovery. Use appropriate recovery and monitoring approaches as approved by the institutional ethics board.

4. OPD is a colored substrate which will spontaneously darken and form dark precipitates that will interfere with absorbance measurements if left in solution for several hours. It is important to prepare this substrate immediately before use rather than leaving in storage.

5. Eosinophils that have been stored on ice or at room temperature prior to stimulation must be prewarmed for at least 15 min to allow membranes to reach a physiological temperature and facilitate receptor-stimulated degranulation responses.

6. An intratracheal instillation apparatus can be made in-house. Wrap two ends of a thin (20–23 gauge) wire around two arms of an extension clamp. Make sure that the wire is taut. Secure the extension clamp with the wire on a ring stand. Anesthetized mice are hung by their front teeth on the wire between the two arms of the extension clamp.

7. During washing for ELISA technique, avoid reusing the same paper towels from previous steps. This will cause contamination of neighboring wells with samples or materials that could cause a spurious signal to appear in the final absorbance measurement.

Acknowledgements

This work was supported by funding from an NSERC Discovery Grant and a CIHR operating grant (MOP 89748) to PL. We would like to acknowledge the outstanding support of our technician, Renjith Pillai, for assisting with experimental details.

References

1. Hogan SP, Rosenberg HF, Moqbel R et al (2008) Eosinophils: biological properties and role in health and disease. Clin Exp Allergy 38:709–750

2. Rosenberg HF, Dyer KD, Foster PS (2013) Eosinophils: changing perspectives in health and disease. Nat Rev Immunol 13:9–22

3. Rothenberg ME, Hogan SP (2006) The eosinophil. Annu Rev Immunol 24:147–174

4. Winder SJ, Ayscough KR (2005) Actin-binding proteins. J Cell Sci 118:651–654

5. Schweizer RC, van Kessel-Welmers BA, Warringa RA et al (1996) Mechanisms involved in eosinophil migration. Platelet-activating factor-induced chemotaxis and interleukin-5-induced chemokinesis are mediated by different signals. J Leukoc Biol 59:347–356

6. Garcia-Zepeda EA, Rothenberg ME, Ownbey RT et al (1996) Human eotaxin is a specific chemoattractant for eosinophil cells and provides a new mechanism to explain tissue eosinophilia. Nat Med 2:449–456

7. Dyer KD, Percopo CM, Xie Z et al (2010) Mouse and human eosinophils degranulate in response to platelet-activating factor (PAF) and lysoPAF via a PAF-receptor-independent mechanism: evidence for a novel receptor. J Immunol 184:6327–6334

8. Heasman SJ, Ridley AJ (2008) Mammalian Rho GTPases: new insights into their functions from in vivo studies. Nat Rev Mol Cell Biol 9:690–701

9. Lacy P, Willetts L, Kim JD et al (2011) Agonist activation of F-actin-mediated eosinophil shape change and mediator release is dependent on Rac2. Int Arch Allergy Immunol 156:137–147

10. Muniz-Junqueira MI, Barbosa-Marques SM, Junqueira LF Jr (2013) Morphological changes in eosinophils are reliable markers of the severity of an acute asthma exacerbation in children. Allergy 68:911–920

11. Adamko DJ, Wu Y, Gleich GJ et al (2004) The induction of eosinophil peroxidase release: improved methods of measurement and stimulation. J Immunol Methods 291: 101–108

12. Kim JD, Willetts L, Ochkur SI et al (2013) An essential role for Rab27a GTPase in eosinophil exocytosis. J Leukoc Biol 94(6):1265–1274

13. Lee NA, McGarry MP, Larson KA et al (1997) Expression of IL-5 in thymocytes/T cells leads to the development of a massive eosinophilia, extramedullary eosinophilopoiesis, and unique histopathologies. J Immunol 158:1332–1344

14. Levi-Schaffer F, Lacy P, Severs NJ et al (1995) Association of granulocyte-macrophage colony-stimulating factor with the crystalloid granules of human eosinophils. Blood 85: 2579–2586

15. Ochkur SI, Kim JD, Protheroe CA et al (2012) A sensitive high throughput ELISA for human eosinophil peroxidase: a specific assay to quantify eosinophil degranulation from patient-derived sources. J Immunol Methods 384: 10–20

16. Ochkur SI, Kim JD, Protheroe CA et al (2012) The development of a sensitive and specific ELISA for mouse eosinophil peroxidase: assessment of eosinophil degranulation ex vivo and in models of human disease. J Immunol Methods 375:138–147

Chapter 12

Human Eosinophil Adhesion and Receptor Expression

Colleen S. Curran

Abstract

Eosinophils migrate from the bone marrow in response to cytokines and chemokines which induce the expression and activation of adhesion receptors. In understanding the recruitment of eosinophils, protocols to identify eosinophil adhesion and receptor expression have been identified. In this summary, the eosinophil peroxidase and fluorescent labeling assays are described as measurements of indirect and direct eosinophil adhesion, respectively. Additional protocols that identify eosinophil receptor expression via immunofluorescent microscopy and flow cytometry are also described.

Key words Receptor, Adhesion, Peroxidase, Flow cytometry, Microscopy, Eosinophil

1 Introduction

Tissue eosinophilia occurs in response to normal organ development and chronic inflammation [1, 2]. The recruitment of eosinophils is regulated by cell surface receptors and the adhesive interactions associated with these receptors [3]. Cytokines, chemokines, free radicals, and cell-to-cell contact are able to modulate the expression of eosinophil adhesion receptors which thereby affects the adhesive interactions of eosinophils with extracellular matrix proteins and additional cells in the microenvironment [3–5]. To explore the mechanisms involved in adhesion and receptor expression, four protocols are described.

The first protocol involves the indirect detection of eosinophil adhesion via the eosinophil peroxidase (EPO) assay. This assay was originally characterized as a method to differentiate eosinophils from neutrophils in a mixed population [6]. Modification of this protocol has allowed for the indirect measurement of eosinophil adhesion in certain publications [4, 5, 7–9]. Specifically, eosinophils cultured in a plate coated with a substrate, such as fibronectin, will differentially adhere to the substrate depending on the receptor expression or the use of blocking antibodies [4, 5, 9]. To identify adherence, the plate is washed and aliquots of the original eosinophil

Garry M. Walsh (ed.), *Eosinophils: Methods and Protocols*, Methods in Molecular Biology, vol. 1178,
DOI 10.1007/978-1-4939-1016-8_12, © Springer Science+Business Media New York 2014

suspension are added to the plate in the form of a standard curve. Residual eosinophils in the sample wells and suspended eosinophils in the standard curve are lysed, thereby releasing EPO. Oxidation of O-phenylenediamine dihydrochloride (OPD) by EPO in the presence of hydrogen peroxide (H_2O_2) creates OPD diimine colored derivatives that can be detected at an absorbance level of 490 nm [6]. The average absorbance of the samples relative to the standard curve provides an indirect measurement of eosinophil adherence.

The second protocol involves the direct detection of eosinophil adhesion through carboxy fluorescein diacetate succinimidyl ester (CFSE) labeling. The acetylated form of CFSE is known to rapidly cross the plasma membrane where the acetate groups are subsequently cleaved by intracellular esterases and the amino-reactive succinimidyl side chain covalently couples to intracellular proteins [10]. The loss of the acetate groups encourages the dye to concentrate within cells which can then be used to measure eosinophil adherence [5, 10], similar to the EPO assay. This method, however, also eliminates the possibility of nonspecific EPO release and adhesion to the wells during culture as previously described [11].

The third and fourth protocols identify eosinophil receptor expression via immunofluorescent microscopy and flow cytometry, respectively. Primary and isotype control antibodies are fluorescently labeled and commonly used to detect eosinophil receptor expression on cells fixed to slides or suspended (live or fixed) in flow cytometry buffer [4, 5, 12]. A significant increase in fluorescence intensity of the primary antibody compared to the isotype is indicative of receptor identification and expression.

In summary, these protocols provide the basic tools in assessing eosinophil adhesion and receptor expression.

2   Materials

2.1   EPO

1. 55 mM Tris buffer: 1 L of 55 mM Tris base in deionized water, pH 8.0. Store at 4 °C.

2. 1 % Triton X100 in Tris buffer: Add 0.1 mL of Triton X100 to 9.9 mL of Tris buffer, and mix thoroughly. Store at 4 °C.

3. 50 mM OPD in Tris buffer: Add 90.5 mg of OPD to 10 mL of Tris buffer. Aliquot 0.5 mL of 50 mM OPD in Tris buffer into 1.5 mL labeled Eppendorfs and store at −80 °C.

4. 4 M H_2SO_4: Stock acid is 18 M. Always handle with acid-proof gloves and under a fume hood. Clean up spills immediately. Add 100 mL concentrated acid to 350 mL dH_2O (never add water to acid), label, and store at room temperature in a glass bottle.

5. Tris-buffered saline (TBS): 1 L of 10 mM Tris base, 150 mM NaCl, pH 8.0. Sterile filter, and store at 4 °C.

6. Coating substrates: Adhesion molecules or extracellular matrix proteins to encourage eosinophil adhesion (e.g.: fibronectin, vascular cell adhesion molecule-1 (VCAM-1)) compared to a nonspecific protein control (e.g.: fatty acid-free bovine serum albumin (BSA)).

7. Blocking antibodies: Commercial antibodies can be purchased that block the receptor interaction of interest as well as the associated isotype control.

8. Hanks' balanced salt solution (HBSS): Commercial HBSS with Ca^{2+}, Mg^{2+}, but without phenol red.

9. 0.12 % H_2O_2 (make fresh for each experiment just prior to use): Add 30 µL of commercial 30 % H_2O_2 to 25 mL of 55 mM Tris buffer. Measure the absorbance of 0.12 % H_2O_2 against a Tris buffer blank on a spectrophotometer at 230 nm. The absorbance at 230 nm should be between 0.7 and 0.9. Calculate the concentration by Beer's law: absorbance = εbc where $\varepsilon = 81.1$ M/cm, $b = 1$ cm, and $c =$ unknown. Thus, $Abs_{230}/81.1 = $ M concentration of H_2O_2. Keep on ice until use.

10. 96-Well plate (*see* **Note 1**).

11. Media: 0.1 % Human serum albumin in HBSS (*see* **Note 2**).

12. Cell stimulants: Commercially available human interleukin-5 (IL-5) or human granulocyte-macrophage colony-stimulating factor (GM-CSF).

13. Eosinophils: For a full 96-well plate, 1×10^6 human primary blood eosinophils in 10 mL media are required.

14. Spectrophotometer capable of assessing the absorbance of H_2O_2 at 230 nm and the absorbance of OPD diimine colored derivatives at 490 nm in a 96-well plate.

2.2 Fluorescent Labeling

1. CFSE.

2. TBS: Prepare 1 L of 10 mM Tris base, 150 mM NaCl, pH 8.0. Sterile filter, and store at 4 °C.

3. Phosphate-buffered saline (PBS): 1 L sterile PBS—136.89 mM NaCl, 2.68 mM KCl, 10.14 mM Na_2HPO_4, and 1.76 mM KH_2PO_4 at a pH of 7.4.

4. Coating substrates: Adhesion molecules or extracellular matrix proteins to encourage eosinophil adhesion (e.g.: fibronectin, VCAM-1) compared to a nonspecific protein control (e.g.: fatty acid-free BSA).

5. Blocking antibodies: Commercial antibodies can be purchased that block the receptor interaction of interest and an isotype control.

6. HBSS: Commercial HBSS with Ca^{2+}, Mg^{2+}, but without phenol red.

7. Media: 10 % Fetal bovine serum (FBS) in RPMI (*see* **Note 2**).

8. Cell stimulants: Commercially available human IL-5 or human GM-CSF.

9. Eosinophils: For a full 96-well plate, 2×10^6 human primary blood eosinophils in 10 mL media are required.

10. Fluorescent plate reader capable of assessing a 96-well plate at an excitation of 485 and emission of 528.

2.3 Immunofluore-scent Microscopy

1. Cover slips, microslides, tweezers, 6-well tissue culture plate.

2. TBS: 2 L of 10 mM Tris base, 150 mM NaCl, pH 8.0 (*see* **Note 3**).

3. Tris-buffered saline with 0.05 % Tween-20 (TBST): Add 0.5 mL Tween to 1 L of TBS.

4. Paraformaldehyde (PFA) 4 %: Suspend in TBS, and store 4–8 mL aliquots at –20 °C.

5. 0.1 % Triton X100: Add 10 μl of Triton X100 to 10 mL TBS, and mix thoroughly.

6. Blocking buffer: 0.1 mL of 1 % BSA in TBST by adding 1 g BSA to 100 mL TBST.

7. Antibodies: Commercial primary antibodies that bind to the receptor of interest (e.g.: mouse anti-human CD11b), isotype control antibodies (e.g.: normal mouse IgG), and fluorescent secondary antibodies that bind to the primary antibodies (*see* **Note 4**).

8. Secondary antibody serum 4 %: To effectively block secondary antibody nonspecific binding, commercially available serum from the antibody source is added to the blocking buffer at 40 μL/mL (e.g.: if the secondary is donkey-anti-mouse IgG, the secondary antibody serum is donkey).

9. Nucleic acid stain: Commercially available 4′,6-diamidino-2-phenylindole (DAPI 1:10,000) to identify the eosinophil bilobed nucleus.

10. Cytospin centrifuge (*see* **Note 5**).

11. Eosinophils: 50,000 Cells/cover slip.

12. Mounting media: Fluoro-Gel w/Tris buffer from Electron Microscopy Sciences.

13. Fluorescent microscope.

2.4 Flow Cytometry

1. Round-bottom 12×75 mm flow cytometry tubes.

2. 1.7 mL Eppendorf tubes.

3. PBS: 1 L Sterile PBS containing 136.89 mM NaCl, 2.68 mM KCl, 10.14 mM Na_2HPO_4, and 1.76 mM KH_2PO_4 at a pH of 7.4.

4. Wash buffer: 1 % BSA in PBS.

5. Primary antibodies (directly conjugated or purified).

6. Secondary antibodies, if necessary.

7. Propidium iodide (PI) staining solution for live cell examination.

8. Eosinophils: 1×10^6/sample and 1×10^6/flow cytometry control.

9. Cell stimulants: Commercially available human IL-5 or human GM-CSF.

10. Flow cytometer and analysis software.

3 Methods

3.1 EPO Activity as an Indirect Measure of Adherence

1. Suspend substrates at 10 µg/ml in TBS pH 8.0 and aliquot 0.1 mL to each sample well of a 96-well plate for 4 h at 37 °C, 5 % CO_2.

2. Suspend isolated eosinophils at a concentration of 1×10^5/ml, keeping an excess of 0.6 mL of the eosinophil suspension on ice for use in a standard curve.

3. Make aliquots of eosinophils to be treated with blocking antibodies or isotype control (10 µg/ml), and incubate antibodies with eosinophils for 5 min at room temperature.

4. Aspirate wells coated with substrate.

5. Aliquot 0.1 mL of eosinophils per well in triplicate ±100 pM IL-5 or GM-CSF.

6. Incubate the 96-well plate at 37 °C, 5 % CO_2, for 1 h.

7. Warm HBSS in a 37 °C water bath during the incubation time.

8. Prepare 10 mL of the OPD substrate solution. In a 15 mL confocal tube, add all the reagents except for the OPD which should be thawed and added to the tube just prior to aliquoting to the plate. To adjust the H_2O_2 to a 1 mM final concentration in substrate: (0.001 M) (10 mL/plate)/M concentration of H_2O_2 = mL of 0.12 % H_2O_2 in Tris buffer needed in 10 mL substrate.

   Example OPD substrate solution:

H_2O_2:	0.974 mL (example derived value)
1 % Triton	1.000 mL (this is a fixed value)
Tris 55 mM (pH 8)	7.826 mL (value depends on the amount of H_2O_2)
OPD 50 mM	0.200 mL (this is a fixed value that is always left out until last minute)
	10.000 mL

9. After 1-h incubation, invert the plate, and vigorously pat the inverted plate dry on paper towel 2–3 times.

10. Add 0.2 mL of warm HBSS to each well, invert the plate, and vigorously pat the inverted plate dry on paper towel 2–3 times.

11. Add 0.1 mL of warm HBSS to each of the incubated wells and the standard dilution wells B10–H12.

12. Add 0.2 mL of the eosinophil suspension to wells A10, A11, and A12, and serially dilute 0.1 mL through row G, leaving wells H10, H11, and H12 as blanks.

13. Add 0.2 mL of OPD to OPD substrate solution, and vortex.

14. Add 0.1 mL of the OPD substrate solution to each well on the plate.

15. Incubate the plate for 30 min at room temperature.

16. Add 0.05 mL H_2SO_4 to each well to stop the reaction.

17. Read the plate immediately on a 96-well spectrophotometer at an absorbance of 490 nm.

18. Calculate an indirect measurement of eosinophil adherence by examining the means of the samples relative to the standard curve (*see* **Note 6**).

3.2 Fluorescent Labeling as a Measure of Adherence

1. Suspend substrates at 10 μg/ml in TBS pH 8.0 and aliquot 0.1 mL to each sample well of a 96-well plate for 4 h at 37 °C, 5 % CO_2.

2. Label eosinophils with 2 μM CFSE according to the manufacturer's protocol. Suspend CFSE in DMSO at a concentration of 5 mM, and store 1 μL aliquots at −80 °C. Place 2.5 mL of sterile PBS in a 15 mL tube and warm to 37 °C in a water bath. Suspend 2×10^6 eosinophils in 100 μL of 10 % FBS RPMI. Add 1 μL of 5 mM CFSE and the 100 μL aliquot of eosinophils to the tube containing 2.5 mL of warm PBS. Place the tube in a 37 °C water bath for ~7 min, occasionally inverting the tube. Add 10 mL of 10 % FBS RPMI, and submerge tube in ice for 1 min. Centrifuge ($400 \times g$, 5 min, room temperature), decant, resuspend cells in 5 mL of 10 % FBS RPMI, and repeat twice. Suspend CFSE-labeled eosinophils in 100 μL of 10 % FBS RPMI, and add this cell suspension to 10 mL of HBSS for a serum concentration of 0.1 % and cell suspension of 2×10^5/ml.

3. Suspend CFSE-labeled eosinophils at a concentration of 2×10^5/ml, keeping an excess of 0.6 mL of the eosinophil suspension on ice for use in a standard curve.

4. Make aliquots of eosinophils to be treated with blocking antibodies or isotype control (10 μg/ml), and incubate antibodies with eosinophils for 5 min at room temperature.

5. Aspirate wells coated with substrate.

6. Aliquot 0.1 mL of eosinophils per well in triplicate ±100 pM IL-5 or GM-CSF.

7. Incubate the 96-well plate at 37 °C, 5 % CO_2, for 1 h.

8. Warm HBSS (*see* **Note 7**) in a 37 °C water bath during the incubation time.

9. After the 1-h incubation, invert the plate, and vigorously pat the inverted plate dry on paper towel 2–3 times.

10. Add 0.2 mL of warm HBSS (*see* **Note 7**) to each well, invert the plate, and vigorously pat the inverted plate dry on paper towel 2–3 times.

11. Add 0.1 mL of warm HBSS (*see* **Note 7**) to each of the incubated wells and the standard dilution wells B10–H12.

12. Add 0.2 mL of the eosinophil suspension to wells A10, A11, and A12, and serially dilute 0.1 mL through row G, leaving wells H10, H11, and H12 as blanks.

13. Read the plate immediately on a fluorescent plate reader capable of assessing a 96-well plate at an excitation of 485 and emission of 528.

14. Calculate the direct measurement of eosinophil adherence by examining the means of the samples relative to the standard curve (*see* **Note 6**).

3.3 Immunofluorescent Microscopy Staining and Fixation

1. Cytospin 50,000 eosinophils in a 50–100 µL aliquot of media onto cover slips ($400 \times g$, 5 min) (*see* **Note 5**).

2. Transfer cover slips into a 6-well plate, and add 1 mL of room-temperature 4 % PFA for 10 min.

3. Aspirate the PFA and wash 3×5 min in 1 mL TBS at room temperature (RT).

4. Add 1 mL 0.1 % Triton X100 to each well, and incubate for 10 min at RT.

5. Wash wells 2×5 min in 1 mL TBS at RT.

6. Wash wells for 5 min in 1 mL TBST at RT.

7. Block for 30 min in 1 % BSA and 4 % secondary antibody serum TBST at RT.

8. Remove blocking buffer, add 0.5 mL of primary antibody in 1 % BSA and 4 % secondary antibody serum TBST at a concentration recommended by the manufacturer, and place the 6-well plate on a shaker for 1 h at RT (*see* **Note 8**).

9. Remove the primary antibody and wash 3×10 min with 1 mL TBST at RT.

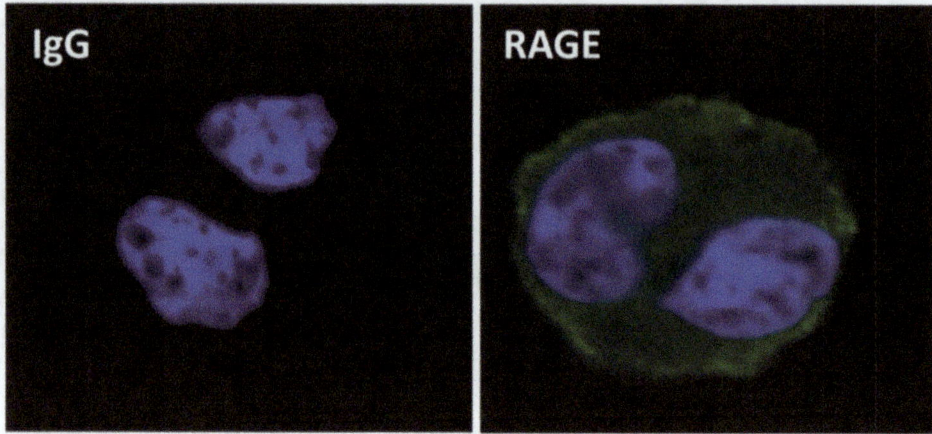

Fig. 1 Immunofluorescence detection of the receptor for advanced glycation end product (RAGE) protein in human eosinophils. Human primary blood eosinophils were cytospun onto cover slips, fixed, permeabilized, and immunostained using goat polyclonal IgG or RAGE antibodies. DAPI nucleic acid stain depicts the eosinophil bilobed nuclei, 100× images

10. Remove the TBST, add the secondary antibody and DAPI (0.5 mL/well in 1 % BSA and TBST) to the cover slips, and place the plate on a shaker for 1 h at RT and in the dark (covered with foil) (*see* **Note 8**).

11. Remove the secondary antibody/DAPI and wash 3×10 min with 1 mL TBST at RT.

12. Remove the TBST, and add 1 mL of deionized water.

13. Clean microslides with 70 % ethanol and kimwipes. Label the microslides.

14. Fill a beaker with deionized water so that the cover slips can be dipped into the water.

15. Place a droplet of mounting media onto a labeled microslide. With tweezers, take the respective cover slip and dip the cover slip in deionized water. Use a kimwipe to gently absorb any excess water on the edge of the cover slip, and place the cover slip atop the mounting media, cell side down.

16. Allow the microslides to dry overnight in the dark.

17. Analyze microslides on a fluorescent microscope (*see* Fig. 1).

3.4 Staining Cell Surface Receptors for Flow Cytometry

1. Culture eosinophils at $1–2×10^6$ cells/mL (*see* **Note 9**), and add a stimulant (optional) for 1–24 h to modify or identify a cell surface receptor (*see* **Note 10**).

2. Label a set of Eppendorf tubes and flow tubes similar to the examples below: (*See* **Note 11**).

One color/receptor detection:

Tube	Treatment	CD69-PE	IgG-PE	PI
Controls:				
A	GM-CSF	------	------	------
B		------	------	++++
C	GM-CSF	++++	------	------
D	GM-CSF	++++	------	++++
Samples:				
1		++++	------	++++
2		------	++++	++++
3	GM-CSF	++++	------	++++
4	GM-CSF	------	++++	++++

Multiple color/receptor detection:

Tube	Treatment	CD11b-PE	CD49d-APC	PI
Controls:				
A	GM-CSF	------	------	------
B		------	------	++++
C	GM-CSF	++++	------	------
D	GM-CSF	------	++++	++++
Samples:				
1		++++	------	++++
2		------	++++	++++
3	GM-CSF	++++	------	++++
4	GM-CSF	------	++++	++++

3. Lift cells from the tissue culture dish by pipetting up and down gently. Transfer cells to a respectively labeled Eppendorf tube (*see* **Note 12**). Wash the wells with ice-cold PBS, and also transfer this volume to respective tubes.

4. Centrifuge ($400{\times}g$, 5 min, $4\,^{\circ}C$), and resuspend cells in 100 µL of wash buffer (*see* **Note 13**).

5. Add the primary antibody at a concentration suggested by the manufacturer or $1\ \mu g/1 \times 10^6$ cells, flick the tube a few times to mix, and keep on ice for 30 min in the dark (covered with foil) if the antibody is fluorescently conjugated.

6. Add 1 mL of wash buffer centrifuge ($400 \times g$, 5 min, 4 °C), and resuspend cells in 100 µL of wash buffer.

7. If the primary was not fluorescently conjugated, add a secondary antibody, flick the tube a few times to mix, and keep on ice for 30 min in the dark (covered with foil).

8. Add 1 mL of wash buffer centrifuge ($400 \times g$, 5 min, 4 °C), and resuspend cells in 100 µL of wash buffer.

9. Add 200 µl PBS to the Eppendorf, transfer cells to flow tubes, and store on ice.

10. Just prior to processing the cells on the flow cytometer, add 3 µg of PI to all tubes but tubes A and C.

11. Analyze data (*see* Figs. 2, 3, and 4).

4   Notes

1. Use tissue culture plates if the aim is to test if eosinophils adhere to a cell line. The incubation time required to reach a confluent layer of cells in the bottom of the wells will need to be determined. Cell lines that are too confluent may become detached during washing. Non-tissue culture plates are recommended for adherence to substrates.

2. Eosinophils can also be adequately cultured in 0.1–10 % FBS in RPMI or DMEM depending on the endpoints sought. The

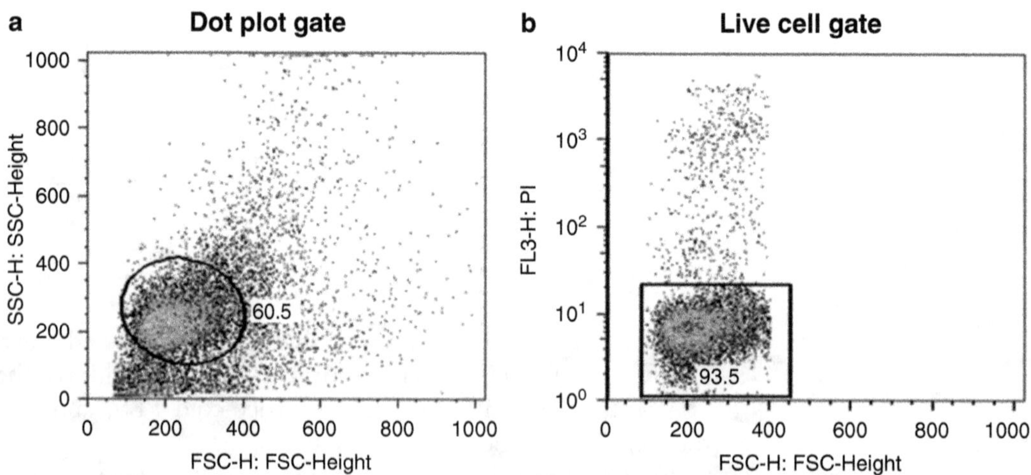

Fig. 2 Eosinophil viability gating. Human blood eosinophils (2×10^5/ml) were cultured above 0.5 % w/v agarose, 48-well plate, ±100 pg/ml GM-CSF. After 3 h, cells were harvested and 10,000 live events were assessed on a FACScan flow cytometer (Becton–Dickinson). Data were analyzed on a log scale with FlowJo data analysis software (TreeStar). A dense population of cells was isolated (**a**) and negatively selected for propidium iodide (PI) stain (**b**)

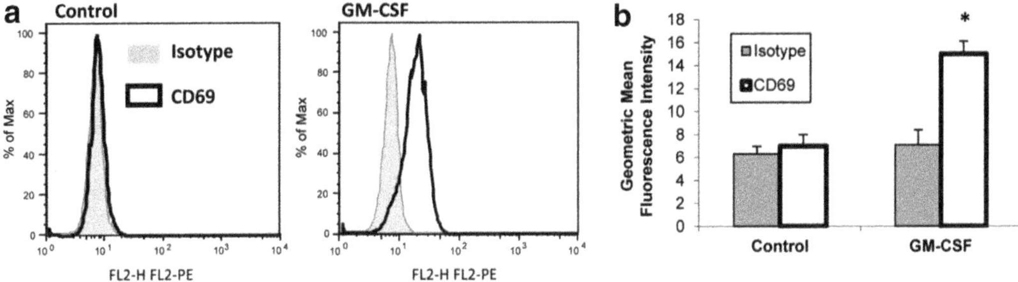

Fig. 3 Eosinophil CD69 expression (one color/receptor detection). Human blood eosinophils (2×10^5/ml) were cultured above 0.5 % w/v agarose, 48-well plate, $\pm$100 pg/ml GM-CSF. After 3 h, cells were harvested and 10,000 live events were assessed on a FACScan flow cytometer (Becton–Dickinson). CD69-positive gates were established on GM-CSF-treated samples and copied to all other samples. Control samples involving media alone were compared against GM-CSF treatment. Representative histograms are displayed from one representative experiment (**a**). The CD69 geometric means $\pm$ SEM are charted (**b**), $N=4$, $^*p<0.0001$ vs. CD69 control

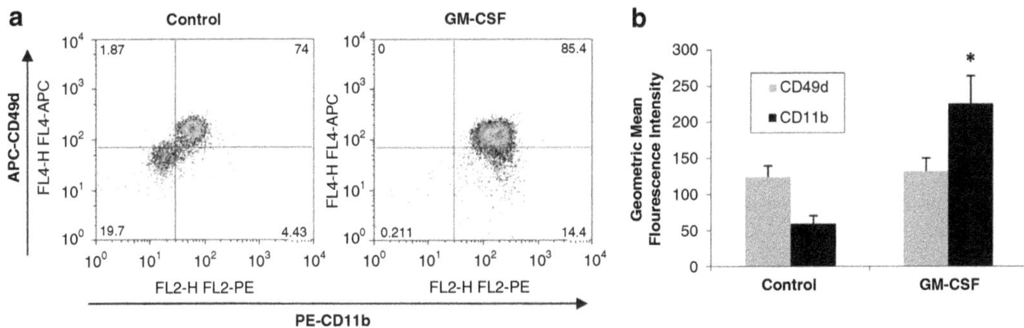

Fig. 4 Eosinophil CD49d and CD11b expression (multiple color/receptor detection). Purified human blood eosinophils (2×10^6 cells/mL) were cultured in plates coated with 10 µg/mL fibronectin. Cells were treated with buffer control or 100 pM GM-CSF for 24 h. Live cells were gated (**a**) and charted (**b**) for integrin expression. CD11b and CD49d are identified via the geometric mean fluorescent intensity $\pm$SEM, $N=4$, $^*p=0.0008$ versus control

excess eosinophil suspension would need to be resuspended in HBSS prior to adding to the plate for the standard curve.

3. PBS may be used instead of TBS throughout the experiment. To prepare 1 L of PBS mix 136.89 mM NaCl, 2.68 mM KCl, 10.14 mM Na_2HPO_4, and 1.76 mM KH_2PO_4 at a pH of 7.4.

4. Note that eosinophil granules tend to have increased autofluorescence at higher excitations (e.g.: 594) which may cause problems in identifying the fluorescence of the antibody of interest.

5. Cells may also be cultured atop cover slips inside the 6-well plate. To encourage adhesion, coat the cover slips with 0.5–1 mL of a substrate (e.g.: fibronectin) at 10 µg/mL in TBS at 37 °C, 5 % CO_2, for 4 h. Aspirate wells, and culture at least 2×10^5

eosinophils/2 mL media ± cell stimulant (e.g.: 100 pM GM-CSF or IL-5) at 37 °C, 5 % CO_2, for 1 h. Aspirate wells, and rinse cover slips with 1 mL PBS prior to adding 4 % PFA.

6. Some reviewers may prefer the assessment of eosinophil adherence as a percentage of total EPO. In this case, the mean sample absorbance would be divided by the mean total absorbance of eosinophils (undiluted wells of the standard curve). By creating a standard curve, both options are possible.

7. TBS can be used instead of HBSS if necessary.

8. To conserve antibody, take a sheet of heavy glass (similar to the size of the plate) and lay a piece of parafilm on top of the glass. Use a kimwipe to firmly wipe the parafilm onto the glass. Draw six wells on the parafilm, and label the wells similar to the 6-well plate. Aliquot 100 µL of antibody in blocking buffer into the labeled parafilm "wells." Pick up a respective cover slip from the 6-well plate with tweezers, carefully noting which side the cells are on, and place the cover slip on top of the 100 µL antibody aliquot/droplet. Place the entire glass sheet containing the cover slips atop wet paper towel and inside of a plastic container and seal to keep moist for 1 h. To subsequently wash cover slips, return the cover slips to the 6-well plate.

9. Cells can be assessed without culturing and at a lower concentration (2×10^5 cells/sample).

10. Eosinophils can be difficult to lift from tissue culture plates, particularly after treating with a stimulant. To avoid this problem, eosinophils can be cultured above wells coated with 0.5 % agarose or a substrate (e.g.: 10 µg/mL fibronectin).

11. Under multiple color/receptor detection, lack of isotype controls is generally accepted. If individual receptor assessment is also desired, isotypes can be added to the sample section by replacing the dashed lines with the respective isotype antibody for that column.

12. Eosinophils can be directly transferred to flow tubes instead of the Eppendorfs for staining. Tubes are centrifuged ($400 \times g$, 5 min, 4 °C), supernatant is discarded to waste, and the tube is inverted onto paper towel to remove residual supernatant. Eppendorfs may be easier to handle in maintaining a volume of 100 µL.

13. If preferred, cells can be fixed at this point by adding 100 µL of 4 % PFA suspended in PBS to samples for a 2 % final concentration. Tap the tubes gently or pipet up and down to mix the PFA with the cells. Incubate tubes (10 min, room temperature), wash cells with 1 mL wash buffer, and store at 4 °C or proceed with staining, leaving out the PI stain.

References

1. Kita H (2011) Eosinophils: multifaceted biological properties and roles in health and disease. Immunol Rev 242(1):161–177
2. Woodruff SA, Masterson JC, Fillon S, Robinson ZD, Furuta GT (2011) Role of eosinophils in inflammatory bowel and gastrointestinal diseases. J Pediatr Gastroenterol Nutr 52(6):650–661
3. Lampinen M, Carlson M, Håkansson LD, Venge P (2004) Cytokine regulated accumulation of eosinophils in inflammatory disease. Allergy 59:793–805
4. Johansson MW, Han ST, Gunderson KA, Busse WW, Jarjour NN, Mosher DF (2012) Platelet activation, P-selectin, and eosinophil β1-integrin activation in asthma. Am J Respir Crit Care Med 185(5):498–507
5. Curran CS, Bertics PJ (2012) Lactoferrin regulates an axis involving CD11b and CD49d integrins and the chemokines MIP-1α and MCP-1 in GM-CSF-treated human primary eosinophils. J Interferon Cytokine Res 32(10):450–61
6. Strath M, Warren DJ, Sanderson CJ (1985) Detection of eosinophils using an eosinophil peroxidase assay. Its use as an assay for eosinophil differentiation factors. J Immunol Methods 83:209–215
7. Curran CS, Evans MD, Bertics PJ (2011) GM-CSF production by glioblastoma cells has a functional role in eosinophil survival, activation, and growth factor production for enhanced tumor cell proliferation. J Immunol 187(3):1254–1263
8. Nagata M, Yamamoto H, Shibasaki M, Sakamoto Y, Matsuo H (2000) Hydrogen peroxide augments eosinophil adhesion via beta2 integrin. Immunology 101(3):412–418, PMID: 11106946
9. Bates ME, Sedgwick JB, Zhu Y, Liu LY, Heuser RG, Jarjour NN, Kita H, Bertics PJ (2010) Human airway eosinophils respond to chemoattractants with greater eosinophil-derived neurotoxin release, adherence to fibronectin, and activation of the Ras-ERK pathway when compared with blood eosinophils. J Immunol 184(12):7125–7133, PMID:20495064
10. Quah BJ, Parish CR (2012) New and improved methods for measuring lymphocyte proliferation in vitro and in vivo using CFSE-like fluorescent dyes. J Immunol Methods 379(1–2): 1–14, PMID:22370428
11. Adamko DJ, Wu Y, Gleich GJ, Lacy P, Moqbel R (2004) The induction of eosinophil peroxidase release: improved methods of measurement and stimulation. J Immunol Methods 291(1–2):101–108, PMID: 15345309
12. Bertram CM, Misso NL, Fogel-Petrovic M, Figueroa CD, Foster PS, Thompson PJ, Bhoola KD (2009) Expression of kinin receptors on eosinophils: comparison of asthmatic patients and healthy subjects. J Leukoc Biol 85(3):544–552

Chapter 13

Adhesion of Eosinophils to Endothelial Cells or Substrates Under Flow Conditions

Viktoria Konya, Miriam Peinhaupt, and Akos Heinemann

Abstract

Recruitment of eosinophils into the lung tissue is a critical event in allergic inflammatory reactions. Extravasation of eosinophils from the bloodstream is a highly dynamic multistep process that involves capture, rolling, activation, firm adhesion, and transendothelial and subendothelial migration of the cells. It is assumed that the rate-limiting step in this cascade is the capture and firm adhesion of cells to the endothelium. As such it is most critical to study endothelial–leukocyte interaction using assays which are capable of mimicking physiological flow conditions. Previously, various parallel flow chamber setups had been used for studying leukocyte adhesion to endothelial cells. Here we describe a highly reproducible technique for investigating eosinophil adhesion to endothelial cell layer or adhesion molecule/extracellular matrix protein coating in biochips by using a semiautomated microfluidic platform and live-cell imaging. In detail, we show eosinophil adhesion to endothelial cells activated by tumour necrosis factor (TNF) alpha, and adhesion to fibronectin of eosinophils stimulated by prostaglandin (PG) D2.

Key words Physiological flow conditions, Cellular interaction, Inflammation, Adhesion molecules, Endothelial cells, Sheer rate, Leukocyte trafficking

1 Introduction

Eosinophil leukocyte extravasation is a hallmark of allergic inflammation; however, eosinophils also mediate non-allergic inflammatory reactions and are part of innate immunity against certain microbes [1]. Interaction of eosinophils with the endothelial cells, gatekeepers of the vascular wall, is defined as a very complex multistep event (Fig. 1a). Thus, therapies targeting specific steps of eosinophil accumulation in inflammatory tissues may be effective in controlling eosinophil-associated disorders [2]. In the course of eosinophil trafficking, majorly involved chemokines are the eotaxins (CCL11, CCL24, and CCL26) [3], or the arachidonic acid product prostaglandin (PG) D_2 [4, 5], among others. Key cytokines in eosinophil-related pathologies are interleukin (IL)-5, IL-4, and IL-13 [2]. Stimulated eosinophils change the conformation of their

Garry M. Walsh (ed.), *Eosinophils: Methods and Protocols*, Methods in Molecular Biology, vol. 1178,
DOI 10.1007/978-1-4939-1016-8_13, © Springer Science+Business Media New York 2014

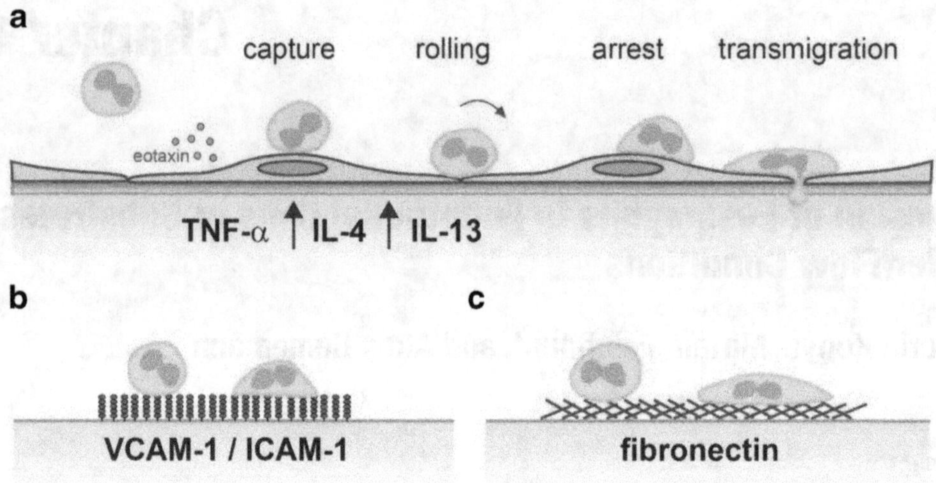

Fig. 1 Eosinophil adhesion cascade. (**a**) Eosinophils circulating in the bloodstream get captured by selectin molecules of, e.g., TNF-α-, IL-4-, or IL-13-activated endothelium. The selectin-mediated weak adhesion allows rolling of eosinophils on the endothelial cell surface to the site of inflammation. The preferred site is identified by chemotaxis towards the eosinophil-specific chemoattractants, such as the eotaxins which are released by inflammatory cells or activated endothelial cells. At the preferred spot the eosinophils are arrested by firm adhesion through the interaction of integrins and endothelial cell adhesion molecules; subsequently activated eosinophils crawl to the rearranged endothelial junctions and transmigrate into the tissue. (**b**) Eosinophil adhesion to substrates can also be studied, including immobilized endothelial adhesion molecules such as VCAM-1 or ICAM-1 or (**c**) extracellular matrix components like fibronectin which might also serve as binding partners for eosinophil integrins

specific integrins, which additionally get rapidly upregulated on the cell surface. Essential eosinophil-expressed integrins are very late antigen 4 (VLA4 or α4β1 or CD49d/Cd29) and Mac-1 (αMβ2 or CD11b/CD18) [6]. Eosinophil infiltration is regulated by specific interactions between eosinophil integrins and endothelial adhesion molecules; additionally extracellular matrix elements can also serve as binding partners for the integrins (Fig. 1b, c) [7]. Important endothelial adhesion molecules are vascular cell adhesion molecule (VCAM)-1 and intercellular adhesion molecule (ICAM)-1.

Studying cellular interactions under physiological flow conditions provides relevant information about the specific regulation of this multicascade event. Furthermore, selective antagonists and inhibitors can be tested as possible interventions against eosinophil recruitment. Previously, different parallel flow chamber setups were applied to investigate the interaction of eosinophils and other leukocytes with endothelial cells [8, 9]. Disadvantages of these systems include the requirement for large quantities of eosinophils and high volumes of reagents for running the experiments. This challenge has been solved by the development of the VenaFlux Microfluidic Platform which enables growing of endothelial cells on tiny substrates or even in the microchannels of sophisticated biochips [10]. The dimensions of the microchannels mimic those of postcapillary vessels.

This microfluidic platform has already been used for studying eosinophil trafficking in different setups. Eosinophil adhesion to VCAM-1- or ICAM-1-coated surfaces was investigated [11–13]. Our laboratory studied interaction of eosinophils with human lung microvascular endothelial cells [14, 15]. Additionally, this platform has been used by us and others for studying endothelial interactions of other leukocytes such as neutrophils or monocytes in various settings [16–19] and adhesion of thrombocytes to collagen and subsequent thrombogenesis in whole blood [20, 21]. Thus, this translational tool provides a promising, physiologically relevant approach to basic cell biology as well as for drug development.

2 Materials

2.1 Cells

1. Freshly isolated human peripheral blood eosinophils: Blood was taken after informed consent from healthy non-atopic volunteers not taking any medication, according to a protocol approved by the Institutional Review Board of the Medical University of Graz. Preparations of polymorphonuclear leukocytes (PMNL) containing neutrophils and eosinophils were performed as described previously [22]. Eosinophils were purified from PMNL by using CD16 microbeads and negative magnetic selection (Miltenyi Biotec, Bergisch-Gladbach, Germany), with resulting purity and viability of >95 %.

2. Human lung microvascular endothelial cells (HMVEC-L) were obtained as cryopreserved tertiary cultures from Lonza (Verviers, Belgium) and were maintained in EGM-2 MV Bullet Kit medium (Lonza) containing 5 % FCS, hFGF-B, VEGF, IGF-1, hEGF, ascorbic acid, hydrocortisone, and GA-100. All culture surfaces were pre-coated with 1 % gelatin for 1 h at 37 °C to promote endothelial cell attachment and growth. The medium was changed every 2 days, and cells were passaged upon reaching 90 % confluence (5–6 days); the cultures were used between five and ten passages [22].

2.2 Instruments

1. VenaEC biochip comprises a "substrate" to accommodate the cultured endothelial cells and a "top" part containing two open channels on its bottom side, which form two microcapillaries as they are assembled.

2. Vena8 Endothelial+ biochip with eight channels enables cultivation of endothelial cells directly in the channels.

3. Vena8 biochip contains eight channels optimal for coating with recombinant adhesion molecules or extracellular matrix components.

    All biochips are commercially available at Cellix Ltd, Trinity Health Centre, St James Hospital, Dublin, Ireland.

4. VenaFlux™ Microfluidic Platform consisting of Mirus nanopump, Zeiss Axiovert 40 CFL microscope, Zeiss A-Plan 10×/0.25 Ph1 lens, Hamamatsu ORCA-03G digital camera plus A3472-06 AC Adaptor, and Cellix VenaFlux Assay 2.1.b Software—Cellix Ltd, Unit 1, Longmile Business Centre, Longmile Road, Dublin 12, Ireland. Detailed description of the microfluidic platform is published elsewhere [10]. The image analysis software DucoCell developed by Cellix Ltd. was used for quantifying eosinophil adhesion.

2.3 Reagents

1. 1 % Gelatin dissolved in 0.9 % NaCl, kept at room temperature.

2. 50 µg/ml Fibronectin (for coating of VenaEC or Vena8 Endothelial+ biochips) and 20 µg/ml fibronectin (for coating of Vena8 biochips) dissolved in PBS without Ca^{2+} and Mg^{2+} stored in aliquots at –20 °C.

3. 10 % BSA dissolved in PBS without Ca^{2+} and Mg^{2+}, always freshly prepared.

4. HEPES-buffered saline solution (HBSS) stored at 4 °C.

5. Trypsin/EDTA and trypsin-neutralizing solution (TNS), both stored in aliquots at –20 °C.

6. TNF-α 10–50 pM dissolved in water containing 1 % BSA stored in aliquots at –70 °C.

7. PGD_2 100 nM solved in ethanol stored in aliquots at –70 °C.

8. Distilled water for washout steps of the microfluidic pump.

9. 70 % Ethanol for washout steps of the microfluidic pump.

10. Washing buffer freshly prepared; PBS without Ca^{2+} and Mg^{2+} containing 0.1 % BSA, 10 mM HEPES, and 10 mM glucose at pH 7.4.

11. Laminar flow bench.

12. Neubauer hemocytometer.

13. Water bath.

14. Centrifuge.

15. Sterile 35 mm Petri dishes, sterile 75 cm^2 cell culture flasks, sterile tubes for centrifugation (15 and 50 mL), sterile 1.5 mL Eppendorf tubes, sterile graded pipettes (10 mL), and Pasteur pipettes.

16. Incubator (5 % CO_2, 95 % relative humidity, 37 °C).

17. Vacuum pump.

---

3 Methods

In summary, the semiautomated microfluidic platform described herein enables investigation of eosinophil adhesion to endothelial cell layer or, alternatively, to immobilized adhesion molecules or

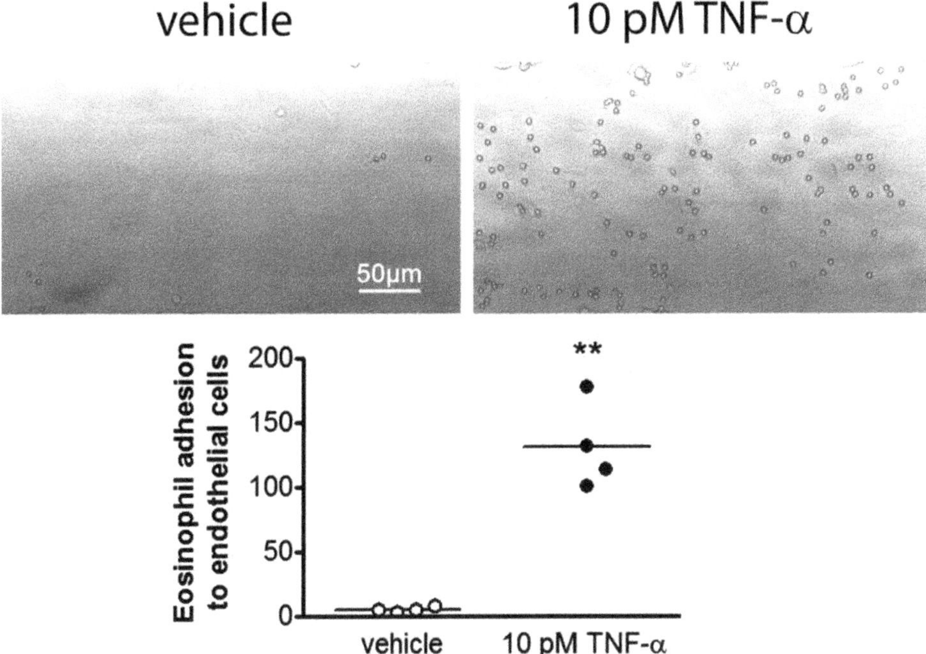

Fig. 2 Eosinophil adhesion to endothelial cells. Human lung microvascular endothelial cells were grown into monolayer on VenaEC biochips. Adhesion of human eosinophils was stimulated by 10 pM TNF-α pretreatment of the endothelial cells for 4 h. Representative images were taken after superfusing eosinophils for 2 min of 0.5 dyn/cm^2 sheer rate. Image quantification was performed by using DucoCell software; data are shown as mean, $n=4$. *$P<0.005$, vehicle versus TNF-α

extracellular matrix components in various settings. There are different biochips available for application with the microfluidic platform such as VenaEC, Vena8 Endothelial+, and Vena8 biochips. Biochips can be seeded with endothelial cells of interest or the Vena8 biochips can be coated with recombinant human adhesion molecules or extracellular matrix elements (Figs. 2 and 3, respectively). Sheer rate of the perfusion can be selected in a wide range as steady or pulsatile flow. For studying eosinophil adhesion the sheer rate of 0.5 dyn/cm^2 and steady flow is used as it mimics physiological condition. Eosinophil adhesion experiments under flow conditions are generally brief, since initial interaction occurs within 1–2 min. Cellular interaction can be observed for longer periods if rolling, firm arrest, shape change, or transendothelial migration of eosinophils are investigated. The described microfluidic platform includes live-cell imaging tools, which allow image quantification of adhered cells and that of dynamic cellular changes like shape change or rolling of eosinophils.

3.1 Application of VenaEC Biochip

1. Place VenaEC substrates in sterile 35 mm Petri dishes or in 6-well plate wells with the tissue culture-treated site (TS) facing upwards.

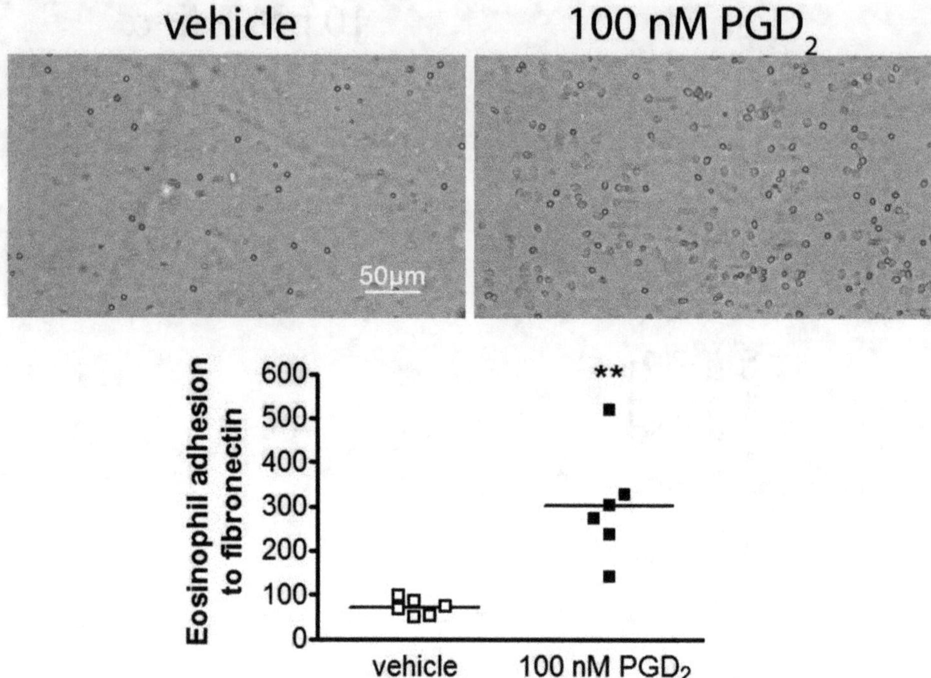

Fig. 3 Eosinophil adhesion to fibronectin. Vena8 biochips were coated with 20 µg/ml fibronectin overnight at 4 °C. Human eosinophil adhesion was triggered by 100 nM PGD$_2$ treatment. Representative images were taken after perfusing eosinophils for 5 min of 0.5 dyn/cm^2 sheer rate. Image quantification was performed by using DucoCell Software; data are shown as mean, $n=6$. *$P<0.005$, vehicle versus PGD$_2$

2. UV sterilize substrates in the laminar flow bench for at least 40 min.

3. Depending on the endothelial cell type to be used, coat the substrates with 1 % gelatin or 50 µg/mL fibronectin in 1 mL solution per well for approximately 2 h at 37 °C. Alternatively, substrates can be coated overnight at 4 °C.

4. In the meantime detach endothelial cells from the cell culture flasks according to your normal protocol for harvesting cells. For these assays, our HMVEC-L are grown in 75 cm^2 cell culture flasks. We wash the endothelial cells with 5 mL HBSS, followed by adding 4 mL trypsin/EDTA for 90 s. Trypsin is deactivated by adding 4 mL trypsin-neutralizing solution. Harvested cells are collected in sterile 50 mL tubes, and cell culture flasks are washed once more with 5 mL HBSS. The collected cells are centrifuged at 220×g for 5 min at room temperature.

5. After centrifugation remove supernatant from the tubes, and resuspend the cell pellet in 1 mL of the endothelial cell culture medium. We use EGM2-MV, a specific medium for human microvascular endothelial cells.

6. Count cells by using a Neubauer hemocytometer.

7. Wash off the coating solution in the 35 mm Petri dishes containing the VenaEC substrates with 1.5 mL HBSS.

8. Prepare the required volume of cell suspension for the seeding, and seed endothelial cells in 2 mL per Petri dish. The required seeding density depends on the respective cell type. We seed generally 4×10^5 HMVEC-L per substrate (4×10^4 cells/cm^2). HMVEC-L with the abovementioned seeding density require approximately 2 days for forming confluent monolayers.

9. On the day of the experiment, treat endothelial cells with the respective pro-inflammatory cytokine. For instance, we use 10–50 pM of TNF-α for stimulation in 2 mL medium per substrate for 4 h at 37 °C.

10. Human peripheral blood eosinophils are isolated in the meantime (*see* details in **item 1** of Subheading 2.1 and in Chapter 2). Prepare 3×10^6 eosinophils in 3 mL washing buffer (*see* **Note 1**).

11. Activate the VenaFlux platform. Switch on the cage heater which is set for 37 °C. Switch on the Mirus pump, the Hamamatsu ORCA-03G digital camera, and then the computer. Start the VenaFlux Assay Software, and select your protocol. Protocols are set up based on the dimensions of the respective biochip such as channel width, diameter, and length (*see* Table 1).

12. Wash the pump three times with distilled water, once with 70 % ethanol, and once more with distilled water.

13. Prepare the "top part" of the VenaEC biochip. The silicon gaskets of the lid are protected with a hard plastic plate. Carefully remove this layer so that the two open channels get exposed. Place the lid in PBS for approximately an hour before assembling the biochip.

14. Place one substrate with the endothelial monolayer on the metal insert which fits to the slot in the center of the frame.

Table 1
Dimensions of the respective biochips

	VenaEC	Vena8 Endothelial+	Vena8
Number of channels	2	8	8
Volume/channel	1.44 µl	2.69 µl	0.8 µl
Width	600 µm	800 µm	400 µm
Diameter	120 µm	120 µm	100 µm
Length	20 mm	20 mm	20 mm

Pipette approximately 100 μL medium on the substrate to avoid drying out of the endothelial cell layer.

15. Insert the pump tubing into the input ports on one side of the top part, add 100 μL medium to the other end of the channels, and dispense some medium through the channel by starting the pump before clamping. Note: This step is to avoid formation of air bubbles in the endothelial cell channels. Air bubbles might impair or even destroy the endothelial cell layer.

16. Carefully place the "top part" which is already connected to the pump on the top of the substrate (*see* **Note 2**).

17. Finally, place the top part of the frame on its lower part containing the assembled VenaEC biochip and tighten the magnetic screws in order to properly clamp the biochip. Place the whole frame onto the microscope stage, find the channels, and focus on the endothelial cells (*see* **Note 3**).

18. Start the flow assay with washing both endothelial cell channels in order to remove dead cells. Use 10 dyn/cm² for the first 10 s to get the perfusion started, and then continue with reduced sheer rate of –0.5 dyn/cm² for at least 1 min.

19. Prepare the freshly isolated human eosinophils at a density of 3×10^6 cells/mL in endothelial medium. To this end, place 300 μL aliquots of the previously prepared eosinophil suspension (3×10^6 in 3 mL washing buffer) into 1.5 mL Eppendorf tubes. Centrifuge eosinophils at $300 \times g$ for 5 min.

20. Resuspend eosinophils in 100 μL of endothelial cell medium, which results in an eosinophil density of 3×10^6 cells/mL. In case that stimulation of eosinophil adhesion is desired, prepare chemoattractants such as eotaxin in the concentration range of 1–10 nM or PGD_2 (30–300 nM) and incubate cells for 5 min at 37 °C.

21. Pipette 100 μL of eosinophil cell suspension into the left reservoir of the VenaEC biochip while the pump tubing is inserted on the right end of the first channel, and start the perfusion. Apply high starting sheer rate of 10 dyn/cm² for the first 10 s in order to get eosinophils into the channels, then reduce sheer rate to 0.5 dyn/cm², and keep perfusion running for at least 2.5–3 min. Flow assays can be performed longer such as for 5–20 min if observation of crawling or transendothelial migration of eosinophils is desired (*see* **Note 4**).

22. Focus on the eosinophils adhering to the endothelial cell layer. Images can be taken throughout the experiment or only in the last 1 min in the whole length of the channel (*see* **Note 5**).

23. Optionally, short videos can be acquired throughout the whole time of the assay by taking advantage of the live-cell imaging system (*see* **Note 6**).

24. After finishing one experiment in the first channel of the VenaEC chip, the same steps (from **step 19** of Subheading 3.1 on) are performed with the second channel.

25. After completing assays on one VenaEC biochip, disassemble the frame and then disassemble the biochip. Discard the substrate, and keep the "top part." Wash thoroughly the "top part," and use it for the next experiments performed on the same day.

As an example eosinophil adhesion to TNF-α-stimulated HMVEC-L is shown in Fig. 2.

3.2 Application of Vena8 Endothelial+ Biochip

1. Place Vena8 Endothelial+ biochips in sterile 10 cm Petri dishes.

2. UV sterilize chips in the laminar flow bench for at least 40 min.

3. Depending on the endothelial cell type you are using, coat the channels with 1 % gelatin or 50 μg/mL fibronectin in 12 μL solution per well for approximately 1–1.5 h at 37 °C. Alternatively, channels can be coated overnight at 4 °C (*see* **Note 7**).

4. After the incubation time, remove coating solution by using a vacuum pump and wash the channels twice with HBSS. Finally, remove HBSS from the channels by the vacuum pump and keep the channels dry (*see* **Note 7**).

5. Prepare endothelial cells for seeding of the microchannels, and perform steps already described in **steps 4–6** of Subheading 3.1. In case stimulation of endothelial cells is desired, endothelial cells should be treated with the respective pro-inflammatory cytokine, e.g., TNF-α 10–50 pM for 4 h prior to harvesting and seeding.

6. Prepare the required volume of cell suspension for the seeding, and seed endothelial cells in 5 μL per channel. The required seeding density depends on the respective cell type. We seed generally 7.5×10^4 HMVEC-L per channel having in total 1.5×10^6 cells/100 μL in EGM2-MV medium (*see* also **item 2** of Subheading 2.1) (*see* **Note 7**).

7. Keep the Vena8 Endothelial+ biochip with the seeded endothelial cells in the CO_2 incubator for 20 min.

8. Check attachment of endothelial cells to the bottom under the microscope. If cells have settled fill up reservoirs with 40–60 μL of medium on both sides of all eight channels. Place Vena8 Endothelial+ biochip into the CO_2 incubator, and incubate cells for approximately 2.5–3 h. Confluent monolayers will be formed within this incubation time (*see* **Note 8**).

9. Human peripheral blood eosinophils are isolated in the meantime (*see* details in **item 1** of Subheading 2.2 and in Chapter 2). Prepare 3×10^6 eosinophils in 3 mL washing buffer (*see* details in **item 10** of Subheading 2.3).

10. Start the VenaFlux platform. Switch on the cage heater which is set for 37 °C. Switch on the Mirus pump, the Hamamatsu ORCA-03G digital camera, and then the computer. Start the VenaFlux Assay Software, and select your protocol. Protocols are set up based on the dimensions of the respective biochip such as channel width, diameter, and length (*see* Table 1).

11. Wash the pump three times with distilled water, once with 70 % ethanol, and once more with distilled water.

12. Place Vena8 Endothelial+ biochip on the frame, fix the whole frame on the microscope stage, find the channels, and focus on the endothelial cells.

13. Start the Vena Flux Assay Software for washing all eight channels with the endothelial cell monolayers. Use -10 dyn/cm^2 for the first 10 s to get the perfusion started, and then continue with reduced sheer rate of -0.5 dyn/cm^2 for at least 1 min.

14. Prepare the freshly isolated human eosinophils, and perform the perfusion assay in the same way as it is described in **steps 19–22** of Subheading 3.1.

15. After completing an experiment with the first channel of the Vena8 Endothelial+ biochip repeat the same steps for the rest of the channels as described in **step 13** of Subheading 3.2.

16. In the end discard the Vena8 Endothelial+ biochip.

3.3 Application of Vena8 Biochip

1. Place Vena8 biochips in sterile 10 cm Petri dishes.

2. UV sterilize chips in the laminar flow bench for at least 40 min.

3. Perform coating of the microchannels by pipetting 10 μL of coating solutions with the recombinant human adhesion molecule or extracellular matrix component of interest, e.g., ICAM-1 (10 μg/mL), VCAM-1 (10 μg/mL), or fibronectin (20 μg/mL) or as control with 10 % BSA. Incubate Vena8 biochips with the coating solution for 1 h in the CO$_2$ incubator at 37 °C. Alternatively, coating can be performed overnight at 4 °C.

4. After the incubation time, remove coating solution by using a vacuum pump and wash the channels with HBSS. Perform coating of all microchannels with 10 % BSA to occupy nonspecific binding sites for a further 30 min at 37 °C. Finally, wash all channels with HBSS (*see* **Note 9**).

5. In the meantime human peripheral blood eosinophils are isolated (*see* details in **item 1** of Subheading 2.1 and in Chapter 2). Prepare cell suspension of 3×10^6 eosinophils in 3 mL washing buffer (*see* details in **item 10** of Subheading 2.3).

6. Start the VenaFlux platform. Switch on the cage heater which is set for 37 °C. Switch on the Mirus pump, the Hamamatsu ORCA-03G digital camera, and then the computer. Start the VenaFlux Assay Software, and select your protocol.

Protocols are set up based on the dimensions of the respective biochip such as channel width, diameter, and length (*see* Table 1).

7. Wash the pump three times with distilled water, once with 70 % ethanol, and once more with distilled water.

8. Place Vena8 biochip on the frame, and fix the whole frame on the microscope stage. Find the first channel.

9. Prepare the freshly isolated human eosinophils, and perform the perfusion assay in the same way as it is described in **steps 19–22** of Subheading 3.1.

10. After completing an experiment with the first channel of the Vena8 biochip repeat the same steps for the rest of the channels as described in **step 13** of Subheading 3.2.

11. In the end discard the Vena8 biochip.

As an example PGD_2-stimulated eosinophil adhesion to fibronectin-coated Vena8 microchannels is shown in Fig. 3.

3.4 Image Analysis

In general image analysis is done by the DucoCell Software, which is the accompanying software for cell adhesion quantification provided in the VenaFlux™ Microfluidic Platform. Alternatively, ImageJ, a freely available image analysis tool, could be used (*see* **Note 10**).

1. Load your image as Bitmap (.bmp) file in the DucoCell Software.

2. Under "Image Setup" menu click on "open calibration" and use a calibration file specific to each biochip subtype. Or create your own calibration file by drawing a calibration line vertically across the image. Click on "set calibration," and define the parameters; check the "use line" button, and set the diameter value of the respective microchannel as µm, e.g., 400 for Vena8 biochip. Additionally set your used "magnification X" to, e.g., 10. Uncheck "draw calibration line," and click on "save calibration file." The calibration is now set for all images.

3. If processing numerous images, all images should have a standardized size. To this end, click on the "show/move mask" button; optionally by clicking on "set mask size" the parameters of the mask can be changed. Having set the optimal mask size, click on "apply mask" (*see* **Note 11**).

4. The image will appear in the previously defined size with the exclusion of the channel walls. In order to quantify eosinophil adhesion, click on the "Detect" main menu. By clicking on "detect cells," adhered cells will be automatically selected and by checking single eosinophils all individual cell properties will be listed in an extra table chart.

5. In case that not all eosinophils are selected or not only eosinophils but also image areas with higher contrast, e.g., endothelial cells below the adhered eosinophils are marked, parameters such as "cell diameter," "contrast level," and "cell area erode" should be optimized. Save the ideal settings by clicking on "save detection settings." Optionally, previously set detection criteria can be used by loading detection settings (*see* **Note 12**).

6. Optionally, cell sorting can be performed by clicking on "Sort Cells" main menu. This feature enables exclusion or inclusion of cells with defined parameters set as "sorting rules." Sorting rule can be any cell parameter like cell diameter, form factor, or ellipticity (*see* **Note 13**).

7. After completing analysis of the first image, load the next images and perform steps listed from **step 3** of Subheading 3.4 on.

8. Collected data can be exported by clicking on "Export Results" main menu. Select "export cell properties table" check box which enables you to get all adhesion events listed with all parameters of the individual cells. These results can now be exported as text file by clicking the "export" button. In case that only cell count of adhered eosinophils per image is desired, this can be seen on the "Cell Properties" dialog bar on the right side of the screen (*see* **Note 14**).

4   Notes

1. Washing buffer is used to keep optimal conditions for the eosinophils; the lack of Mg^{2+} and Ca^{2+} avoids activation of the cells.

2. Once the "top part" of the biochip is placed on the substrate do not move it; otherwise you scratch the endothelial layer.

3. Close the frame tight enough; otherwise the channel will be leaky during the flow, but not too tight; otherwise you might impair the lumen of the channels.

4. Take care of the correct settings for video acquisition.

5. Taking images at predefined time points enables relevant comparison of different conditions.

6. Settings for the video such as frame delay and number of frames depend on personal preferences.

7. Difficulties with formation of air bubbles might occur. Try to avoid creating air bubbles; otherwise there will be endothelial cell-free regions in the channel.

8. The time required for formation of confluent endothelial cell monolayer is highly dependent on the used cell type and the cell seeding density.

9. Try to avoid formation of air bubbles in the microchannels.

10. See more detailed information in the DucoCell Manual provided by Cellix Ltd.

11. Cropping the area of interest in the image is important for proper image analysis due to possible unspecific adhesion of eosinophils to the channel walls. Additionally, at the channel walls contrast/brightness of the image can be different compared to the central part of the image, which would create difficulties at the automatic counting of the adhered cells.

12. Adjacent eosinophils and bigger aggregates of cells might be automatically detected as one cell; such aggregates can be split into individually detected cells by checking "separate cells" or if required by selecting the "separate more" check box.

13. If running flow assays for longer periods than 10–15 min, the big majority of stimulated eosinophils will get polarized in shape and flatten to the bottom of the channel. By using sorting options eosinophils with shape change or crawling eosinophils can be quantified.

14. There are several possibilities for visualizing statistics of the results by using options like "export histogram" or "export scatterplot."

Acknowledgments

This work was supported by the Austrian Science Fund FWF (Grant P25531 to V.K., P22521 to A.H.) and the Jubiläumsfonds of the Austrian National Bank (14263 to A.H.). M.P. was funded by the Ph.D. Program DK-MOLIN (W1241). The authors would like to thank Wolfgang Platzer and Iris Red for professional technical assistance.

References

1. Kita H (2013) Eosinophils: multifunctional and distinctive properties. Int Arch Allergy Immunol 161(Suppl 2):3–9

2. Fulkerson PC, Rothenberg ME (2013) Targeting eosinophils in allergy, inflammation and beyond. Nat Rev Drug Discov 12:117–129

3. Pease JE, Williams TJ (2001) Eotaxin and asthma. Curr Opin Pharmacol 1:248–253

4. Schratl P, Royer JF, Kostenis E et al (2007) The role of the prostaglandin D2 receptor, DP, in eosinophil trafficking. J Immunol 179:4792–4799

5. Schratl P, Sturm EM, Royer JF et al (2006) Hierarchy of eosinophil chemoattractants: role of p38 mitogen-activated protein kinase. Eur J Immunol 36:2401–2409

6. Barthel SR, Johansson MW, McNamee DM et al (2008) Roles of integrin activation in eosinophil function and the eosinophilic inflammation of asthma. J Leukoc Biol 83:1–12

7. Gonlugur U, Efeoglu T (2004) Vascular adhesion and transendothelial migration of eosinophil leukocytes. Cell Tissue Res 318:473–482

8. Patel KD (1998) Eosinophil tethering to interleukin-4-activated endothelial cells requires both P-selectin and vascular cell adhesion molecule-1. Blood 92:3904–3911

9. Cuvelier SL, Patel KD (2001) Shear-dependent eosinophil transmigration on interleukin 4-stimulated endothelial cells: a role for endothelium-associated eotaxin-3. J Exp Med 194:1699–1709

10. Williams V, Kashanin D, Shvets IV et al (2002) Microfluidic enabling platform for cell-based assays. J Lab Autom 7:135–141, http://jla.sagepub.com/content/7/6/135.full.pdf+html

11. Wu P, Mitchell S, Walsh GM (2005) A new antihistamine levocetirizine inhibits eosinophil adhesion to vascular cell adhesion molecule-1 under flow conditions. Clin Exp Allergy 35:1073–1079

12. Robinson AJ, Kashanin D, O'Dowd F et al (2008) Montelukast inhibition of resting and GM-CSF-stimulated eosinophil adhesion to VCAM-1 under flow conditions appears independent of cysLT(1)R antagonism. J Leukoc Biol 83:1522–1529

13. Robinson AJ, Kashanin D, O'Dowd F et al (2009) Fluvastatin and lovastatin inhibit granulocyte macrophage-colony stimulating factor-stimulated human eosinophil adhesion to inter-cellular adhesion molecule-1 under flow conditions. Clin Exp Allergy 39:1866–1874

14. Konya V, Philipose S, Balint Z et al (2011) Interaction of eosinophils with endothelial cells is modulated by prostaglandin EP4 receptors. Eur J Immunol 41:2379–2389

15. Schroder R, Xue L, Konya V et al (2012) PGH1, the precursor for the anti-inflammatory prostaglandins of the 1-series, is a potent activator of the pro-inflammatory receptor CRTH2/DP2. PLoS One 7:e33329

16. Choi EY, Chavakis E, Czabanka MA et al (2008) Del-1, an endogenous leukocyte-endothelial adhesion inhibitor, limits inflammatory cell recruitment. Science 322:1101–1104

17. Demyanets S, Konya V, Kastl SP et al (2011) Interleukin-33 induces expression of adhesion molecules and inflammatory activation in human endothelial cells and in human atherosclerotic plaques. Arterioscler Thromb Vasc Biol 31:2080–2089

18. Kuckleburg CJ, Tilkens SB, Santoso S et al (2012) Proteinase 3 contributes to transendothelial migration of NB1-positive neutrophils. J Immunol 188:2419–2426

19. Konya V, Ullen A, Kampitsch N et al (2013) Endothelial E-type prostanoid 4 receptors promote barrier function and inhibit neutrophil trafficking. J Allergy Clin Immunol 131(532–40):e1–e2

20. Philipose S, Konya V, Sreckovic I et al (2010) The prostaglandin E2 receptor EP4 is expressed by human platelets and potently inhibits platelet aggregation and thrombus formation. Arterioscler Thromb Vasc Biol 30:2416–2423

21. Philipose S, Konya V, Lazarevic M et al (2012) Laropiprant attenuates EP3 and TP prostanoid receptor-mediated thrombus formation. PLoS One 7:e40222

22. Konya V, Sturm EM, Schratl P et al (2010) Endothelium-derived prostaglandin I(2) controls the migration of eosinophils. J Allergy Clin Immunol 125:1105–1113

Chapter 14

Human Eosinophil Transmigration

Stanislawa Bazan-Socha, Joanna Zuk, Bogdan Jakiela, and Jacek Musial

Abstract

In this chapter we describe an optimized eosinophil transmigration assay. Transmigration of purified human peripheral blood eosinophils can be studied using special insert with membrane coated with extracellular matrix components or membrane covered with cells growing as a confluent monolayer, such as vascular endothelial cells of any origin or airway epithelial cells. In our opinion, eosinophil transmigration assay performed through monolayer of human microvascular endothelial cells of lung origin is a suitable tool to estimate the full migratory potential of eosinophils in studies on the pathology of asthma or other respiratory diseases, where eosinophils play important effector functions. This experimental system is easy to perform, simple for optimization, and comparable to in vivo processes occurring during eosinophil migration to the inflammatory sites in lungs.

Key words Eosinophil, Transmigration assay, Endothelial cell monolayer, Inflammation

1 Introduction

Eosinophils are one of the major effector cells in many chronic inflammatory diseases, including airway inflammation in asthma [1]. However, mechanisms involved in eosinophil recruitment to the lungs as well as the pathways of its activation have not been fully elucidated [2]. Cell migration through a blood vessel wall into the inflammatory site is a multistep process, mediated by a variety of cell-surface receptors and their extracellular matrix ligands [1, 2]. For this reason, in order to study migratory properties of eosinophils it is recommended to perform a functional assay, in which effector cells migrate through a porous membrane covered with endothelial cells, a simplified model of a blood vessel wall. Transmigration assay using transwell inserts has been used to study infiltration properties of immune cells in many different systems [3]. Recently we optimized such an experimental approach using cell culture plastic inserts equipped with porous membranes (3 µm in diameter), covered by confluent monolayer of human microvascular

Garry M. Walsh (ed.), *Eosinophils: Methods and Protocols*, Methods in Molecular Biology, vol. 1178, DOI 10.1007/978-1-4939-1016-8_14, © Springer Science+Business Media New York 2014

endothelial cells (HMVEC) seeded on collagen IV-pre-coated surface [4] or seeded directly on the plastic membrane [5]. Such assay is capable to analyze not only the function of specific surface receptors involved in transmigration but also the interactions between migrating cells and extracellular matrix or endothelial cells as well as cell motility towards chemotactic gradients. The assay evaluating transmigration of human peripheral blood eosinophils across the membrane covered with cell monolayer was found to be easy to perform and repetitive. Moreover, it can be adopted in experiments with various extracellular matrix compounds or inserts covered with any in vitro-cultured cells growing as a monolayer, such as vascular endothelial cells of any origin or airway epithelial cells. Any compounds with hypothetical inhibitory or excitatory properties on eosinophils or cells used as a transmigration barrier as well as any eosinophil chemoattractant may be tested in these experiments, as required by the investigator. Moreover, transmigrated and non-transmigrated cells could also be further analyzed using, e.g., flow cytometry (*see* **Note 1**).

2   Materials

2.1   Cell Culture Supplies, Compounds, and Cells Used for Insert's Membrane Covering

1. Transparent cell culture inserts: Incorporating polyethylene terephthalate (PET) track-etched membranes, 3.0 μm pore size, low pore density, 0.3 cm^2 diameter. Using these inserts live cultures can be observed with routine light phase-contrast or bright-field microscopy (Fig. 1).

2. Flat-bottom 24-well tissue culture plates suitable for the above inserts.

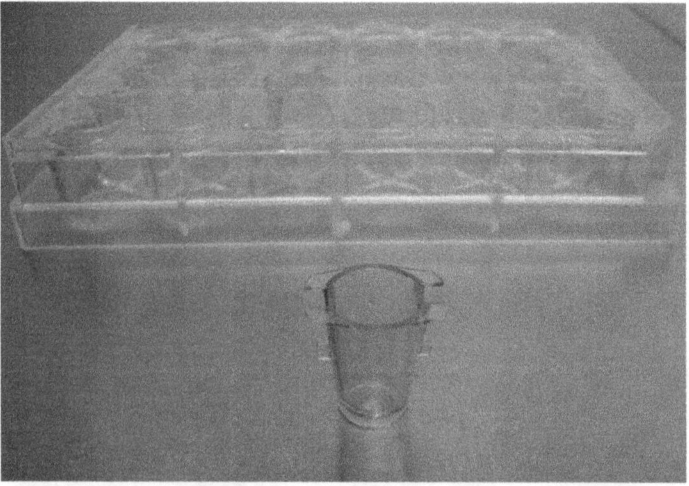

Fig. 1 Cell culture plastic insert and suitable for its cell culture plate used in eosinophil transmigration assay

3. FluoroBlok inserts: 3.0 μm Pore size, low pore density—for fluorescence detection of transmigration assay (*see* **Note 1**).

4. 50 and 15 ml Falcon tubes.

5. Collagen IV: 10 g/ml Reconstituted in 10 mM acetic acid (*see* **Note 2**).

6. Acetic acid: Diluted in deionized water to 10 mM (store at 4 °C).

7. Lung-derived human microvascular endothelial cells (L-HMVEC), purchased from Lonza, Walkersville Inc., USA (*see* **Note 2**).

8. EGM-2-MV—cell culture medium for L-HMVEC (Lonza, Walkersville Inc., USA).

9. 75 cm^2 Tissue culture flasks.

10. Trypsin/EDTA solution for L-HMVEC detachment.

11. Trypsin-neutralizer solution.

12. Sterile tweezers.

2.2 Transmigration Assay

1. Culture medium RPMI 1640 supplemented with 4 mM L-glutamine, 100 IU/ml penicillin, and 100 μg/ml streptomycin.

2. Calcein AM: 5 μg/ml Dissolved in supplemented RPMI 1640 (*see* **Note 1**). Filter with 0.2 μm syringe filter before use.

3. Fetal calf serum.

4. TNFα: 3 ng/ml in EGM-2-MV.

5. FGF: 5 ng/ml in EGM-2-MV.

6. VEGF: 2.2 ng/ml in EGM-2-MV.

7. L-Glutamine: 4 mM in RPMI 1640.

8. Penicillin: 100 IU/ml in RPMI 1640.

9. Streptomycin: 100 μg/ml in RPMI 1640.

10. Eotaxin (0.1 μg/ml in RPMI 1640).

11. Trypan blue: 0.8 mM Solution in PBS.

12. Giemsa: Eosinophil staining.

13. May Grünwald solution: Eosinophil staining.

3 Methods

3.1 Insert Preparation for ECM Work

1. Remove from packages in sterile conditions using sterile tweezers, and gently position in the wells (*see* **Notes 3** and **4**). Use care when handling inserts, as membranes are very thin and easily damaged (*see* **Note 5**).

2. Fill upper chamber with 0.1 ml of a collagen IV solution (*see* **Notes 2** and **6**). Position inserts in well to ensure regular distribution of fluid (*see* **Note 3**). Bottom chamber remains empty (Fig. 2a).

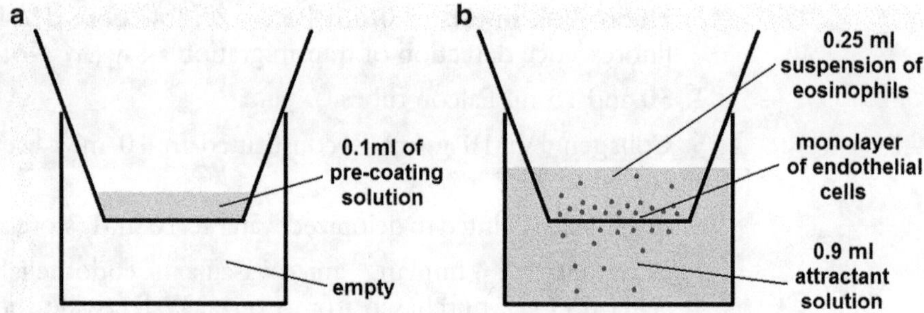

Fig. 2 Scheme of insert's membrane pre-coating (**a**) and eosinophil transmigration assay (**b**)

3. Incubate for 1–3 h at 37 °C.

4. Gently remove solution from inserts by aspiration, and air-dry membranes at room temperature. Avoid touching the membrane with a pipette tip during aspiration (*see* **Note 7**). This procedure creates a thin layer of matrix protein coating.

5. Rinse membranes twice with 0.2 ml of EGM-2-MV culture medium if insert is to be used for further endothelial cell seeding or PBS (if using matrix protein coating alone) (*see* **Note 7**).

6. After washing with PBS, membranes are blocked for 30 min at 37 °C with 0.1 ml of 0.1 % bovine serum albumin in PBS.

7. After removal of fluid and single PBS washing the system is ready for transmigration assay.

3.2 Endothelial Cell Monolayers on Insert Membranes

1. Pre-warm all buffers and media in incubator for 20 min before using.

2. Culture L-HMVEC cells in 75 cm^2 cell culture flasks in EGM-2-MV growth medium at 37 °C/5 % CO_2, with media changes every 2–3 days until 80–90 % confluent. Cells are used between passages 5 and 9.

3. For cell passage wash cells twice with 5–10 ml of calcium-free PBS and incubate with 5 ml of trypsin/EDTA solution at room temperature or in cell culture incubator. As soon as cells start to detach (usually 2–3 min) tap the flask gently and inhibit trypsin by adding 15 ml trypsin-neutralizer solution.

4. Place cells in a 50 ml Falcon tube, and wash flask with 30 ml EGM-2-MV medium. Add to tube, and centrifuge at $300 \times g$ for 7–10 min at room temperature. Resuspend cells by gently flicking tube, and wash once with EGM-2-MV medium at $300 \times g$ for 7–10 min at room temperature.

5. Three confluent 75 cm^2 flasks of L-HMVEC are required for all inserts on 24-well plate.

6. Resuspend cells in growth medium, and seed cells onto the insert membranes at optimal density of $0.7-1 \times 10^5$ L-HMVEC in 0.3 ml of growth medium per insert (*see* **Note 5** and **8**). Leave the lower chamber empty. Make sure that inserts are properly positioned to provide regular distribution of cells (*see* **Note 3**).

7. Leave the plate for 24 h at 37 °C and 5 % CO_2 for cells to become confluent. Bottom of the well below the insert is usually wet, but if the fluid penetrates through the insert to the lower chamber, it should not be used for further experiments (*see* **Note 5**).

   Optional: After 24 h replace EGM-2-MV with fresh EGM-2-MV medium containing one stimulating agent or the mixture of stimulating agents: 3 ng/ml TNFα, 5 ng/ml FGF, and 2.2 ng/ml VEGF in 0.3 ml of EGM-2-MV medium—for L-HMVEC stimulation. Leave the plates with this stimulating cocktail for next 3 h at 37 °C and 5 % CO_2, then remove medium, and replace with 0.3 ml of fresh EGM-2-MV medium.

8. Move inserts to the new 24-well plate. Now, the system is ready for transmigration assay (*see* **Note 9**).

3.3 Eosinophil Isolation

Take at least 40 ml of peripheral blood to isolate eosinophils (*see* **Note 9**)—purified as detailed in Chapter 2. Eosinophils are used immediately after isolation procedure (*see* **Notes 9** and **10**) with greater than 90 % purity and viability. Suspend isolated eosinophils in supplemented RPMI 1640 medium (with or without FCS, depending on your experimental system) at a concentration of 10^6/ml. Incubate cells with study reagents (e.g., with anti-adhesive proteins) for 30 min at room temperature prior to starting transmigration assay.

3.4 Transmigration Assay

1. Pipette 0.25 ml of eosinophil suspension in RPMI 1640 into the upper insert chamber.

2. Put 0.9 ml of RPMI 1640 with selected chemical attractant solution to the lower chamber (we used eotaxin 0.1 μg/ml in RPMI 1640 or 10 % FCS) (Fig. 2b).

3. Incubate plate at 37 °C and 5 % CO_2 for 3–4 h.

4. After incubation discard inserts (*see* **Note 11**) and collect medium from the lower compartment (migrated cells). Count eosinophils using a hemocytometer, and confirm cell purity by a cytospin preparation and May-Grunwald-Giemsa staining and viability using trypan blue.

   Calculate the percentage of transmigrated eosinophils using the formula (number of migrated eosinophils)/(total eosinophil added to the upper chamber) $\times 100$ (%) (*see* **Note 12**).

3.5 Transmigration Assay Using Fluorescently Labeled Eosinophils

If the number of eosinophils available for transmigration assay is very high or if using an eosinophilic cell line, use FluoroBlok inserts with fluorescence detection of transmigrated cells (*see* **Note 1**).

1. Incubate eosinophils with calcein for 45 min at room temperature in 15 ml tube.

2. Add 10 ml of RPMI medium with 10 % of FCS, and centrifuge at $350 \times g$ for 10 min at room temperature.

3. Wash cells three times with 10 ml of RPMI 1640 with 10 % of FCS; centrifuge cells at $350 \times g$ for 10 min at room temperature.

4. Perform transmigration assay as described in Subheading 3.4.

5. Read plate during transmigration assay using fluorescence plate reader and appropriate fluorescence filters after 2, 3, 4, and 6 h. Fluorescence signal would be detected from upper and lower compartments: "top" and "bottom" in the settings of the reader, but only signal from the lower chamber ("bottom") is pivotal for you.

4 Notes

1. FluoroBlok inserts allow automation and simultaneous detection of fluorescent-labeled eosinophils from upper and lower chambers in repeated manner using fluorescence plate reader. It also provides information about the spatial and temporal dynamics in eosinophil transmigration during the whole assay. The main disadvantage of this protocol is the necessity to intensively wash off the excess dye with at least three centrifugation steps resulting in significant loss of the stained eosinophils. This method would be suitable for studying of eosinophils obtained from subjects with high blood eosinophilia and improved cell yield during isolation, e.g., Churg–Strauss syndrome or hypereosinophilic syndrome, but not from those with normal or low blood eosinophil count.

2. We do not recommend using of inserts covered with extracellular matrix components only, as it does not allow for fine discrimination in experiments with inhibitors of transmigration (e.g., between control cells and cells incubated with anti-adhesive proteins). Additionally, such system reflects merely the interaction of cells with components of tissue matrix, but not initial (decisive) stages of eosinophil migration across cell barrier. In our hands the most repeatable experiments were performed with inserts covered with monolayer of L-HMVEC on collagen IV or if cells were seeded directly onto the uncoated membrane.

3. Always ensure that the insert is inserted into the well correctly; that is, position insert with the flanges resting in the notches

on the top edge of each well. This will position inserts diagonally with the membrane in a horizontal position; otherwise fluid or cell distribution will be irregular.

4. All steps of eosinophil transmigration assay must be under aseptic conditions using a laminar flow cabinet.

5. All manipulations with inserts must be performed very gently. Insert membranes are very thin and delicate and can be easily damaged inadvertently. Remember: Inserts with damaged membrane should never be used in experiments; otherwise your results will be unreliable.

6. Seeding HMVEC directly on plastic membrane (without any pre-coating) decreases the number of manipulations and risk of insert damage. In our study results were similar if cells were seeded on collagen IV or directly without any pre-coatings.

7. If you use vacuum for removing fluid from inserts, do it very gently, use gel loading tips, and never touch directly the membrane, but adhere the tip to the insert's wall—it will help to avoid membrane damage.

8. Each investigator should determine the optimal seeding density depending on the type of cells used and their growing properties.

9. Eosinophils for transmigration assay must be used immediately after blood purification. For this reason, blood for eosinophil isolation should be drawn only if a transmigration system is ready for use with confluent L-HMVEC monolayer on inserts' membranes.

10. After blood isolation and before transmigration assay eosinophils should be stored on ice.

11. Before removing inserts after transmigration assay, shake plate gently for 1–2 min in order to detach eosinophils that transmigrated but are still adhered to the lower membrane.

12. Eosinophils after transmigration assay could be studied, e.g., by flow cytometry (cells that transmigrated versus those that did not transmigrated or versus control sample with eosinophils that were not studied in transmigration assay, but stored in the same condition). In order to achieve enough cells for these subsequent experiments all experimental settings should be repeated in several wells, because the number of transmigrated eosinophils in a single well is very limited.

Acknowledgment

This work was supported by the State Committee for Scientific Research: registration number N N402 186835.

References

1. Bousquet J, Chanez A, Vignola J et al (1994) Eosinophil infiltration in asthma. Am J Respir Crit Care Med 150:33–38
2. Bazan-Socha S, Bukiej A, Marcinkiewicz C et al (2005) Integrins in pulmonary inflammatory diseases. Curr Pharm Des 11:893–901
3. Yamamoto H, Sedgwick JB, Vrtis RF et al (2000) The effect of transendothelial migration on eosinophil function. Am J Respir Cell Mol Biol 23:379–388
4. Bazan-Socha S, Zuk J, Plutecka H et al (2012) Collagen receptors $\alpha1\beta1$ and $\alpha2\beta1$ integrins are involved in transmigration of peripheral blood eosinophils, but not mononuclear cells through human microvascular endothelial cells monolayer. J Physiol Pharmacol 63:373–379
5. Bazan-Socha S, Zuk J, Macinkiewicz C, et al. (2013) Collagen receptors: $\alpha_1\beta_1$ and $\alpha_2\beta_1$ integrins are involved in eosinophil transmigration through human microvascular endothelial cell lung monolayer. Abstract presented on EAACI conference, Milan, 22–26 June 2013. Abstract number: 523.

Chapter 15

Measurement of Eosinophil Kinetics in Healthy Volunteers

Neda Farahi, Chrystalla Loutsios, Rosalind P. Simmonds, Linsey Porter, Daniel Gillett, Sarah Heard, A. Michael Peters, Alison M. Condliffe, and Edwin R. Chilvers

Abstract

Radiolabelled leukocyte scans are widely used in nuclear medicine to locate sites of infection and inflammation. Radiolabelling of leukocyte subpopulations can also yield valuable information on cell trafficking and kinetics in vivo, but care must be taken to minimize inadvertent cell activation ex vivo. Here, we describe the use of autologous indium[111]-labelled eosinophils to measure eosinophil intravascular life-span and monitor their distribution and fate using gamma camera imaging in healthy non-atopic individuals.

Key words Granulocytes, Eosinophils, Radiolabelling, Imaging, Cell trafficking

1 Introduction

There is now a substantial body of data on the biology of eosinophils in terms of their development and release from the bone marrow, the mechanism of priming, and the impact of eosinophil-derived products [1–5]. However, much less is known about the distribution, life-span, and fate of these cells in vivo. A number of groups have attempted to study the kinetics of circulating eosinophils, but, due to their low abundance, this work to date has been limited to patients with hypereosinophilia or undertaken in murine models [6–9]. Recently, the development of clinical grade CD16 immunomagnetic beads has offered an opportunity to study the kinetics of eosinophils in healthy volunteers [10].

Ex vivo labelling of mixed leukocytes using radioisotopes such as indium[111] or technetium[99m] is widely used to monitor leukocyte distribution and life-span. As well as monitoring leukocyte trafficking in healthy individuals this approach can also be used to detect sites of infection and inflammation [11]. More recently, technetium[99m]-labelled neutrophils, purified by discontinuous plasma-Percoll gradients, have been used to quantify neutrophil migration into the

Garry M. Walsh (ed.), *Eosinophils: Methods and Protocols*, Methods in Molecular Biology, vol. 1178,
DOI 10.1007/978-1-4939-1016-8_15, © Springer Science+Business Media New York 2014

lungs of patients with chronic obstructive pulmonary disease [12]. Scott Harris and colleagues have utilized the inflammatory biomarker fludeoxyglucose (^{18}F) coupled with positive emission tomography (PET) imaging to indirectly monitor eosinophilic airway inflammation [13].

Two methodological approaches to determine eosinophil kinetics in vivo are discussed in this chapter. Firstly, the measurement of intravascular life-span of minimally manipulated eosinophils is described. In this case a mixed leukocyte population is radiolabelled before re-injection and eosinophils are then isolated from postinjection blood samples. The advantage of this approach is that there is reduced handling of eosinophils, which minimizes their activation and maintains their viability. The second approach utilizes clinical grade CD16 immunomagnetic beads to isolate purified eosinophils, which are subsequently labelled with a radio-isotope and re-injected, and real-time images acquired using gamma cameras. This technique yields information on the sites of eosinophil margination and migration and their physiological fate in vivo. Whilst the data described in this chapter have been obtained from healthy volunteers, the methods may also be useful to monitor eosinophil activity in disease.

Prior to commencement of this study ethical approval should be obtained and authorization given from the regulatory body responsible for the administration of radioactive materials (e.g., ARSAC in the UK). A dosimetric assessment should also be undertaken by a medical physicist to determine the effective dose to the volunteer.

2   Materials

All procedures for cell isolation should be performed in a sterile environment, ideally within a hospital radiopharmacy department, using a negative pressure isolator with integrated centrifuge and wearing appropriate clothing (sterile surgical gowns, masks, gloves, foot covers, and caps). All materials and disposables must be sanitized using 70 % ethanol. Isolation and radiolabelling procedures for granulocytes require aseptic conditions and should follow the European Association of Nuclear Medicine guidelines on the Preparation of Radiopharmaceuticals [14]. Cross contamination or mix-up of blood should be prevented at all times. Exposure to gamma radiation should be minimized by the use of lead shielding and monitoring of radiation exposure. Radioactive contamination will be avoided effectively by the use of appropriate clothing for sterile work as described above. The effective doses to those performing the separation and labelling procedures are minimal, but the advice of a radiation protection supervisor or radiation protection advisor should be sought and an appropriate radiation risk assessment made prior to starting work.

2.1 Mixed Leukocyte Isolation and Radiolabelling

1. Sterile plasticware.
2. 50 mL Syringes.
3. 19 G Cannula.
4. Luer-lock 10 mL syringes.
5. 30 mL Universal tubes.
6. Kwill tubes and luer-lock syringe cap.
7. 5 % Hydroxyethyl starch.
8. 10 MBq indium^{111}-chloride.
9. 0.1 mL Tropolone 0.054 % w/v.
10. Radionuclide calibrator.

2.2 Neutrophil and Eosinophil Isolation from Mixed Leukocytes

1. RoboSep™ automated cell separator with RoboSep filter tips, RoboSep™ buffer (500 mL), and HetaSep™ (100 mL) (StemCell Technologies, Vancouver, Canada).
2. EasySep™ human eosinophil enrichment and human neutrophil enrichment kits (StemCell Technologies).
3. 3 % Acetic acid (v/v in PBS).
4. 5 % Acid citrate dextrose.
5. Hemocytometer.
6. 50 mL Polypropylene tubes, 15 mL polypropylene tubes.
7. Gamma counter.

2.3 Eosinophil Separation

1. 2.2 mL Clinical grade CD16 beads (CliniMACS, Miltenyi Biotec, Bisley, UK), CliniMACS PBS buffer (1 L), VarioMACS magnet, and three LS columns (Miltenyi Biotec).
2. Percoll Plus (GE Healthcare, Chalfont St Giles, UK), 5 M sodium chloride, and water for injection.
3. 5 % Hydroxyethyl starch and 5 % acid citrate dextrose.
4. 10 MBq indium^{111}-chloride, 0.2 mL tropolone 0.054 % w/v.
5. Sterile plasticware: 30 mL Universal tubes, 15 mL sterile tubes, kwill tubes, and 10 mL luer-lock syringes and luer-lock syringe cap.
6. Radionuclide calibrator and gamma counter.

2.4 Eosinophil Imaging

1. Double-headed gamma camera fitted with medium-energy parallel-hole collimator.
2. Xeleris™ image processing workstation with software version 3.0423 or other equivalent image processing workstation.
3. 19 G Cannula, luer-lock extension tube (2.5 × 4.0 mm, length 25 cm, and volume 1.6 mL).
4. Three-way stopcock.
5. 25 mL Saline 0.9 % w/v for flush.

3 Methods

3.1 Mixed Leukocyte Isolation and Radiolabelling

Carry out all procedures at room temperature unless otherwise specified. Bring all reagents to room temperature 1 h before starting the procedure. Lead shielding must be in place around the workbench and surrounding the RoboSep to reduce exposure to gamma radiation.

1. Collect 2×40 mL of blood from the volunteer. Each syringe contains 8 mL of 5 % acid citrate dextrose and 5 mL 5 % hydroxyethyl starch.

2. Transfer the blood into 4×30 mL universal tubes and leave to sediment for up to 45 min.

3. Remove the upper layer containing the mixed leukocytes using a 10 mL syringe fitted with a kwill tube and transfer into 2×30 mL universal tubes.

4. Centrifuge the mixed leukocytes for 5 min at $150 \times g$ (with low brake).

5. Remove the supernatant (consisting of platelet-rich plasma) from each of the two tubes. Remove as much plasma as possible, but leave the mixed leukocyte pellet in at least 0.5 mL of plasma. It is important not to disturb the cell pellet at this stage.

6. Centrifuge the supernatant at $1,300 \times g$ for 5 min. Attach a kwill tube to a 10 mL syringe, and transfer the supernatant (cell-free plasma) into a universal tube.

7. Label each of the two leukocyte pellets by carefully adding 0.1 mL of tropolone solution to the mixed leukocyte suspension, followed by the addition of the 5 MBq indium[111]-chloride solution, and carefully add this to the mixed leukocyte suspension. Cap the universal tube securely, gently mix, and measure the cell suspension activity in the tube.

8. Incubate the mixed leukocyte suspension containing indium[111]-tropolone for 10 min.

9. After the incubation, add 5 mL of cell-free plasma to the labelled cells in each of the two tubes to remove any unbound label. Invert the tubes gently twice and centrifuge at $150 \times g$ for 5 min (with low brake).

10. Remove the supernatant, measure the activity in each tube, and record the values. Measure the activity remaining in each tube, and record the values. Using these values, calculate the labelling efficiency (*see* **Note 1**).

11. Attach a kwill to a 10 mL syringe, and draw up 3 mL of cell-free plasma. Gently resuspend and draw up the labelled mixed leukocyte suspension from a universal tube. Repeat for the second tube, and combine the labelled mixed leukocytes.

Cap the syringe securely with a luer-lock syringe cap. Remove 10 % of the labelled mixed leukocytes in a separate tube for use as a standard (*see* **Note 2**).

12. The activity in the syringe is measured to recheck before re-injection into an antecubital vein.

13. At each time point (45 min, 2 h, 4 h, 6 h, 9 h, 24 h, 48 h, and 72 h postinjection) collect 40 mL blood. Sediment blood for 30 min using HetaSep (8 mL of HetaSep per 40 mL blood). In parallel a full blood count sample should be obtained at each time point to determine circulating neutrophil and eosinophil numbers.

14. Remove the upper layer of mixed leukocytes and decant into fresh 50 mL tubes. Top up to 50 mL using RoboSep buffer, and mix gently. Centrifuge for 10 min at $250 \times g$, and gently resuspend the cell pellet by flicking before adding 50 mL of RoboSep buffer.

15. Count the mixed leukocytes using a hemocytometer by diluting a 10 µL sample 1:2 with 3 % acetic acid to exclude the red blood cells. Remove 80 % of the mixed leukocytes for eosinophil isolation and 20 % of the mixed leukocytes for neutrophil isolation. Centrifuge both samples for 10 min at $250 \times g$.

16. Resuspend each sample in RoboSep buffer at a concentration of 50×10^6 cells per mL. The maximum volume per sample is 6.5 mL.

17. Place samples in the specified quadrants of the RoboSep cell separator, and insert filter tips, RoboSep buffer, polypropylene tubes, neutrophil enrichment kit, and eosinophil enrichment kit in the designated areas (*see* **Note 3**).

18. Follow on-screen instructions to start the RoboSep cell separation, which will finish after 1 h.

19. Remove the isolated neutrophils and eosinophils and centrifuge at $250 \times g$ for 10 min before resuspension in 1 mL of RoboSep buffer. Determine the cell counts in each sample (in duplicate).

20. Repeat **steps 1–7** for each time point that blood is collected. At the end of the procedure, transfer each 1 mL sample into a gamma counter tube and determine the counts per minute (cpm), reading each sample for at least 1,500 s (*see* **Note 4**).

21. Each sample is corrected for indium[111] physical decay (67.3 h) to the time of re-injection.

Percentage granulocyte recovery is calculated using the following formula [15]:

Granulocyte recovery (%) = granulocyte-associated activity (cpm/mL) × blood volume (mL)/injected granulocyte-associated activity (cpm/mL).

The pre-injection sample is divided by the blood volume. Blood volume is calculated using the prescribed formula (*see* **Note 5**). The age, height, and weight of the volunteer must be obtained to calculate the blood volume. A graph of neutrophil or eosinophil recovery vs. time can then be plotted and the intravascular life-span calculated as the area under the curve divided by the 45-min recovery (*see* Fig. 1).

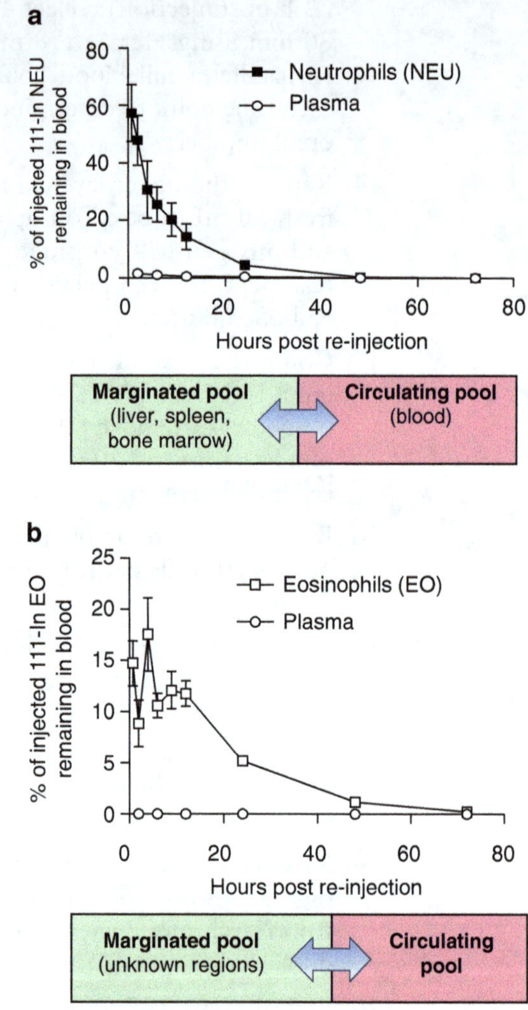

Fig. 1 After re-injection of indium[111]-labelled mixed leukocytes, 40 mL blood samples were taken. (**a**) Neutrophils and (**b**) eosinophils were isolated from blood samples using RoboSep before measurement of cell-associated radioactivity. Data represent the mean ± SEM of seven independent experiments. *$P < 0.05$, compared with 2- and 6-h values (one-way ANOVA test). The schematic diagrams illustrate that neutrophils are distributed equally between the marginated pool and the circulating pool as the neutrophil recovery after 45 min is 57 %. The recovery of eosinophils after 45 min is 15 %, indicating greater distribution in the circulating pool compared to the marginated pool. This research was originally published in *Blood*. Farahi et al. Use of indium[111]-labelled autologous eosinophils to establish the in vivo kinetics of human eosinophils in healthy subjects. Blood. 2012; 120:4068–71. © The American Society of Hematology

3.2 Eosinophil Isolation and Imaging

1. Collect 160 mL of blood in 4×50 mL syringes in 8 mL of 5 % acid citrate dextrose.

2. Follow **steps 2–4** as described in Subheading 3.1.

3. Centrifuge 40 mL of blood at $1,300 \times g$ for 10 min (low brake). Collect the upper layer of supernatant (cell-free plasma) and set aside for the preparation of the plasma-Percoll gradients.

4. While the red cells are sedimenting the plasma-Percoll gradients can be prepared. To prepare the iso-osmotic Percoll (IOP) solution dilute 3 mL of 5 M sodium chloride with 7 mL of water for injection. Three solutions of plasma-Percoll are prepared: 50 % IOP, 60 % IOP, and 65 % IOP (*see* Table 1) for volumes.

5. Add 2 mL of the 65 % IOP to a 15 mL tube, and use a pen to mark the height of the column. Gently overlay in a dropwise manner the 60 % IOP followed by the 50 % IOP. Mark the volume level of each solution on the tube.

6. Gently resuspend the leukocyte pellet in cell-free plasma and make up to a final volume of 2 mL.

7. Withdraw the leukocyte/CFP mixture in a 10 mL syringe and add slowly to the 15 mL tube containing the IOP solutions.

8. Centrifuge the gradients with no brake for 5 min at $150 \times g$.

9. Remove the peripheral blood mononuclear cells at the upper interface (*see* Fig. 2) using a 10 mL syringe with a kwill tube attached. Using a fresh 10 mL syringe and kwill tube remove the granulocyte layer at the lower gradient interface.

10. Centrifuge the granulocytes with low brake for 5 min at $150 \times g$.

11. Prepare a solution of CliniMACS buffer containing 0.5 % CFP (at least 80 mL).

12. Incubate the granulocytes with 2.7 mL of CliniMACS buffer containing CFP and 0.35 mL of CD16 beads. Leave to incubate for 30 min at room temperature, gently inverting by hand every 5 min.

13. Place all three LS columns into the magnet, and rinse each with 3 mL of the CliniMACS buffer containing CFP.

Table 1
Plasma-Percoll concentrations

Final Percoll concentration (%)	Iso-osmotic Percoll (mL)	Cell-free plasma (mL)
65	2.6	1.4
60	2.4	1.6
50	2.0	2.0

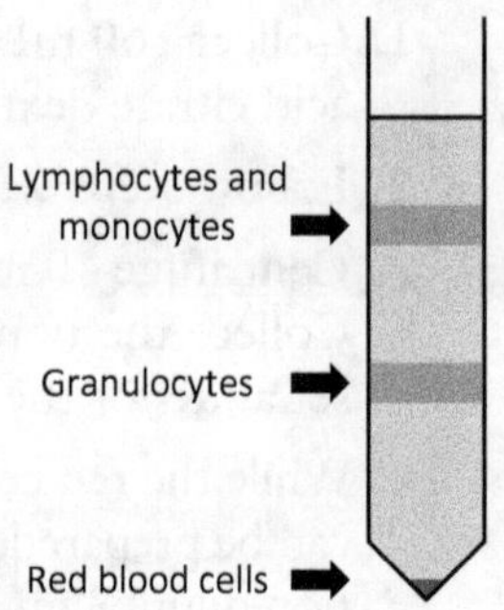

Fig. 2 Plasma-Percoll gradient following centrifugation

14. Following the incubation place equal volumes of the granulo-cyte/CD16 bead mixture into each LS column. After the mixture elutes through the column, add another 3 mL of CliniMACS buffer containing CFP to each column. Follow with two additional 3 mL washes using the CliniMACS buffer containing CFP.

15. Centrifuge collected samples at $150 \times g$ for 5 min (low brake).

16. Remove supernatant and discard. Centrifuge eosinophils at $150 \times g$ for 5 min (low brake) with cell-free plasma.

17. Proceed with radiolabelling and calculation of radiolabelling efficiency as described in Subheading 3.1, **steps 7–11**.

18. Assay the radiolabelled eosinophils prior to re-injection to ensure that they are within the approved activity range for the study; 2.5–10 MBq should give adequate image quality for quantification in the organs as detailed below.

     The next stage requires a minimum of two people—one to administer the radiolabelled eosinophils and the other to operate the gamma camera.

19. With the volunteer lying supine, the gamma camera is positioned to obtain simultaneous anterior and posterior images of the chest and upper abdomen. Place a cannula in an antecubital vein, and position both arms on armrests perpendicular to the patient.

20. For administration, connect an extension tube to a cannula and a three-way tap with a 20 mL saline flush and the shielded, radiolabelled eosinophils. Attach the administration syringe to the tap such that it is in-line with the extension tube—this will give the best flow and minimize cell damage. All syringes and connectors should be luer lock.

21. The radiolabelled eosinophils are administered as a bolus, followed immediately with a 20 mL saline flush—in a continuous and smooth manner.

22. Images are recorded as soon as the bolus of labelled eosinophils is administered. To obtain continuous imaging from the point

Table 2
Gamma camera imaging parameters

Parameters	indium[111]
Pixel size	~4 mm
Energy peak	171, 245 keV
Window width	±10 %
Collimator	Medium energy general purpose (MEGP)
Auto contour (if available)	Yes

Table 3
Imaging frame times

Time after administration (min)	Planar	
	Number of planar frames	Frame duration (s)
0	120	1
2	114	20
45	–	–
120	30	20
240	30	20
360	30	20
1,440	30	20
2,880	30	20

of administration images should be acquired at the following intervals: one image every second for the first 2 min followed by one image every 20 s for 38 min (*see* Tables 2 and 3).

23. At later time points (e.g., 2, 4, 6, and 24 h post-re-injection) images can also be acquired. The length of these later acquisitions may vary, but images obtained every 20 s for a 10-min duration should provide sufficient data. Depending on the radiolabel used the images at the later time points may not be of sufficient quality for analysis. For indium[111]-labelled eosinophils the last image should be obtained no later than 48 h post-re-injection.

24. Following acquisition of all images, image analysis can be performed using a Xeleris™ image processing workstation or similar. On the planar images regions of interest (*see* Fig. 3) are drawn around the organs of interest, e.g., right and left lungs,

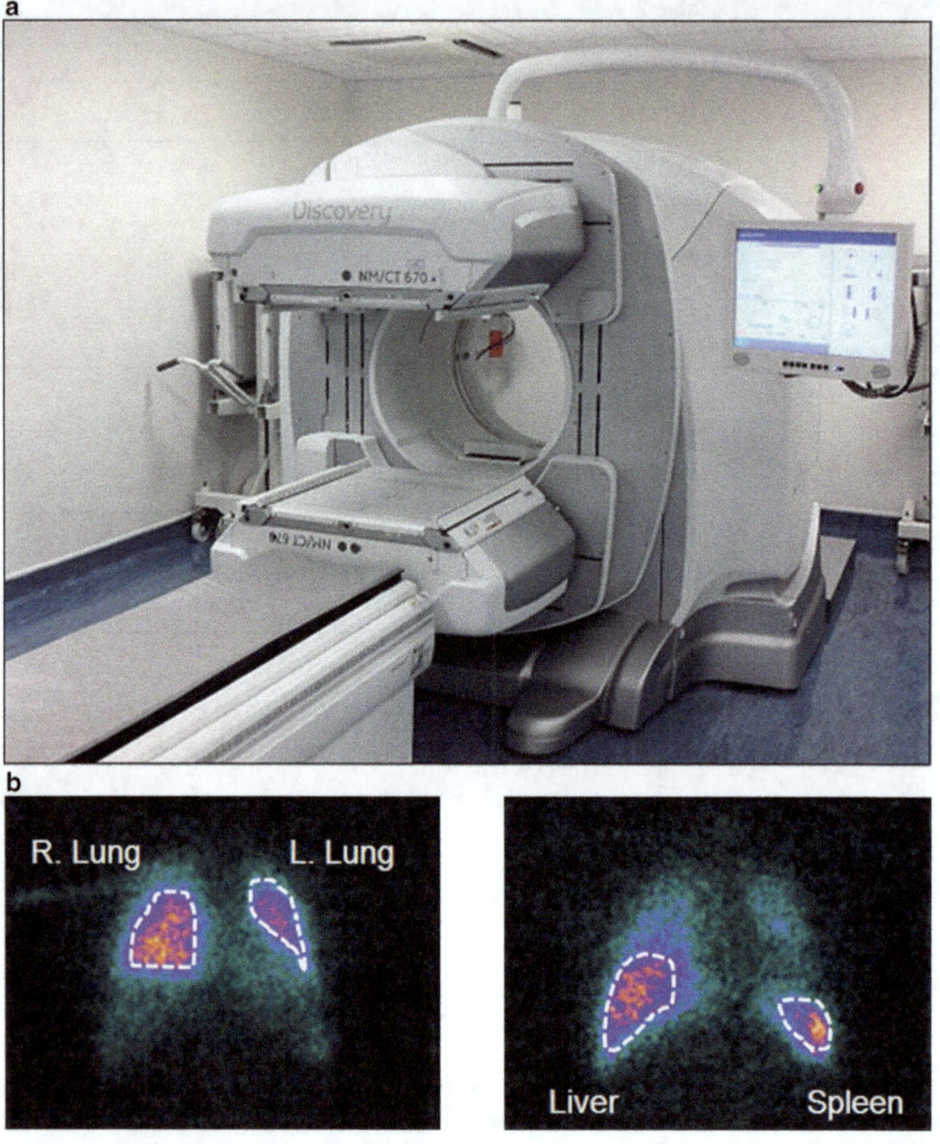

Fig. 3 Imaging of radiolabelled eosinophils using gamma camera imaging. (**a**) Collimated gamma camera. (**b**) Representative *anterior* images showing regions of interest in the liver, spleen, right lung, and left lung after re-injection of indium[111]-labelled eosinophils. This research was originally published in *Blood*. Farahi et al. Use of indium[111]-labelled autologous eosinophils to establish the in vivo kinetics of human eosinophils in healthy subjects. Blood. 2012; 120:4068–71. © The American Society of Hematology

right ventricle, spleen, and liver. The counts in each organ recorded over time are corrected for physical decay of indium[111] (67.3 h). Record the number of pixels for each organ and express as counts/pixel/MBq injected.

4   Notes

1. The percentage labelling efficiency is calculated as follows:
   Activity on cells/(sum of the activity on cells and the supernatant activity) × 100.

2. The standard sample is used to isolate the neutrophils and eosinophils using the RoboSep cell separator (*see* Subheading 3.2) and also provides the activity of the injected neutrophils and eosinophils.

3. Ensure that there are sufficient volumes of the neutrophil and eosinophil enrichment kit. The magnetic particles within the enrichment kit must be resuspended gently 2–3 times with a 1 mL pipette prior to use.

4. The neutrophils and eosinophils isolated from the injected sample will have high counts that may exceed the upper limit of the gamma counter settings (known as "dead time"). To ensure that this does not happen, these samples should be serially diluted as follows: 1:10, 1:100, and 1:1,000 in PBS in a total volume of 1 mL. All of these dilutions are counted, but the 1:1,000 dilution should be sufficient to use in calculations as the readings will not exceed the upper limit of detection.

5. Blood volume (in litres) is calculated as follows [16]: If male,

$$\frac{(1486+1578)\times\left(\text{weight}^{0.425}\times\text{height}^{0.725}\times0.007184\right)-825)}{1,000}.$$

   If female,

$$\left(\left(\left(1.06\times\text{age}\right)+\left(\left(822+1395\right)\times\left(\left(\text{weight}^{0.425}\right)\times\left(\text{height}^{0.725}\right)\times0.007184\right)\right)\right)\right)/1,000.$$

Acknowledgements

This work was supported by Asthma UK [08/11]; the Medical Research Council [grant number MR/J00345X/1]; the Wellcome Trust [grant number 098351/Z/12/Z]; Biotechnology and Biological Sciences Research Council [grant number BB/H531100/1]; Papworth Hospital R&D; and Cambridge National Institute for Health Research Biomedical Research Centre.

References

1. Humbles AA, Lloyd CM, McMillan SJ et al (2004) A critical role for eosinophils in allergic airways remodeling. Science 305:1776–1779

2. Kampen GT, Stafford S, Adachi T et al (2000) Eotaxin induces degranulation and chemotaxis of eosinophils through the activation of ERK2 and p38 mitogen-activated protein kinases. Blood 95:1911–1917

3. Sehmi R, Wood LJ, Watson R et al (1997) Allergen-induced increases in IL-5 receptor α-subunit expression on bone marrow-derived CD34+ cells from asthmatic subjects. A novel marker of progenitor cell commitment towards eosinophilic differentiation. J Clin Invest 100:2466–2475

4. Holgate ST (2000) Epithelial damage and response. Clin Exp Allergy 30:37–41

5. Kingham PJ, McLean WG, Walsh MT et al (2003) Effects of eosinophil on nerve cell morphology and development: the role of reactive oxygen species and p38 MAP kinase. Am J Physiol Lung Cell Mol Physiol 285:L915–L924

6. Herion JC, Glasser RM, Walker RI et al (1970) Eosinophil kinetics in two patients with eosinophilia. Blood 36:361–370

7. Dale DC, Hubert RT, Fauci A (1976) Eosinophil kinetics in the hypereosinophilic syndrome. J Lab Clin Med 87:487–495

8. Yamauchi K, Suzuki Y (1989) Kinetics of indium-III–labelled eosinophils in two patients with eosinophilia. Eur J Nucl Med 15:274–278

9. Runge VM, Rand TH, Clanton JA et al (1985) 111In-labeled eosinophils: localization of inflammatory lesions and parasitic infections in mice. Int J Nucl Med Biol 12:135–144

10. Farahi N, Singh NR, Heard S et al (2012) Use of 111-Indium-labelled autologous eosinophils to establish the in vivo kinetics of human eosinophils in healthy subjects. Blood 120:4068–4071

11. Peters AM, Saverymuttu SH (1987) The value of Indium-labelled leucocytes in clinical practice. Blood Rev 1:65–76

12. Ruparelia P, Szczepura KR, Summers C et al (2011) Quantification of neutrophil migration into the lungs of patients with chronic obstructive pulmonary disease. Eur J Nucl Med Mol Imaging 38:911–919

13. Harris RS, Venegas JG, Wongviriyawong C et al (2011) 18F-FDG uptake rate is a biomarker of eosinophilic inflammation and airway response in asthma. J Nucl Med 52:1713–1720

14. Elsinga P, Todde S, Penuelas I et al (2010) Eur J Nucl Med Mol Imaging 37:1049–1062

15. Weiblen BJ, Forstrom L, McCullough J (1979) Studies of the kinetics of indium-111-labeled granulocytes. J Lab Clin Med 94:246–255

16. Allen TH, Peng MT, Chen KP (1956) Prediction of blood volume and adiposity in man from body weight and cube of height. Metabolism 5:328–345

Chapter 16

Assays of Eosinophil Apoptosis and Phagocytic Uptake

David A. Dorward, Sidharth Sharma, Ana L. Alessandri,
Adriano G. Rossi, and Christopher D. Lucas

Abstract

Eosinophilic inflammation plays an important role in driving a variety of inflammatory and allergic conditions. Delineating the mechanisms by which these terminally differentiated granulocytes undergo programmed cell death (apoptosis) and their subsequent clearance by surrounding phagocytes are central to understanding disease pathogenesis and development of novel pharmacological agents. Dysregulation of the processes of either apoptosis or phagocytosis can result in chronic inflammation and disease progression due to either increased eosinophil life-span or cell necrosis with loss of cell membrane integrity and release of toxic intracellular mediators. A variety of in vitro methods have therefore been developed to understand these mechanisms in isolated primary human eosinophils. Here we describe the key assays used to study eosinophil apoptosis and the intracellular signalling pathways involved as well as phagocytic clearance of these cells.

Key words Eosinophil, Apoptosis, Caspase, Phagocytosis, Mitochondria

1 Introduction

Allergic diseases including asthma, eczema, and rhinitis are characterized by increased eosinophil accumulation at sites of inflammation [1]. Recruited as part of a process including Th2 lymphocyte infiltration and immunoglobulin E (IgE)-mediated mast cell activation eosinophils are central to disease pathogenesis. Their subsequent release of reactive oxygen species, proteases, and inflammatory mediators including cytokines can result in increased inflammation, tissue damage, and organ dysfunction. In order to attenuate this inflammatory process eosinophil apoptosis and the subsequent non-phlogistic clearance of apoptotic cells are essential in ensuring resolution of the inflammatory process. A delay in either of these components results in ongoing tissue injury and chronic inflammation [2].

The circulating life-span of eosinophils is short with an intravascular presence of around 18–25 h, prior to migration into tissues, with the thymus and gastrointestinal tract the usual destination of

Garry M. Walsh (ed.), *Eosinophils: Methods and Protocols*, Methods in Molecular Biology, vol. 1178,
DOI 10.1007/978-1-4939-1016-8_16, © Springer Science+Business Media New York 2014

eosinophils in health [3]. Here their life-span is thought to be several days. Eosinophils isolated from peripheral blood undergo constitutive apoptosis, although at a much slower rate than the closely related neutrophil granulocyte. The eosinophil half-life in vitro is approximately 48 h following isolation [4–6]. The process of eosinophil apoptosis is dependent upon the activation of cysteine-aspartic proteases (caspases) which are contained as inactive zymogens within the cell with eosinophils containing caspases 3, 6, 7, 8, and 9. Caspase cleavage occurs due to activation of either the extrinsic or the intrinsic pathways of apoptosis [2]. The extrinsic pathway relies on the ligation of "death receptors" such as the tumor necrosis factor receptor (TNF-R), the Fas receptor (FasR), and the TNF-related apoptosis-inducing ligand receptor (TRAIL-R) [7]. Cross-linking of these receptors causes clustering and, through associations with internal adaptor proteins, allows the formation of pro-caspase complexes, caspase-8 cleavage, and subsequent apoptosis. The intrinsic pathway is activated when the cell faces withdrawal of survival factors, genotoxic stress, exposure to ultraviolet radiation, or chemotherapeutic agents allowing pro-apoptotic members of the B cell lymphoma 2 (Bcl-2) family to dissociate from their anti-apoptotic regulators and translocate to the mitochondria. Resultant increased mitochondrial membrane permeability and pore formation lead to cytochrome c release into the cytosol with cleavage of pro-caspase-9 to active caspase-9, thereby committing the cell to caspase-3-mediated apoptosis. The process of apoptosis results in morphological and biochemical changes including cell shrinkage, nuclear condensation, and apoptotic body formation; increased mitochondrial permeability with loss of membrane potential; DNA fragmentation; caspase activation; and externalization of phosphatidylserine on the plasma membrane.

Eosinophil life-span can be modulated through alterations in the balance of pro-survival and pro-apoptotic signals and proteins. Apoptosis can be delayed by a variety of factors including cytokines (interleukin-5 (IL-5), GM-CSF, eotaxin, and interferon-γ), hypoxia, bacterial exotoxins [8] and DNA which also serve to induce eosinophil migration and activation into areas of inflammation. Conversely apoptosis can be accelerated by IL-4; FAS ligand; ligation of CD69, CD45, and CD30 cell surface receptors; and intracellular oxidant production with pharmacological agents including corticosteroids, theophyllines, and cyclin-dependent kinase inhibitors [9].

Numerous changes in cell surface marker expression and the secretion of soluble factors that occurs during apoptosis facilitate the phagocyte uptake of these cells by surrounding macrophages and dendritic cells as well as nonprofessional phagocytes including epithelial cells [10, 11]. Important alterations to the cell membrane include phosphatidylserine exposure, changes in ICAM-1 epitopes, modification in glycosylation patterns, and charge and expression of calreticulin. Phagocytosis is a key event in macrophage phenotypic switching from a pro-inflammatory to a pro-resolving phenotype with release of anti-inflammatory cytokines and lipids (including IL-10, transforming growth factor-β (TGF-β), and resolvins) [12]. Failure in clearance of apoptotic effete cells however results in eventual disintegration of the cell membrane (termed secondary necrosis) with release of toxic intracellular contents, tissue damage, and perpetuation of the inflammatory response.

Eosinophils form approximately 1–3 % of the granulocyte population in the peripheral blood of a non-atopic individual; therefore enrichment following conventional granulocyte isolation methods is essential [13, 14]. Negative selection (anti-CD16) is most widely used. Eosinophil life-span can be influenced by a number of factors, therefore ensuring that eosinophil activation is prevented during isolation and culture is vital for in vitro study. Factors which may alter constitutive eosinophil life-span and affect interpretation of results include the method of isolation, serum presence, temperature, pH level, oxygen tension, and cell density [2].

As described the molecular and morphological changes that occur during the process of apoptosis allow in vitro study through a variety of different assays and approaches ranging from assessment of externalization of phosphatidylserine by flow cytometry and nuclear condensation by light microscopy to assessment of DNA fragmentation by hypodiploid peak analysis and mitochondrial membrane permeability with chromogenic dyes. This chapter therefore describes the methodologies used to examine components of the apoptotic process and subsequent phagocytic clearance of these cells.

2   Materials

2.1   Culture of Human Eosinophils In Vitro

1. Iscove's Modified Dulbecco's Medium (IMDM).
2. Penicillin/streptomycin 100×.
3. 10 % Autologous serum (*see* **Note 1**).
4. 96-Well flat-bottomed plate.

2.2   Cytocentrifuge Preparations of Eosinophils for Light Microscopy

1. Cytocentrifuge chambers, filter cards, glass slides, and cover slips.
2. Methanol, Diff-Quik™ stains.
3. DPX mounting medium.

2.3 Preparation for Electron Microscopy

1. 3 % Glutaraldehyde, 25 % stock solution diluted in 0.1 M sodium cacodylate buffer (pH 7.2).
2. 1 % Osmium tetroxide in 0.1 M sodium cacodylate.
3. 100, 90, 70, and 50 % normal-grade acetones and analar acetone.
4. Araldite resin.
5. Reichert OmU4 ultramicrotome.

2.4 Annexin V/ Propidium Iodide Staining

1. 96-Well flat-bottomed plate.
2. Annexin V-conjugated fluorescein isothiocyanate (FITC).
3. Annexin binding buffer (Hanks' balanced salt solution (HBSS) with 2.5 mM Ca^{2+}): Store at 4 °C.
4. Stock solution of 1 mg/ml propidium iodide in sterile ddH_2O.

2.5 Alterations in Mitochondrial Permeability

1. MitoCapture™ Mitochondrial Apoptosis Detection Fluorometric Kit (Biovision, Milpitas, CA 95035 USA) contains: MitoCapture™ reagent (store at −20 °C), incubation buffer (store at 4 °C).

2.6 Western Blotting for Intracellular Proteins That Regulate Apoptosis

1. Tris-buffered saline (TBS 10×): NaCl (87.66 g), Tris base (24.22 g), distilled water (ddH_2O, 800 ml), pH adjusted to 7.4 with HCl and then made to 1 l with ddH_2O, dilute 1:10 with ddH_2O prior to use for 1× TBS.
2. Protease inhibitor buffer (*see* **Note 2**): 780 μl 1× TBS added to 20 μl protease inhibitor cocktail, supplemented with 4-(2-aminoethyl)benzenesulfonyl fluoride hydrochloride (AEBSF; 20 μl—400 mM stock in H_2O), aprotinin (20 μl—0.15 μM stock in H_2O), leupeptin (20 μl—20 mM stock in H_2O), pepstatin A (40 μl—0.75 μM stock in methanol), sodium vanadate (20 μl—1 M stock in H_2O, pH 10, boiled), benzamidine (20 μl—0.5 M stock in H_2O), levamisole (20 μl—2 M stock in H_2O), β-glycerophosphate (60 μl of 3.33 M stock in H_2O).
3. 10 % Nonidet P-40 (NP-40) detergent in 1× TBS.
4. BCA protein assay.
5. Sample buffer (for 4×): 50 % Glycerol (4 ml), 20 % SDS (4 ml), Tris–HCl (2.5 ml 1 M, pH 6.8), 1 % (w/v in ethanol) bromophenol blue (20 μl), β-mercaptoethanol (400 μl—add in fume hood).
6. Benchmark™ prestained molecular weight standards (Invitrogen).
7. 12 % SDS gel.
8. Running buffer (10×): Tris base (121 g), SDS (10 g), Hepes (238 g), ddH_2O (800 ml), once dissolved made up 1 l (ddH_2O); diluted 1:10 (ddH_2O) for 1× solution prior to use.

9. Transfer buffer (10×): Tris base (30.3 g), glycine (144.12 g), ddH$_2$O (800 ml), once dissolved made up 1 l (ddH$_2$O).

10. Transfer buffer (1×): 10× Transfer buffer (100 ml), methanol (200 ml), ddH$_2$O (700 ml).

11. Polyvinylidene difluoride (PVDF) membrane.

12. Blocking buffer: 1× TBS: 0.1 % Tween®20 (polysorbate 20), 5 % dried milk powder.

13. Primary antibodies: Mcl-1 (1:500; Santa-Cruz, Biotechnology, CA, USA), GAPDH (1:10,000; Sigma), cleaved caspase-3 (1:1,000, Cell Signalling, Danvers, MA, USA), cleaved caspase-9 (1:1,000; Cell Signalling),

14. Secondary antibodies: Corresponding horseradish-peroxidase-conjugated antibodies (1:2,500, Dako, Cambridgeshire, UK).

15. ECL prime, light-sensitive film, X-ray developer.

2.7 Fluorimetric Caspase kit

1. Homogeneous Caspases Assay Kit (Roche Diagnostics Ltd, Lewes, UK): 1× Incubation buffer, stock caspase substrate solution (500 µM DEVD-R110 in DMSO), positive control (lysate from apoptotic camptothecin-treated U937 cells), and R110 standard for calibration curve construction (1 mM in DMSO).

2.8 Caspase Profiling Plate

1. ApoAlert™ Caspase Profiling Plate (Clontech, Saint-Germain-en-Laye, France) contains 96-Well microplate with immobilized substrates for caspase 2 (VDVAD-AMC), caspase 3 (DEVD-AMC), caspase 8 (IETD-AMC), and caspase 9 (LEHD-AMC) in 24 wells each, lysis buffer, 2× reaction buffer, 100× DTT solution, and inhibitors of caspases 2, 3, 8, and 9.

2.9 Gel Electrophoresis for DNA Fragmentation

1. Wizard® genomic DNA purification kit.

2. 5× TBE running buffer: Tris base (54 g), boric acid (27.5 g), EDTA (20 ml—0.5 M pH 8.0), ddH$_2$O (800 ml), pH adjusted to 8.3 and then made to 1 l with ddH$_2$O and 0.5× TBE.

3. SeaKem LE agarose for DNA electrophoresis.

4. GelRedTM Nucleic Acid Gel Stain.

5. 6× Blue/orange loading dye.

2.10 Propidium Iodide Staining for Hypodiploid Nuclei

1. 96-Well flat-bottom plate.

2. PI solution: Propidium iodide (250 µl—10 mg/ml in ddH$_2$O), sodium citrate (2.2 ml—2.2 g in 10 ml ddH$_2$O), Triton X-100 (50 µl), ddH$_2$O (made up to 50 ml total volume). Store solution at 4 °C in the dark.

2.11 TUNEL Staining

1. 96-Well flat-bottom flexible plate.

2. In Situ Cell Death Detection Kit, Fluorescein (Roche Diagnostics Ltd) contains 10× enzyme solution (TdT) in storage

buffer and 1× labelled nucleotide mixture in reaction buffer. This protocol also requires PBS (wash buffer), 3 % H_2O_2 in methanol (blocking solution), 4 % paraformaldehyde in PBS at pH 7.4 (fixation buffer; freshly prepared), and 0.1 % Triton X-100 in 0.1 % sodium citrate (permeabilization buffer; freshly prepared).

2.12 Flow Cytometry-Based Phagocytosis Assay

1. 5-Chloromethylfluorescein diacetate (CMFDA; CellTracker™ Green, Invitrogen).

2. pHrodo™ Red succinimidyl ester (Invitrogen).

3. 0.25 % Trypsin/1 mM ethylenediaminetetraacetic acid solution.

---

3 Methods

3.1 Assessing Morphological Changes of Apoptosis Using Light Microscopy

Apoptotic eosinophils are distinguishable from viable cells, under light microscopy, by their characteristic morphological appearances of nuclear condensation and cell shrinkage (Fig. 1a, c).

1. Suspend eosinophils (of at least 97 % purity—determined by cytocentrifuge preparation as described below) at 4×10^6 cells/ml in IMDM supplemented with 10 % autologous serum and penicillin/streptomycin (1×) (*see* **Note 1**).

2. In a 96-Well flat-bottomed plate add 75 μl of eosinophil suspension. Add 15 μl of apoptosis-modifying agents (10× concentration) or vehicle control and 60 μl IMDM with 10 % autologous serum to each well. (NB: If two agents are used only 45 μl of IMDM is required for total volume of 150 μl.)

3. Cover the plate with a lid, and incubate at 37 °C in a 5 % CO_2 incubator for the required amount of time.

4. Gently pipette the cell suspension in the well to resuspend adherent cells and load 200 μl into a cytospin chamber.

5. Cytocentrifuge at 300 rpm ($30 \times g$) for 3 min.

6. Air-dry for 5 min.

7. Fix in methanol for 2 min.

8. Stain in Diff Quik™ solution 1 or equivalent acid dye for 2 min.

9. Stain in Diff Quik™ solution 2 or equivalent basic dye for 2 min.

10. Rinse with distilled water.

11. Air-dry slides before mounting with a drop of DPX and cover slip. View slides using a light microscope with a 40× or a 100× (oil) objective, and count >300 cells per slide (*see* **Note 3**).

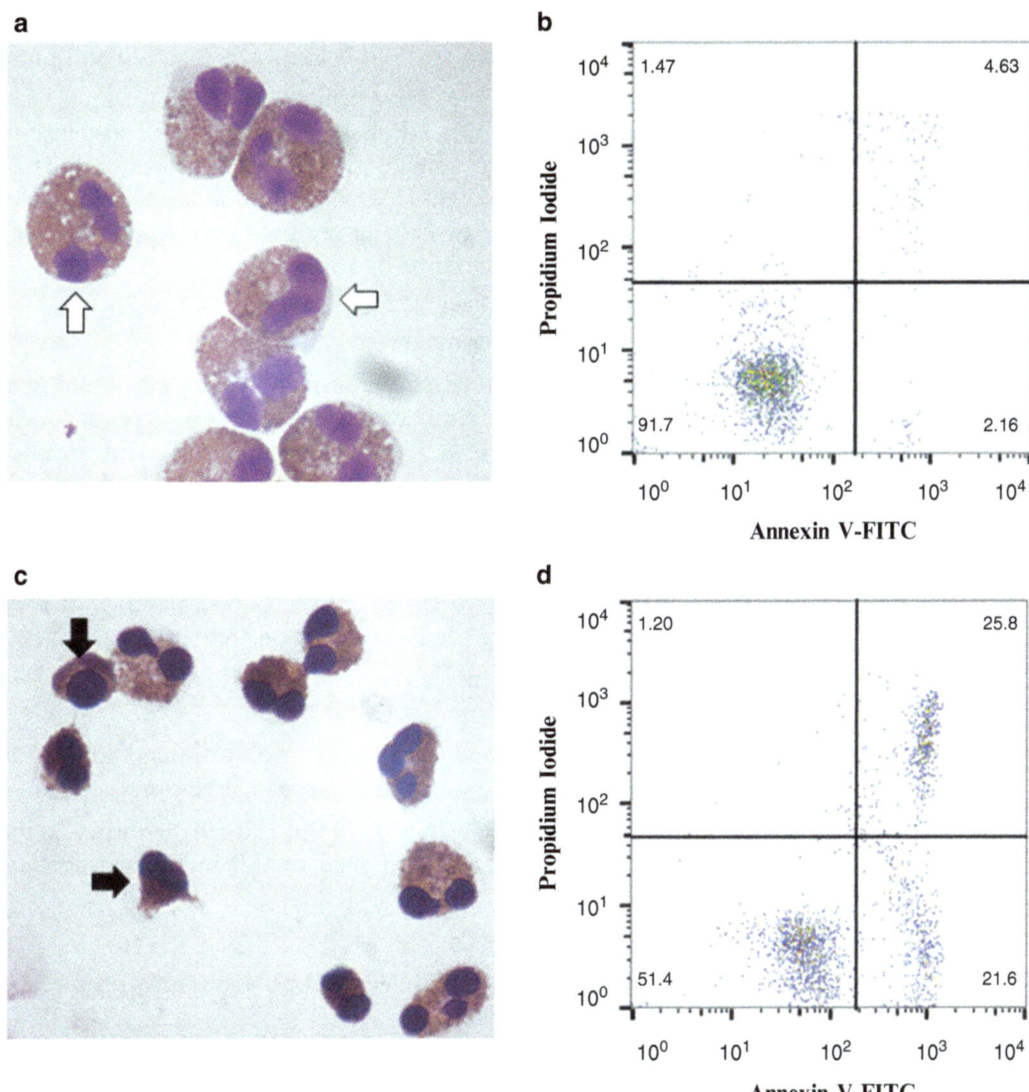

Fig. 1 Determining eosinophil apoptosis by light microscopy and flow cytometry. Viable eosinophils isolated from peripheral venous human blood have eosinophilic cytoplasmic staining, abundant granules, and bilobed nucleus (*white arrow*) (**a**). Flow cytometric analysis of cell death immediately following isolation demonstrates that the majority of cells are viable (AnnV^{-ve}/PI^{-ve}) (**b**). Apoptotic eosinophils in vitro display characteristic morphological changes of cell shrinkage, membrane blebbing, nuclear condensation, darkening of cytoplasmic staining, and nuclear condensation (*black arrows*) (**c**). Similarly increased apoptotic (AnnV^{+ve}/PI^{-ve}) and necrotic (AnnV^{+ve}/PI^{+ve}) staining is seen with flow cytometry (**d**). All images 1,000× magnification

3.2 Analysis of Eosinophil Morphology by Electron Microscopy

Although conventional light microscopy provides information regarding the general morphological changes that occur during apoptosis it is electron microscopy that allows detailed structural analysis of these processes.

1. Suspend eosinophils (at least 97 % purity) at 4×10^6 cells/ml in IMDM supplemented with 10 % autologous serum and penicillin/streptomycin (1×) (*see* **Note 1**).

2. In a 96-Well flat-bottomed plate add 75 μl of cell suspension, 15 μl of apoptosis-modifying agents (10× concentration) or vehicle control, and 60 μl IMDM with 10 % autologous serum to each well. (NB: If two agents are used only 45 μl of IMDM is required for total volume of 150 μl.)

3. Cover and incubate at 37 °C in a 5 % CO_2 incubator for duration of the experiment.

4. Gently pipette the cell suspension in the well to resuspend adherent cells, combine the contents of five replicate wells together into a 500 μl Eppendorf tube, and centrifuge for 5 min at $300 \times g$.

5. Resuspend in 3 % glutaraldehyde in 0.1 M sodium cacodylate buffer, pH 7.3, for 2 h.

6. Centrifuge at $300 \times g$ for 5 min, and resuspend in 0.1 M cacodylate. Incubate for 10 min (repeat three times).

7. Postfix in 1 % osmium tetroxide in 0.1 M sodium cacodylate for 45 min.

8. Centrifuge for 5 min at $300 \times g$, and resuspend in 0.1 M cacodylate. Incubate for 10 min (repeat three times).

9. Dehydrate sequentially in 50, 70, 90, and 100 % normal-grade acetones (10 min each) and then for 10 min analar acetone (repeat twice).

10. Embed in araldite resin.

11. Cut 1 μm sections on Reichert OmU4 ultramicrotome and stain with toluidine blue.

12. Select appropriate areas for further study using a light microscope.

13. From those areas cut ultrathin (60 nm) sections and stain with uranyl acetate and lead citrate.

14. View section with a Philips CM120 transmission electron microscope.

3.3 Annexin V/
Propidium Iodide
Staining and Flow
Cytometric Analysis
of Apoptosis

Externalization of phosphatidylserine to the outer surface of the cell membrane is a key component in the apoptotic process, in particular allowing the recognition apoptotic cells by surrounding phagocytes. Annexin V (AnnV), in the presence of Ca^{2+}, binds phosphatidylserine, and when fluorescently conjugated (commonly AnnV-FITC) it can be used to identify apoptotic cells. Discrimination between viable, apoptotic, and necrotic cells is possible by using AnnV together with propidium iodide (PI) in a simple flow cytometry assay. PI, a nucleophilic dye, is excluded from cells with an intact cell membrane; however during necrosis when membrane integrity is lost PI enters the cell and binds nuclear material with a consequent increase in fluorescence.

1. Suspend eosinophils (of at least 97 % purity) at 4×10^6 cells/ml in IMDM supplemented with 10 % autologous serum and penicillin/streptomycin (1×) (*see* **Note 1**).

2. In a 96-Well flat-bottomed plate add 75 μl of cell suspension, 15 μl of apoptosis-modifying agents (10× concentration) or vehicle control, and 60 μl IMDM with 10 % autologous serum to each well. (NB: If two agents are used only 45 μl of IMDM is required for total volume of 150 μl.)

3. Cover and incubate at 37 °C in a 5 % CO_2 incubator for duration of the experiment.

4. Gently pipette the cell suspension in the well to resuspend adherent cells, and pipette 50 μl of the cell suspension into a flow tube with 250 μl AnnV buffer (*see* **Note 4**).

5. Incubate on ice for 5 min.

6. Add PI (1 μl of 1 mg/ml solution) to each sample immediately prior to running the sample on a flow cytometer.

7. Analyze on a flow cytometer using FL-1/FL-2 channel analysis. Viable cells are dual AnnV/PI negative; apoptotic cells are AnnV positive and PI negative; necrotic cells are dual AnnV/PI positive (Fig. 1b, d).

3.4 Measuring Mitochondrial Membrane Potential Using MitoCapture™

The formation of pores within the mitochondrial membrane that occurs during the intrinsic apoptotic process results in loss of mitochondrial membrane potential ($\Delta_{\Psi m}$) and facilitates the movement of proteins into the cytoplasm, in particular cytochrome c, with resultant caspase activation. Changes in the mitochondrial membrane potential of eosinophils can be measured using MitoCapture™, a cationic dye which in viable cells accumulates and polymerizes within mitochondria and fluoresces in the red (FL-2) channel—indicated by a fluorescence emission shift from green (535 nm) to red (590 nm). During apoptosis, when $\Delta_{\Psi m}$ is compromised, the dye remains monomeric within the cytoplasm and fluoresces in the green (FL-1) channel. This mitochondrial depolarization can be quantified by flow cytometry as an increase in FL-1 fluorescence (Fig. 2a) or by plate-based fluorometric assay as a decrease in the red/green fluorescence intensity ratio.

1. For each sample dilute 0.5 μl MitoCapture™ reagent in 500 μl pre-warmed (37 °C) MitoCapture™ Incubation Buffer in a 1.5 ml Eppendorf tube. (NB: This protocol relies on the use of a MitoCapture™ mitochondria permeability detection kit.)

2. Suspend eosinophils (at least 97 % purity) at 4×10^6 cells/ml in IMDM (10 % autologous serum).

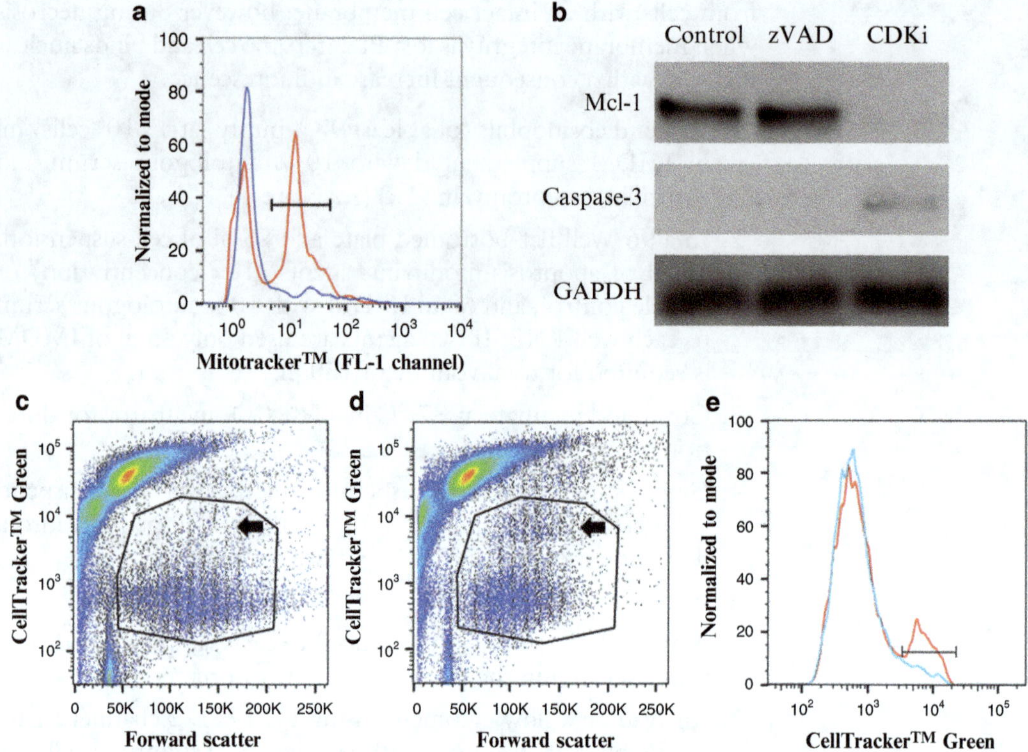

Fig. 2 Assessing intracellular events during apoptosis and phagocytic clearance of apoptotic cells. Loss of mitochondrial membrane potential due to increased membrane permeability during apoptosis is measured by increased fluorescence of Mitotracker™ dye. Representative histogram (**a**) of control (*blue*)- and dexamethasone (*red*)-treated eosinophils after 20-h in vitro culture—apoptotic cells indicated by gate. Changes in expression of intracellular regulators of apoptosis can be assessed by western blot (**b**). Caspase inhibitor zVAD delays apoptosis, maintains Mcl-1 expression, and prevents caspase-3 cleavage, while pro-apoptotic cyclin-dependent kinase inhibitors (CDKi) cause Mcl-1 downregulation and caspase-3 cleavage. Measurement of phagocytosis of apoptotic cells by monocyte-derived macrophages (gated) is demonstrated by increased CellTracker™-green fluorescence from phagocytosed apoptotic eosinophils by dexamethasone-treated macrophages (**d**) relative to control (**c**) (*black arrows*). Overlay histogram demonstrates population of macrophages containing apoptotic cells (**e**, gated)

3. In a 96-well flat-bottomed plate add 75 μl of cell suspension, 15 μl of apoptosis-modifying agents (10× concentration) or vehicle control, and 60 μl IMDM with 10 % autologous serum to each well. (NB: If two agents are used only 45 μl of IMDM is required for total volume of 150 μl.)

4. Cover and incubate at 37 °C in a 5 % CO_2 incubator for duration of the experiment.

5. Add 150 μl of cell suspension to 500 μl diluted MitoCapture™ reagent.

6. Incubate on shaking heat block at 37 °C, 300 rpm, for 15 min.

7. Centrifuge at $300 \times g$ for 5 min, and discard supernatant.

8. Resuspend cells in 300 µl MitoCapture™ Incubation Buffer.

9. Analyze using a flow cytometer with increased fluorescence in FL-1 channel indicating loss of $\Delta_{\psi m}$ and increased apoptosis.

3.5 Western Blotting for Caspases and Apoptotic Proteins

Caspases are essential throughout the apoptotic process in both the initiation and execution of the cell death process. The detection of the cleaved active forms of these proteins, or the disappearance of their inactive forms, alongside changes in expression of other pro- and anti-apoptotic proteins in response to extrinsic and intrinsic modulators of eosinophil life-span is possible through a variety of assays (Fig. 2b).

1. Suspend eosinophils (at least 97 % purity) at 4×10^6 cells/ml in IMDM (10 % autologous serum). Pipette 750 µl cells into a 2 ml Eppendorf tube and incubate with 150 µl apoptosis-modifying agents and 600 µl IMDM (10 % autologous serum). (NB: If two agents are used only 450 µl of IMDM is required for total volume of 1,500 µl.)

2. Incubate at 37 °C in a shaking heat block for the duration of the experiment.

3. Centrifuge the Eppendorf tube at $16,000 \times g$ for 1 min. Discard the supernatants.

4. Resuspend cell pellets in 90 µl protease inhibitor buffer and incubate on ice for 10 min (*see* **Note 2**).

5. Add 10 µl 10 % NP-40 (diluted in TBS), vortex thoroughly, and incubate for a further 10 min on ice.

6. Centrifuge at 13,000 rpm for 20 min at 4 °C, and transfer the protein-rich supernatant into a 500 µl Eppendorf tube. Freeze samples (−20 °C) until use.

7. Calculate protein concentration of each sample using BCA protein assay as per the manufacturer's instructions.

8. Transfer volume equivalent to 30 µg protein into fresh Eppendorf tubes and make up to total volume of 30 µl with PBS (without cations) and 8 µl of 4× sample buffer.

9. Heat at 95 °C for 5 min.

10. Load samples onto a 12 % polyacrylamide (or equivalent) gel including molecular weight standards. Run at 110 V until the dye front reaches the bottom of the gel.

11. Transfer proteins onto the PVDF membrane at 80 V for 1 h at 4 °C.

12. Wash the membrane in TBS/0.1 % Tween®20 for 5 min on a rocking platform.

13. Block the membrane for 1 h with 10 ml of 5 % dried milk powder in TBS/0.1 % Tween®20 at room temperature on a rocking platform.

14. Wash the membrane in TBS/0.1 % Tween®20 for 5 min (repeat three times).

15. Incubate with primary antibody overnight at 4 °C—concentrations as per Subheading 2.6, **item 13**—in TBS/0.1 % Tween®20 containing 5 % dried milk powder (5 ml).

16. Wash membrane in TBS/0.1 % Tween®20, each for 5 min (repeat three times).

17. Incubate with the corresponding secondary antibody diluted 1:2,500 in TBS/0.1 % Tween®20 containing 5 % dried milk powder (5 ml) for 2 h.

18. Wash membrane in TBS/0.1 % Tween®20 for 5 min (repeat three times).

19. Develop using enhanced chemiluminescence according to the manufacturer's instructions.

20. Strip and reprobe blot with β-actin or GAPDH as a loading control.

3.6 Fluorometric Homogeneous Caspase Assay

As discussed previously apoptosis is a caspase-dependent process; therefore assessment of caspase activity can be used as a marker of apoptotic cell death. Quantification of total caspase activity is possible using commercially available assays (homogeneous caspase assay), but their use is limited given the inability to discriminate between individual caspases. Cleavage of a fluorescently conjugated caspase substrate (e.g., VAD-fmk) to produce a fluorescent product (e.g., FITC, rhodamine 110) enables fluorescent intensity to be measured as a marker of total caspase activity.

1. These instructions are based on the use of Homogeneous Caspases Assay Kit.

2. Suspend eosinophils (at least 97 % purity) at 1×10^6 cells/ml in IMDM (10 % autologous serum).

3. In a black 96-well microplate load 100 μl of cell suspension (1×10^5 cells per well) with apoptosis-modifying agents and incubate at 37 °C for the duration of the experiment.

4. Dilute stock caspase substrate 1:10 in incubation buffer, and add 100 μl freshly prepared 1× caspase substrate to each well. Include negative and positive controls (media alone and cell lysate).

5. Incubate at 37 °C in the dark for at least 1 h.

6. Use a plate reader to measure fluorescence (excitation: 470–500 nm, emission: 500–560 nm).

3.7 Caspase Profiling Assay

Fluorometric assays for specific caspases are similar to the homogeneous assays described above but have a greater degree of specificity between the substrates of individual caspases or groups of caspases. Fluorescently conjugated substrates specific for certain caspases are immobilized in a 96-well plate. When cell lysates are added to the wells, the level of fluorescence emitted is an indicator of the activity of that particular caspase allowing delineation of specific pathways of the apoptotic process.

1. These instructions assume the use of the ApoAlert™ Caspase Profiling Plate.

2. Suspend eosinophils (at least 97 % purity) at 2×10^6 cells/ml in IMDM (10 % autologous serum). In 2 ml Eppendorf tubes pipette 1 ml of cell suspension (2×10^6 cells) and apoptosis-modifying agents and incubate at 37 °C for the desired length of time.

3. Centrifuge at $220 \times g$ for 5 min at 4 °C, and aspirate the supernatant.

4. Resuspend the cell pellet in 400 μl ice-cold 1× lysis buffer; incubate on ice for 10 min.

5. While cells are incubating add 10 μl DTT per 1 ml 2× reaction buffer, and then pipette 50 μl to each well of the 96-well caspase profiling plate.

6. Cover the plate and incubate for 5 min at 37 °C.

7. Vortex the cell lysate, and add 50 μl of lysate to duplicate wells of each caspase substrate.

8. Cover the plate and incubate for 2 h at 37 °C.

9. Use a plate reader to measure fluorescence (excitation: 380 nm, emission 460 nm).

3.8 Assessing Nuclear Changes During Apoptosis: Gel Electrophoresis of DNA

Activation of the apoptotic process results in endonuclease-mediated cleavage of DNA. After early large-scale degradation of DNA (50–200 kbp) endonuclease activity generates single-nucleosome or oligonucleosomal fragments of around 180 bp (or multiples thereof). This cleavage process creates discrete sized lengths of DNA which, when run through gel electrophoresis, produce a characteristic "laddering" effect that is distinct from the "smear" generated by the random DNA cleavage that occurs during cell necrosis.

1. Suspend eosinophils (at least 97 % purity) at 5×10^6 cells/ml in IMDM (10 % autologous serum). In 2 ml Eppendorf tubes pipette 1 ml of cell suspension (2×10^6 cells) and apoptosis-modifying agents and incubate at 37 °C for the desired length of time.

2. Extract genomic DNA using Wizard® Genomic DNA Purification Kit.

3. Run the DNA (23 μl DNA mixed with 7 μl loading dye) on a 2 % agarose gel containing GelRed (5 μl in 50 ml) in 1× TBE buffer at 110 V.

4. Run until the dye front reaches the end of the gel, and visualize the gel under ultraviolet illumination.

3.9 Hypodiploid DNA Content

Endonuclease-mediated cleavage of nuclear DNA during apoptosis causes an apparent decrease in DNA content of triton-permeabilized cells. Nuclear staining using propidium iodide allows detection of this "hypodiploid" cell population. This technique works well with eosinophils, as they are terminally differentiated and do not undergo proliferation meaning only two peaks are visible when DNA content is measured: diploid (viable) cells and hypodiploid (apoptotic) cells.

1. Suspend eosinophils (at least 97 % purity) at 4×10^6 cells/ml in IMDM (10 % autologous serum).

2. In a 96-well flat-bottomed plate add 75 μl of cell suspension, 15 μl of apoptosis-modifying agents (10× concentration) or vehicle control, and 60 μl IMDM with 10 % autologous serum to each well. (NB: If two agents are used only 45 μl of IMDM is required for total volume of 150 μl.)

3. Cover and incubate at 37 °C in a 5 % CO_2 incubator for the duration of the experiment.

4. Gently pipette the well to resuspend adherent cells, and add 50 μl to a flow tube containing 250 μl of PI solution.

5. Incubate in the dark at 4 °C for 15 min.

6. Analyze by flow cytometry (FL-2 channel) to determine the percentage of cells with hypodiploid DNA content.

3.10 TUNEL Staining for DNA Breaks

DNA cleavage can be measured enzymatically as DNA breaks create acceptor sites for enzymes such as terminal deoxyribonucle-otidyltransferase (TdT). TdT together with fluorescein-12-2′ deoxyuridine-5′-triphosphate is used to identify DNA fragmentation in terminal uridine nucleotide end-labelling (TUNEL) staining.

1. These instructions assume the use of In Situ Cell Death Detection Kit, Fluorescein.

2. Suspend eosinophils (at least 97 % purity) at 20×10^6 cells/ml in IMDM (10 % autologous serum).

3. To a 96-well flat-bottom plate add 90 μl of cell suspension and 10 μl of apoptosis-modifying agents (10× concentration) or vehicle control.

4. Cover and incubate at 37 °C in a 5 % CO_2 incubator for the duration of the experiment.

5. To a 96-well U-bottom flexible plate pipette 100 μl of cell suspension and centrifuge at $200 \times g$ for 2 min at 4 °C. Discard the supernatants.

6. Wash the cells three times adding 100 μl PBS per well. Spin the plate at $200 \times g$ for 3 min at 4 °C, discarding the supernatants, and vortex for 5 s.

7. Add 100 μl of fixation solution to each well.

8. Incubate on a shaking heat block for 60 min at 300 rpm at room temperature.

9. Add 200 µl PBS to each well, then spin the plate at $200 \times g$ for 10 min at 4 °C, and discard the supernatant.

10. Resuspend the cells in permeabilization solution and incubate for 2 min on ice.

11. Add 50 µl of nucleotide mixture to two negative control wells.

12. Make the TUNEL reaction mixture by adding the enzyme solution (50 µl) to 450 µl nucleotide mixture.

13. Treat the two positive control wells with DNase I for 10 min at room temperature to introduce DNA strand breaks.

14. Wash the plate twice in PBS (200 µl per well) and then resuspend in TUNEL reaction mixture (50 µl per well).

15. Cover the plate and incubate at 37 °C for 60 min.

16. Wash twice in PBS (200 µl per well), and then transfer to flow cytometry tubes for analysis of fluorescence levels (FL-1).

3.11 Assessing Phagocytic Uptake of Apoptotic Cells: Culture of Monocyte-Derived Macrophages

To assess macrophage phagocytosis of apoptotic eosinophils it is necessary to differentiate blood-derived monocytes into macrophages in in vitro culture. A variety of methods exist in order to, as closely as possible, recapitulate the phenotype of tissue macrophages. Isolation by adherence utilizes monocytes' ability to rapidly attach to tissue culture plastic in preference to neutrophils and lymphocytes. Washing off non-adherent cells after 1 h leaves a relatively homogenous cell population for subsequent culture (*see* **Note 5**).

1. Resuspend peripheral blood mononuclear cells at 4×10^6 cells/ml in IMDM without serum, add 500 µl/well in a 48-well plate, and incubate for 60 min at 37 °C.

2. Wash adherent cells 3–4 times with IMDM and incubate in 500 µl IMDM with 10 % autologous serum at 37 °C (*see* **Note 6**).

3. Culture monocytes for 5–7 days with media changed after day 3 in culture prior to use in subsequent experiments.

3.12 Flow Cytometry-Based Phagocytosis Assay

This assay uses a fluorescent chloromethyl dye that diffuses across cell membranes to label the cytoplasm of live eosinophils without altering their functional activity (Fig. 2c–e). Alone this is a valid method for assessment of phagocytic uptake of apoptotic cells; however CellTracker™-green can also be used alongside a pH-sensitive succinimidyl ester (pHrodo™) to allow definite discrimination of phagocytosis of apoptotic cells. pHrodo™ dyes are non-fluorescent at a neutral pH but fluoresce brightly in acidic conditions (i.e., within the phagolysosome); therefore macrophages display dual fluorescence upon phagocytosis of apoptotic CellTracker™-green-labelled eosinophils.

1. This method assumes the use of adherent monocyte-derived macrophages in Costar® 48-well TC-treated microplates.

2. Suspend eosinophils (at least 97 % purity) at 20×10^6 cells/ml in IMDM (10 % autologous serum) in a 15 ml Falcon® conical polypropylene tube. Add 2μg/ml of 10 mM CMFDA (CellTracker™ Green), pipette gently, and incubate at 37 °C for 30 min.

3. Centrifuge at $220 \times g$ for 5 min, wash cell pellet in PBS, and spin again at $220 \times g$ for 5 min.

4. Resuspend cells at 4×10^6 cells/ml in IMDM (10 % autologous serum). Transfer the eosinophil suspension into Costar® 75 cm² cell culture flask and incubate for 20 h at 37 °C (5 % CO_2).

5. Transfer the eosinophils into a 50 ml Falcon® conical polypropylene tube, wash twice in warm IMDM (50 ml volume per wash) ($220 \times g$ for 5 min), and discard the supernatant. Following each wash, resuspend the eosinophil pellet in 1 ml of warm IMDM to avoid cell clumping. Resuspend the aged eosinophils at 1×10^6 cells/ml in warm HBSS (37 °C).

6. Incubate cells with 20 ng/ml pHrodo™ (30 min, room temperature).

7. Centrifuge at $220 \times g$ for 5 min, wash cell pellet in PBS, and spin again at $220 \times g$ for 5 min.

8. Resuspend cells at 4×10^6/ml in warm IMDM (serum free).

9. Rinse the macrophages with warm IMDM to wash off non-adherent cells.

10. Pipette 500 μl (2×10^6 cells) of labelled aged eosinophils in IMDM (serum free) atop the macrophage monolayer. Incubate for 60 min at 37 °C in a 5 % CO_2 atmosphere. *NB: This is an excess number of apoptotic eosinophils in order to determine macrophage phagocytic capacity and not a surrogate marker of eosinophil apoptosis.*

11. Remove the eosinophil suspension from the plate, and wash macrophages with PBS three times.

12. Incubate the macrophages with 500 μl 0.25 % trypsin/1 mM ethylenediaminetetraacetic acid solution for 10 min at 37 °C followed by 10 min at 4 °C (*see* **Note 7**).

13. Collect the detached macrophages by pipetting vigorously and place in a flow cytometer tube on ice.

14. Analyze samples immediately by flow cytometry.

15. Apoptotic cells and macrophage populations are identified by their distinct forward and side scatter characteristics. By dividing the number of dual CellTracker/pHrodo-positive events in the macrophage gate by the total macrophage number the percentage of macrophages that have internalized apoptotic cells can be calculated.

4 Notes

1. Reference to autologous serum used in the culture of eosinophils denotes autologous plasma-derived serum. It is made by adding 20 mM $CaCl_2$ to platelet-rich plasma (harvested after centrifugation of citrate-anticoagulated blood) and incubated for 1 h at 37 °C in glass tubes. Alternatively, foetal calf serum can be used or eosinophils may be cultured without serum but with a small amount of supplemental protein (e.g., 0.5 % (w/v) serum albumin)—the latter will however accelerate the rate of apoptosis.

2. Eosinophil granules are rich in proteases; therefore, in order to prevent the protein of interest from being degraded, care should be taken to keep all samples on ice during the preparation of lysates. In addition higher protease inhibitor concentrations are necessary than for lysis of other cell types.

3. Supplemental serum can be added to cells in the cytospin chamber to prevent artefacts caused by cell breakage during centrifugation. This however reduces the effectiveness of visualizing secondary necrotic eosinophils, thereby underestimating the rate of eosinophil apoptosis. Secondary necrotic eosinophils appear as cell ghosts with little or no evidence of nuclear staining having undergone "nuclear evanescence," and as such they may, incorrectly, not be included in quantification of morphological changes.

4. Annexin binding buffer should always be used in the preparation of Annexin V as the absence of supplemental Ca^{2+} causes rapid dissociation of Annexin V from phosphatidylserine on the apoptotic cell surface.

5. Purification of monocytes from the mononuclear cell population by adherence is frequently used as described. Isolation is also possible using negative selection of contaminating lymphocytes and neutrophils with magnetic beads (Pan Monocyte Isolation Kit, Miltenyi Biotec, Surrey, UK) according to the manufacturer's instructions [15]. Caution should be taken using anti-CD16-negative selection to remove neutrophils as this may also remove CD16[hi] inflammatory monocytes. Isolated monocytes are plated out at 3×10^5/well in a 48-well plate.

6. Differentiation of monocytes in in vitro culture can also be performed by culturing a combination of IL-4, IL-6, and GM-CSF (as described in ref. 16).

7. Treatment with trypsin–EDTA may lead to clumping of cells leading to blockage of the flow cytometer's sample intake nozzle. Clumping may be minimized by adding 50 μl of bovine serum to each well following incubation with trypsin–EDTA.

Acknowledgements

The authors would like to acknowledge funding from the Wellcome Trust WT096497 (D.A.D.) and WT094415 (C.D.L.) and the Chief Scientist Office, ETM/86 (S.S., A.L.A).

Conflicts of interest: No conflicts of interest are declared.

References

1. Rosenberg HF, Dyer KD, Foster PS (2013) Eosinophils: changing perspectives in health and disease. Nat Rev Immunol 13:9–22

2. Leitch AE, Duffin R, Haslett C, Rossi AG (2008) Relevance of granulocyte apoptosis to resolution of inflammation at the respiratory mucosa. Mucosal Immunol 1:350–363

3. Farahi N, Singh NR, Heard S, Loutsios C, Summers C, Solanki CK, Solanki K, Balan KK, Ruparelia P, Peters AM, Condliffe AM, Chilvers ER (2012) Use of 111-Indium-labeled autologous eosinophils to establish the in vivo kinetics of human eosinophils in healthy subjects. Blood 120:4068–4071

4. Duffin R, Leitch AE, Sheldrake TA, Hallett JM, Meyer C, Fox S, Alessandri AL, Martin MC, Brady HJ, Teixeira MM, Dransfield I, Haslett C, Rossi AG (2009) The CDK inhibitor, R-roscovitine, promotes eosinophil apoptosis by down-regulation of Mcl-1. FEBS Lett 583:2540–2546

5. Park YM, Bochner BS (2010) Eosinophil survival and apoptosis in health and disease. Allergy Asthma Immunol Res 2:87–101

6. Tai PC, Sun L, Spry CJ (1991) Effects of IL-5, granulocyte/macrophage colony-stimulating factor (GM-CSF) and IL-3 on the survival of human blood eosinophils in vitro. Clin Exp Immunol 85:312–316

7. Robertson NM, Zangrilli JG, Steplewski A, Hastie A, Lindemeyer RG, Planeta MA, Smith MK, Innocent N, Musani A, Pascual R, Peters S, Litwack G (2002) Differential expression of TRAIL and TRAIL receptors in allergic asthmatics following segmental antigen challenge: evidence for a role of TRAIL in eosinophil survival. J Immunol 169:5986–5996

8. Wedi B, Wieczorek D, Stunkel T, Breuer K, Kapp A (2002) Staphylococcal exotoxins exert proinflammatory effects through inhibition of eosinophil apoptosis, increased surface antigen expression (CD11b, CD45, CD54, and CD69), and enhanced cytokine-activated oxidative burst, thereby triggering allergic inflammatory reactions. J Allergy Clin Immunol 109:477–484

9. Akakura S, Singh S, Spataro M, Akakura R, Kim JI, Albert ML, Birge RB (2004) The opsonin MFG-E8 is a ligand for the alphav-beta5 integrin and triggers DOCK180-dependent Rac1 activation for the phagocytosis of apoptotic cells. Exp Cell Res 292:403–416

10. Ravichandran KS (2010) Find-me and eat-me signals in apoptotic cell clearance: progress and conundrums. J Exp Med 207:1807–1817

11. Walsh GM, Sexton DW, Blaylock MG, Convery CM (1999) Resting and cytokine-stimulated human small airway epithelial cells recognize and engulf apoptotic eosinophils. Blood 94:2827–2835

12. Serhan CN, Savill J (2005) Resolution of inflammation: the beginning programs the end. Nat Immunol 6:1191–1197

13. Alessandri AL, Duffin R, Leitch AE, Lucas CD, Sheldrake TA, Dorward DA, Hirani N, Pinho V, de Sousa LP, Teixeira MM, Lyons JF,

Haslett C, Rossi AG (2011) Induction of eosinophil apoptosis by the cyclin-dependent kinase inhibitor AT7519 promotes the resolution of eosinophil-dominant allergic inflammation. PLoS One 6:e25683

14. Dorward DA, Lucas CD, Alessandri AL, Marwick JA, Rossi F, Dransfield I, Haslett C, Dhaliwal K, Rossi AG (2013) Technical advance: autofluorescence-based sorting: rapid and nonperturbing isolation of ultrapure neutrophils to determine cytokine production. J Leukoc Biol 94:193–202

15. Marwick JA, Dorward DA, Lucas CD, Jones KO, Sheldrake TA, Fox S, Ward C, Murray J, Brittan M, Hirani N, Duffin R, Dransfield I, Haslett C, Rossi AG (2013) Oxygen levels determine the ability of glucocorticoids to influence neutrophil survival in inflammatory environments. J Leukoc Biol 94(6):1285–1292. doi:10.1189/jlb.0912462

16. Chomarat P, Banchereau J, Davoust J, Palucka AK (2000) IL-6 switches the differentiation of monocytes from dendritic cells to macrophages. Nat Immunol 1:510–514

Chapter 17

Clinical Measurement of Eosinophil Numbers in Eosinophilic Conjunctivitis

Osmo Kari and K. Matti Saari

Abstract

Cytological examination of conjunctival scrapings is a valuable technique in differentiating various types of conjunctivitis. Brush conjunctival cytology is easy to use, and it may show a rich cell sample also from the deeper conjunctival layers. It is atraumatic and suitable for tarsal conjunctival cytology. The Papanicolaou staining can be used for examination of epithelial cells and inflammatory cells. The semiquantitative counting method is rapid to use and gives some information about the severity and nature of the inflammation. Our modified method identifies the presence of eosinophils which are the hallmark both in allergic conjunctivitis and in non-allergic eosinophilic conjunctivitis (NAEC). NAEC is quite common affecting in most cases middle-aged or older people with the majority being women. NAEC is often connected with dry eye which in many cases can be seen in conjunctival cytology.

Key words Conjunctivitis, Counting cell numbers, Dry eye, Eosinophils, Epithelium, Goblet cells, Inflammation, Inflammatory cells

1 Introduction

Eosinophils are active polymorphonuclear leucocytes seen in the conjunctiva in many viral and chlamydial infections as well as in allergic and autoimmune diseases, drug reactions, parasitic infections, some malignancies, metabolic disorders, and in hypereosinophilic syndrome. Eosinophils can be seen in mucous membranes of the conjunctiva, nose, lungs, and gastrointestinal tract. Conjunctival eosinophils are a good indicator of allergic conjunctivitis and the non-allergic eosinophilic conjunctivitis (NAEC) [1, 2]. However, the amount of eosinophils in conjunctival cytology is often sparse which requires some special conditions. For definition of NAEC (Fig. 1), the identification of eosinophils in conjunctival cytology is crucial. In allergic conjunctivitis there are also other inflammatory cells including neutrophils (Fig. 2).

In taking the cytological sample it is very important to obtain sufficient cells for reliable diagnosis. The sampling can be done by

Garry M. Walsh (ed.), *Eosinophils: Methods and Protocols*, Methods in Molecular Biology, vol. 1178, DOI 10.1007/978-1-4939-1016-8_17, © Springer Science+Business Media New York 2014

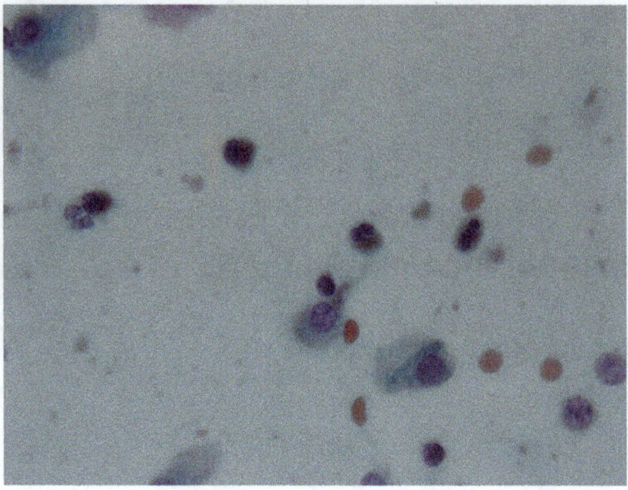

Fig. 1 Brush conjunctival cytology in non-allergic eosinophilic conjunctivitis

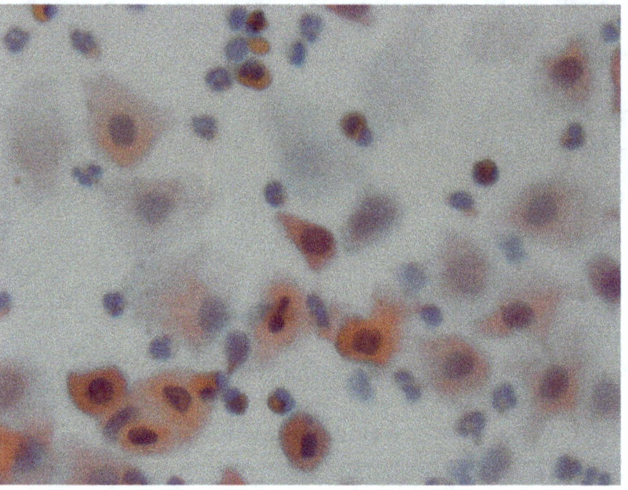

Fig. 2 Brush conjunctival cytology in eosinophilic allergic conjunctivitis

using a spatula [3, 4], cotton wool applicators [3], various plastic devices [5], cellulose acetate filter paper (impression cytology) [6], or brush cytology [7]. Brush cytology is a simple technique providing a good sample of intact cells. It is suitable also for immune histochemistry [8]. The brush cytology is easy to use, atraumatic, and suitable for most adult people. By using local anesthetic drops it can be used also for older children. Because of the small cell number it is good to take the sample both from the upper and lower lid conjunctiva of one or both eyes. In the case that it is not possible to get the sample from the upper lids it is recommended to take the sample from the conjunctiva of both lower lids. It is not recommended to take the sample from the bulbar conjunctiva.

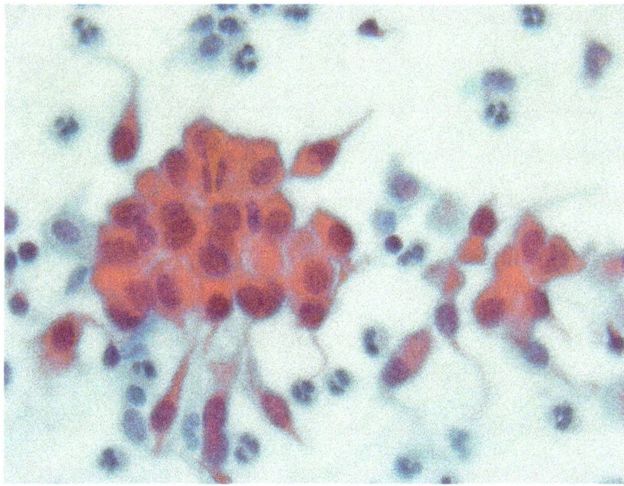

Fig. 3 Conjunctival eosinophils and epithelial metaplasia in chronic conjunctivitis with a dry eye

It is possible to use many staining methods including Wright–May-Grunwald–Giemsa, which stains inflammatory cells and eosinophils [1, 4]. In this staining technique the epithelial cells are not well visualized which makes it difficult to interpret the condition of epithelial cells. Papanicolaou staining is useful also for conjunctival cytology which provides a straightforward and easy-to-use method [9].

The counting of cells and their interpretation are demanding. We nowadays have many technical aids for it, but still the best method is a pure handwork. The small cell number of the specimen demands a careful examination of the whole sample which may be time consuming (*see* **Note 1**). The time-saving semiquantitative counting of cell numbers makes the grading easier [4]. Another reason for screening of the whole sample is if a small number of eosinophils are present (Fig. 3). But even a small number of eosinophils may be significant for the diagnosis of an allergic disease.

The epithelial cells are also active (Fig. 4). Their counting and interpretation help in differential diagnosis of dry eye (*see* **Note 2**).

Brush cytology is an easy and safe method, and it can be used both in private doctor's office and in the hospital. It is also cheap which makes it useful in developing countries. For training purpose it is good practice to evaluate the stained specimens and counting of cell numbers together with a pathologist (*see* **Note 3**). Later on also educated nurses may screen the samples before the doctor's interpretation. In most cases it is used only for the diagnosis of different prolonged conjunctival inflammation. However, it should be kept in mind that in occasional cases we can meet malignancies which demand experience in ocular pathology.

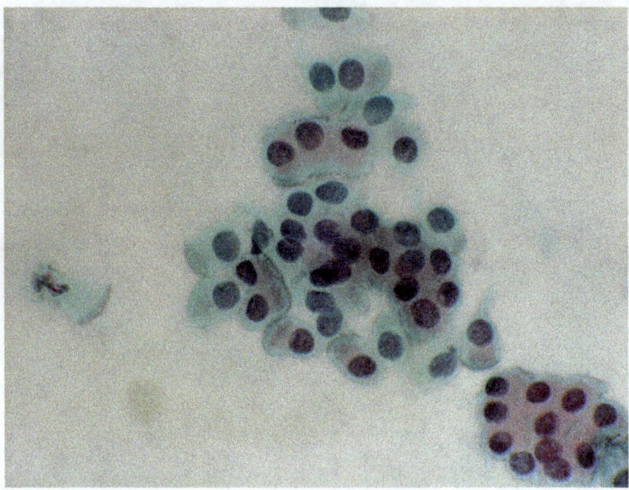

Fig. 4 Epithelial cells in conjunctival brush cytology specimen

2   Materials

2.1   Basic

1. Glass slides (with mat end).

2. Mark pen: Super Pap Pen, for marking the sample place on back side of the glass.

3. Pencil: To write the name, birthday, and the day of the specimen on the mat end of the glass. The name and specimen are on the top side of the glass.

4. Sample brush: Minitip flocked swab 501CS01 (Copan Italy Spa., Brescia, Italy).

5. Local anesthesicum drops (tetracaine or oxybuprocaine).

6. Ethyl alcohol 96 % for fixation.

7. Or fixation spray: For example, Cytofixx Cytology Fixative (CellPath Ltd, Powys, UK).

8. Cuvet: For alcohol fixation.

2.2   Reagents

1. Mayer's hematoxylin–Mayer hemalum solution.

2. OG-6 (orange, for keratin): Cell Bath RBA-4211-00A (Cell Bath Ltd, Newtown, Powys, UK).

3. EA-50—Cell Bath RBA-4212-00A (Cell Bath Ltd, Newtown, Powys, UK).

4. HCl-alcoholdiff.

   - 10 ml Pure HCl + 990 ml 96 % alcohol.

   - HCl.

   - Hydrochloric acid fuming 37 %.

   5. NH_3-alcoholdiff.
- 30 ml Strong ammonia + 970 ml 96 % alcohol.
- NH_3.
- Ammonia solution 25 %.

   6. Absolute ethanolum.

   7. Ethyl alcohol 96 %.

   8. Ethyl alcohol 80 %.
- 80 ml Absolute alcohol + 20 ml aqua.

   9. Ethyl alcohol 70 %.
- 70 ml Alcohol absolutum + 30 ml aqua.

10. Ethyl alcohol 50 %.
- 50 ml Alcohol absolutum + 50 ml aqua.

11. Xylene.

12. Pertex.

3 Methods

Sample brush, Minitip flocked swab 501CS01 (Copan Italy Spa., Brescia, Italy), is used for sampling. The sample is taken from the lower and upper lid tarsal and fornical conjunctiva pulling the brush from inner canthus to outer canthus and rotating it at the same time. It should be done two times to get sufficient cells. In adult persons it can be done in most cases without local anesthetic drop. When local anesthetic drops are used it often irritates the eye and increases lacrimation. If this occurs wait for a minute or two until it stops. Thereafter the specimen is spread on the object glass to marked places by rotating the brush several times to get all the cells. Note that the marking is on the other side of the glass than the specimen. Next the object glass is put for 10 min in 96 % ethyl alcohol or fixed with a special spray, Cytofixx Cytology Fixative (CellPath Ltd, Powys, UK).

After fixation the specimen can be stained at any time.

3.1 Staining

The specimen is fixed on the object glass in 96 % ethanolum for 10 min or with fixation spray.

Object glasses are stained using a modified Papanicolaou staining. Staining is regressive when the nucleus is overstained with hematoxylin, and the excess color is removed with HCl-alcoholdiff. The tint of nucleus is dyed blue and sharpened by using another NH_3-alcoholdiff. OG-6 and EA-50 are used as acid colors for staining the cytoplasm.

Modified Papanicolaou staining is done by using an automatic Dakon DRS machine.

3.2 Cell Counting

The specimen is examined under light microscope with 40× dry and 100× oil objective lenses. All the cells are counted [4]:

1–10 cells: +.

11–40 cells: ++.

41–60 cells: +++.

>60 cells: ++++.

4 Notes

1. All inflammatory cells are counted. Special attention is paid to eosinophils. Often the eosinophils are very sparse, and therefore it is important to examine the whole glass.

2. Papanicolaou staining is good also for the epithelium. Also the epithelial cells, squamous and columnar epithelial cells and mucus-producing goblet cells, are counted. The morphology of epithelial cells is important because of the common dry eye syndrome which is often connected to NAEC. The number of mucus-producing goblet cells gives also some indication for the presence of dry eye.

3. Sometimes the microscopic examination may show mucus in abundance which may be a sign of broken goblet cells.

References

1. Kari O, Haahtela T (1992) Conjunctival eosinophilia in atopic and non-atopic external eye symptoms. Acta Ophthalmol Scand 70:335–340
2. Kari O, Haahtela T, Laine P et al (2010) Cellular characteristics of non-allergic eosinophilic conjunctivitis. Acta Ophthalmol Scand 88:245–250
3. Norn MS (1960) Cytology of conjunctival fluid. Acta Ophthalmol, Suppl., Munksgaard, Copenhagen
4. Kari O (1988) Atopic conjunctivitis. A cytologic examination. Acta Ophtalmol Scand 66:381–386
5. Thatcher RW, Darougar S, Jones BR (1977) Conjunctival impression cytology. Arch Ophtalmol 95:678–681
6. Nelson JD, Havener VR, Cameron JD (1983) Cellulose acetate impression of the ocular surface in dry eye states. Arch Ophthalmol 101:1869–1872
7. Tsubota K, Takamura E, Hasegawa T et al (1991) Detection by brush cytology of mast cells and eosinophils in allergic and vernal conjunctivitis. Cornea 10:525–531
8. Kari O, Määttä M, Tervahartiala T et al (2009) Tear fluid concentration of mmp-8 is elevated in non-allergic eosinophilic conjunctivitis and correlates with conjunctival inflammatory cell infiltration. Graefes Arch Clin Exp Ophthalmol 247:681–686
9. Peuravuori H, Kari O, Peltonen S et al (2004) Group IIA phospholipase A2 content of tears in patients with atopic blepharoconjunctivitis. GraefesArch Clin Exp Ophthalmol 242:986–989

Chapter 18

Qualitative and Quantitative Studies of Eosinophils in Parasitic Infections

Masataka Korenaga and Fabrizio Bruschi

Abstract

Th2 responses such as peripheral and tissue eosinophilia are characteristic features in the host animals infected with *Strongyloides venezuelensis* and *Trichinella spiralis*. Th2 responses are characterized by a specific profile of cytokines and chemokines induced during the course of infection. In this chapter, we describe the methodology that is utilized in our laboratories to study the production of cytokine, chemokine, and antibodies related to the eosinophilia seen in mice infected with the parasites. Furthermore, protocols are described for the different methods used to study eosinophil functions in the blood and tissues of these experimental models of parasitic infections.

Key words *Strongyloides venezuelensis*, *Trichinella spiralis*, Eosinophils, CCL11/eotaxin-1

1 Introduction

Chemokines are derived from heterogeneous sources and serve to direct leukocytes to sites of inflammation. Eosinophilia is strongly linked with parasitic infections. Eotaxin is a fundamental regulator of eosinophil trafficking during both healthy status and inflammation. Expression of CCL11/eotaxin-1 and CCL24/eotaxin-2 in various tissues correlates with the number of eosinophils infiltrating inflammatory tissues. During infection with *T. spiralis*, CCL11/eotaxin-1 is important in intestinal tissue eosinophilia but not in peripheral eosinophilia, while CCL24/eotaxin-2 is only induced in the infected intestine [1]. Increased levels of CCL11/eotaxin-1 have been observed in the sera of patients with *Strongyloides stercoralis* when compared to healthy donors [2]. Eosinophils have been suggested as effector cells for innate immunity to *S. stercoralis* larvae [3] and for adaptive immunity to *S. venezuelensis* [4] and *Strongyloides ratti* [5]. However, the precise role and function of eosinophils still remain uncertain during the course of parasitic helminth infections [6, 7]. We describe here parasitological and immunological methodologies for studying the role of eosinophils in parasitic infections.

Garry M. Walsh (ed.), *Eosinophils: Methods and Protocols*, Methods in Molecular Biology, vol. 1178,
DOI 10.1007/978-1-4939-1016-8_18, © Springer Science+Business Media New York 2014

2   Materials

2.1 Serial Passage and Experimental Infection of Parasites and Antigen Preparation

1. Filter paper (30 × 30 cm, No. 50).

2. 250 µL Glass syringes with a 27G needle (Ishizawa Manufacturing Co., Ltd., Ibaraki, Japan).

3. Penicillin G potassium (10^5 units/mL) and streptomycin sulfate (100 mg/mL, were diluted in sterile saline, aliquoted, and stored at –20 °C.

4. Phosphate-buffered saline (PBS): 9.6 g of the powder containing 8,000 mg sodium chloride, 200 mg potassium chloride, 1,150 mg disodium phosphate (anhydrous), and 200 mg monopotassium phosphate (anhydrous) dissolved in 1 L distilled water; sterilize by autoclaving.

5. A testing sieve (JIS Z8801, aperture 75 µm, wire diameter 52 µm, Iida Manufacturing Co., Ltd. Osaka, Japan).

2.2 Collection of Samples

1. Teflon feeding tube (1.2 × 50 mm), Fuchigami Kiki, Kyoto, Japan.

2. Homogenizer, sonicator, standard centrifuge.

3. TRIzole.

4. Zirconia ball (5 mm in diameter, Asone Corporation, Osaka, Japan).

5. Carnoy's fixative: Ethanol (6 vol.), chloroform (3 vol.), acetic acid (1 vol.).

2.3 Cytospin, Cell Culture, ELISPOT, ELISA, PCR, and Histology

1. Diff-Quik.

2. Hinkelman's solution: 0.5 % w/v Eosin Y, 0.5 % w/v phenol, and 0.185 % v/v formaldehyde in distilled water.

3. Cytocentrifuge.

4. Cell strainer (40 µm Nylon): 48- or 96-well cell culture plate.

5. Cell culture medium: RPMI-1640 medium supplemented with 2 mM L-glutamine, 5 % heat-inactivated fetal bovine serum (FBS), 0.1 mM sodium pyruvate, 100 IU/mL penicillin, 100 µg/mL streptomycin, 15 mM 2-[4-(2-hydroxyethyl)-1-piperazinyl] ethane sulfonic acid (HEPES), and 0.05 mM 2-mercaptoethanol.

6. RPMI-1640 containing 2 % FBS and 30 mg/L DNase I.

7. Tris (2.05 g/L)-buffered ammonium chloride (7.5 g/L).

8. ELISPOT assay multiscreen HA nitrocellulose filter-based 96-well plate (Merck Millipore, Billerica, MA, USA). Capture antibody: 10 µg/mL anti-mouse CCL11/eotaxin (affinity-purified goat IgG). Detection antibody: dilute appropriately anti-mouse CCL11/eotaxin (biotinylated affinity-purified goat IgG).

9. ELISPOT Color-development reagent: Dissolve 8 mg of 4-chloro-1-naphthol in 1 mL of ethanol. Add 20 mL of 50 mM Tris/HCl (pH 7.5). Filter the solution to remove debris. Add 7 μL of 30 % H_2O_2 just before use.

10. Takara PrimerScript RT regent kit (Takara Bio Inc., Shiga, Japan).

11. SYBER Green (FastStart Universal Probe Master (ROX), Roche-Diagnostics, Tokyo, Japan).

12. MixerMill, thermal cycler (PCR system 9700) and Genetic analyzer.

13. The primer set of CCL11/eotaxin-1 and β-actin: CCL11/eotaxin-1: Upper primer; 5′ GGC TTC ATG TAG TTC CAG AT 3′, lower primer; 5′ TTC CTC AAT AAT CCC ACA TC 3′. β-Actin: Upper primer; 5′ AGC ACC ATG AAG ATC AAG 3′, lower primer; 5′ GTA AAA CGC AGC TCA GTA A 3′.

14. ELISA plate: 96-Well plates.

15. PBS/T: PBS containing 0.05 % Tween 20.

16. IgG1 conjugated to peroxidase.

17. TMB: 3,3′, 5,5′-Tetramethylbenzidine liquid substrate system.

18. PD-10 column (Amersham Biosciences Europe, Freiburg, Germany).

19. Water-soluble biotin N-hydroxysuccinimide ester.

20. Murine total IgE ELISA (Alpha Diagnostic, San Antonio, TX).

21. Avidin-peroxidase.

22. Orthophenylenediamine.

23. H_2O_2 (Sigma Aldrich).

24. 0.5 % Alcoholic Congo red solution of Highman.

25. Wright–Giemsa stain.

3 Methods

3.1 Faecal Culture and Inoculation of S. venezuelensis

1. A strain of *S. venezuelensis* has been maintained by serial passage in 7–19-week-old male Wistar rats infected with 40,000 filariform larvae (L3) every 2 weeks. C57BL/6 or BALB/c male mice were infected subcutaneously with 1,000 L3 4 weeks before a challenge infection with the same dose.

2. Collect faeces from cages of rats which were infected with the parasites 6–8 days ago.

3. Spread paste of rat faeces on a sheet of filter paper (7.5 × 30 cm). Fold the sheet of filter paper and place in a 500 mL beaker containing 150 mL of tap water (*see* **Note 1**). Cover the top of beaker with aluminum foil (Fig. 1).

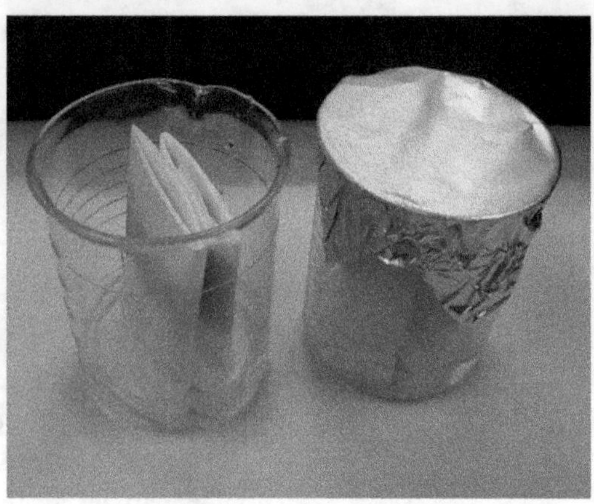

Fig. 1 Faecal culture of *Strongyloides venezuelensis* using a filter paper

4. Incubate the faecal culture at 26–27 °C for 5–7 days.

5. Discard the filter paper, and collect the tap water containing L3. Filtrate debris through double-gauze clothes.

6. Decant and wash with saline. Repeat several times.

7. After washings, add 0.5 mL of conc. penicillin and streptomycin into the decanter. Keep it for at least 60 min and more.

8. Decant and wash with sterile saline.

9. Count the number of L3 in 10 µL of the suspension. Adjust the suspension to 1,000 L3/200 µL.

10. Anesthetize mice with diethyl ether and/or Nembutal, if necessary; shave skin on the trunk region of the mice 1 day before an inoculation. Subcutaneously inoculate 200 µL of the suspension using a glass syringe attached with a needle.

3.2 Experimental Infection with *T. spiralis*

1. A strain of *T. spiralis* has been maintained by serial passage in 7-week-old ddY or CD1 (outbred) mice. Mice are infected orally with 400 muscle larvae.

2. Sacrifice mice with diethyl ether.

3. Eviscerate and cut mouse carcasses into small pieces.

4. Digest them for 1 h for infection or overnight for counting muscle worm burden at 37 °C in a pepsin–HCl digestion fluid, using a magnetic stirrer (*see* **Note 2**).

5. Pour and pass digested carcasses through double-gauze clothes into a 500 mL beaker.

6. Pour the fluid through the testing sieve.

7. Wash the muscle larvae on the sieve with running tap water.

8. Pour the muscle larvae into a funnel on a 50 mL graduated cylinder, and then fill with saline to the top of the cylinder.

9. Decant.

10. Wash and decant with saline.

11. Transfer suspension of muscle larvae to a 20 mL glass vial.

12. Count and adjust the number of larvae.

13. Make aliquots containing 400 muscle larvae per 200 µL of saline in Eppendorf tube (*see* **Note 3**).

14. Inoculate the larvae to mice orally using a feeding tube attached with a tuberculin syringe (*see* **Note 4**).

3.3 Parasite Somatic Crude Antigens

1. Homogenize *S. venezuelensis* L3 or *T. spiralis* muscle larvae using a high-speed homogenizer.

2. Sonicate the homogenate on ice.

3. Centrifuge the suspension at $435,000 \times g$ (100,000 rpm) for 10 min, 4 °C by ultracentrifuge.

4. Measure the protein concentration of the supernatantusing Bio-Rad protein assay.

5. Make aliquots, and store them at −30 °C until use.

3.4 Collection of Samples

1. At given days, sacrifice mice to collect tissues and organs.

2. Anesthetize mice with diethyl ether, take each 5 µL of blood to put into 20 µL of Hinkelman's solution, and count the number of eosinophils in peripheral blood using an improved Neubauer hemocytometer.

3. After sacrifice, to collect sera, make an incision on the inguinal skin to cut the femoral artery and vein to collect blood into Eppendorf tubes. Collect sera after clotting.

4. After sacrifice, to collect bronchus alveolar lavage fluid (BALF), make an incision on the neck to expose the trachea. Put a cotton ligature under the trachea, and make a 0.5–1 mm long incision vertically on the trachea. Insert Teflon feeding tube (*see* **Note 5**) attached with a tuberculin syringe filled with 1 mL of cold PBS. If necessary, use PBS containing 1 % bovine serum albumin (BSA) or normal mouse serum. Tighten the ligature beneath the incision to secure the tubing. Slowly push and pull the piston of the syringe, making sure that both lungs are filled with PBS. BALF should be kept on ice.

5. For RT-PCR, collect a piece of tissues of the lungs, small intestine, spleen, lymph nodes, and skin into a 2 mL screw-capped tube containing cold 0.5–1 mL of TRIzole with a zirconia ball.

6. For pathology, keep the tissues in 5 % buffered formalin until use. When mucosal mast cells are to be examined, tissues are fixed with Carnoy's fixative overnight and processed.

7. After sacrifice, remove the femoral bone, and flush out the bone marrows into an Eppendorf tube using a tuberculin syringe with 25G needle containing 1 mL of cold PBS.

3.5 Cytospin

1. Count the number of cells in cell suspension from BALF, bone marrow washings, etc.

2. Centrifuge cell suspension at $400 \times g$ for 10 min. Keep the supernatant at $-80\ ^\circ C$.

3. Adjust cell suspension at 1×10^6 cells/mL with 30 % normal mouse serum (*see* **Note 6**) in PBS.

4. Apply 100 µL of the suspension to a cytospin apparatus attaching slide glass.

5. Centrifuge at 650 rpm for 3 min.

6. Fix and stain cytospin specimens with Diff-Quik.

3.6 Cell Culture

1. After sacrifice, remove aseptically the spleen, mesenteric lymph nodes, etc. from mice.

2. Squeeze the tissues through a cell strainer with the plunger of a plastic syringe.

3. Rinse with 15 mL of RPMI-1640 containing 2 % FBS and 30 mg/L DNase I.

4. Allow the debris to settle.

5. Transfer cell suspension to a 15 mL tube.

6. Centrifuge $400 \times g$ for 10 min.

7. Resuspend in 2 mL of Tris/ammonium chloride for 2 min on ice to lyse erythrocytes.

8. Wash twice.

9. Resuspend in culture medium.

10. Count the number of cells using 0.1 % trypan blue solution.

11. Adjust cell suspension to 5×10^6 cells/mL (depending on the desired experiment).

12. Apply cells to 96- or 24-well flat-bottom culture plate.

13. Add antigen or supplements (depending on the desired experiment).

14. Incubate the culture plate for 48 h at 37 $^\circ C$ in a CO_2 incubator.

15. Centrifuge the plate at $400 \times g$ for 10 min to obtain supernatant.

16. Store the supernatant at $-80\ ^\circ C$ until use.

3.7 ELISPOT Assay

1. Coat each well of a multiscreen HA nitrocellulose filter-based 96-well plate with 50 µL of capture antibody and incubate at 4 $^\circ C$ overnight.

2. Wash three times with PBS.

3. Block each well with 250 µL RPMI-1640 containing 1% BSA at room temperature for 3 h or at 37 $^\circ C$ for 1 h.

4. Wash with RPMI-1640.

5. Seed cells at concentrations of 10^3, 10^4, and 10^5 cells/well in 100 µL of culture medium.

6. Culture at 37 °C for 2–6 h in a CO_2 incubator.

7. Wash three times with PBS, and wash once with PBS-T.

8. Apply 50 µL/well of detection antibody at 37 °C for 1 h.

9. Wash three times with PBS-T.

10. Apply 50 µL/well of HRP–streptavidin.

11. Wash three times with PBS-T.

12. Apply 150 µL/well of color-development reagent, and incubate at room temperature for 200 µL/well of 10–60 min in the dark.

13. Wash three times with DW.

14. Dry completely.

15. Count the spots using a dissecting microscope.

3.8 RNA Extraction, cDNA Synthesis, and Real-Time Quantitative PCR

1. Extract the total RNA from the lung or any tissues using TRIzole reagent.

2. Put a small piece (less than 50 mg) of the lung tissue into 0.5 mL TRIzole in a 2 mL tube containing a zirconia ball.

3. Shake vigorously the tube using MixerMill (30 cycles/s for 2 min).

4. After cell destruction, store the samples in a deep freezer (−80 °C) until use.

5. Extract RNA followed by the manufacturer's protocol (Invitrogen™).

6. Reverse-transcribe RNA samples (500 ng) to cDNA using Takara PrimerScript RT regent kit. Amplification conditions: 37 °C for 15 min, 85 °C for 5 s, and then 4 °C using a thermal cycler.

7. Perform real-time quantitative PCR (qPCR) in a 25 µL volume using SYBER Green. Amplification conditions: 50 °C for 2 min, 95 °C for 10 min, and 40 cycles of 95 °C for 15 s and 63 °C for 1 min using a genetic analyzer.

8. Calculate the fold changes in mRNA expressions for targeted genes which are relative to the respective vehicle groups of mice after normalization to β-actin using $\Delta\Delta$ Ct method.

3.9 ELISA for Parasite-Specific IgG

1. To detect parasite-specific IgG1 antibody, coat each well of a 96-well plate with 100 µL of the parasite somatic antigen solution (*see* **Note** 7) at 4 °C overnight.

2. Wash four times with PBS/Tween 20.

3. Block with 100 µL/well of 1 % BSA in PBS at 37 °C for 1 h.

4. Wash with PBS/Tween 20.

5. Apply serum samples at 1:10 dilution.

6. Incubate at 37 °C for 1 h.

7. Wash four times with PBS/Tween 20.

8. Apply 100 μL/well of goat anti-mouse IgG1 conjugated to peroxidase at a 1:4,000 (v/v) dilution (*see* **Note 8**).

9. Incubate at 37 °C for 1 h.

10. Wash four times with PBS/Tween 20.

11. Apply 100 μL/well of TMB to the wells. The plate should be kept in the dark during the reaction.

12. Add 100 μL/well of 0.5 M H_2SO_4 to stop the reaction.

13. Read absorbance values using a spectrophotometer at 450 nm.

3.10 Trichinella Spiralis Excretory/ Secretory Preparation and Biotinylation

T. spiralis excretory/secretory (Ts E/S) antigen preparation and biotin labeling are performed according to Del Prete et al. [8], following the following steps:

1. Culture *T. spiralis* muscle larvae, obtained as described above, in RPMI-1640 medium containing streptomycin (500 μg/mL) at 37 °C in a 5 % CO_2 atmosphere.

2. After 18 h, collect the supernatant and desalt it into the appropriate buffer with a PD-10 column.

3. The TsE/S antigen protein concentration is estimated by means of absorbance at 280 nm using a spectrophotometer.

4. Incubate TsE/S antigen (4 mg/mL) in sodium bicarbonate buffer, pH 8.5, with water-soluble biotin *N*-hydroxysuccinimide ester for 2 h at room temperature.

5. Add glycine (10 mg) to stop the reaction, and dialyze extensively biotinylated TsE/S antigen against PBS.

3.11 Measurement of Total and Ts E/S-Specific IgE in Plasma or Serum

Total mouse IgE levels in the plasma or serum are assessed by using a specific ELISA according to the manufacturer's instruction. Ts E/S-specific IgE in plasma or serum samples is determined by means of a modification of the ELISA assay for total IgE:

1. Seed plasma samples diluted 1:2 in PBS in the microplates coated with the anti-mouse IgE derived from the commercial kit for total IgE assay (0.1 mL/well), and incubate it for 4 h at room temperature.

2. Wash microplates with PBS–0.05 % Tween 20.

3. Add biotinylated Ts E/S antigen (10 μg/mL).

4. Keep plates for 4 h at room temperature.

5. Wash microplates with PBS–0.05 % Tween 20.

6. Add avidin-peroxidase to each well.

7. Incubate with orthophenylenediamine for 30 min with H_2O_2; the plate should be kept in the dark during the reaction.

8. Stop the reaction with H_2SO_4.

9. Read OD at 490 nm by a microplate spectrophotometer.

3.12 Histochemical Identification of Eosinophils

Tissue sections are stained with hematoxylin/eosin/azure II which stains eosinophils pink [9] or with 0.5 % alcoholic Congo red solution of Highman or modified Luna's methodology which stains eosinophils orange [10–12]. Wright–Giemsa stain can also be used in some cases [13] to identify all granulocytes (Fig. 2).

1. Collect a sample of tongue or diaphragm at 42 days postinfection with *T. spiralis* from each sacrificed animal, and process them for routine histology of formalin-fixed paraffin-embedded tissues.

2. From each animal cut 5 μm sections of the tongue at different depths.

3. Mount the specimens on glass slides, and then after routine processing, stain with hematoxylin and eosin to evaluate total inflammation or with Congo red which is suitable for eosinophil counts.

4. Observe the slides by a microscope and acquire by a video camera. Image analysis system is accomplished using an appropriate software program (Adobe® Photoshop® CS3). Through software tools, the inflammatory infiltrate around the nurse cell–parasite complex is measured in pixels calculating the difference between the whole area of nurse cell–parasite complex plus surrounding inflammation and the area delimited by the collagen capsule. The inflammatory pixel value, analyzed for more than 300 larvae per experimental group on different sections, is then converted in μm^2 (50 μm^2 = 78,478.8 pixel) [14].

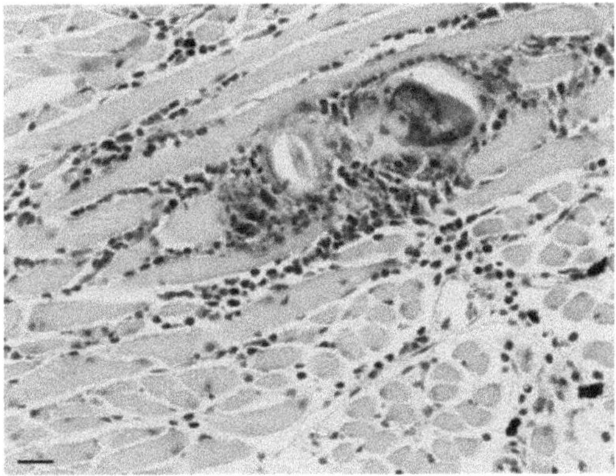

Fig. 2 Tongue tissue of mouse experimentally infected with *Trichinella spiralis* on day 21. Giemsa stain. Bar = 50 μm

3.13 Other Techniques for Blood Eosinophil Count in Rodents

1. Collect peripheral blood in Na-heparin tubes from the retro-orbital venous plexus in anaesthetised animals before infection and at different time points after infection.

2. Obtain blood smears and stain with May-Grünwald method to establish the percentage of eosinophils, and count total leukocytes in parallel by means of a Thoma's chamber or a cell counter after lysis of the erythrocytes with a hypotonic solution of NaCl [9].

3. Alternatively, dilute blood 1/2 with PBS containing 100 U/mL heparin. Dilute the mixture 1/10 in Discombe's fluid (0.05 % eosin Y), and count eosinophils directly in a hemocytometer [15].

3.14 Eosinophil Apoptosis Evaluation

1. Seed cells at a concentration of 1×10^6/mL in 48-well flat-bottom culture plates.

2. Incubate at 37 °C in a humidified atmosphere with 5 % CO_2.

3. Stain the smears obtained from these cells with May-Grünwald–Giemsa.

4. Count a number of apoptotic eosinophils in a total of 200 cells/slide under a light microscope at 1,000× magnification.

5. Use the following criteria to distinguish apoptotic from non-apoptotic cells: in both cases the cytoplasm granules are present. Normal eosinophils have ringlike nuclei, whereas those in apoptosis are smaller than normal and the nuclei are condensed basophilic with a round shape ([16] and Chapter 17).

4 Notes

1. Do not use deionized water.

2. Two hundred mL of 1 % pepsin in 1 % HCl solution per mouse: The solution can be stored in a freezer.

3. Use a yellow tip from which the tip end is cut.

4. Apply again 200 µL saline into the same syringe, and inoculate again. Sometimes the larvae remain inside the syringe.

5. The ball-ended tip of the tubing should be cut to an acute angle.

6. 5–10 % BSA can be used instead of serum to adhere cells to a glass slide.

7. Antigen solution is adjusted to 10 µg/mL in PBS containing 0.1 % normal goat IgG or BSA.

8. Checkerboard titration is necessary for every lot of antibody for appropriate dilution of sera and detection antibody.

References

1. Dixon H, Blanchard C, deSchoolmeester ML, Yuill NC, Christie JW, Rothenberg ME, Else KJ (2006) The role of Th2 cytokines, chemokines and parasite products in eosinophil recruitment to the gastrointestinal mucosa during helminth infection. Eur J Immunol 36:1753–1763

2. Mir A, Benahmed D, Igual R, Borras R, O'Connor JE, Moreno MJ, Rull S (2006) Eosinophil-selective mediators in human strongyloidiasis. Parasite Immunol 28:397–400

3. Galioto AM, Hess JA, Nolan TJ, Schad GA, Lee JJ, Abraham D (2006) Role of eosinophils and neutrophils in innate and adaptive protective immunity to larval *Strongyloides stercoralis* in mice. Infect Immun 74:5730–5738

4. Korenaga M, Hitoshi Y, Yamaguchi N, Sato Y, Takatsu K, Tada I (1991) The role of interleukin-5 in protective immunity to *Strongyloides venezuelensis* infection in mice. Immunology 72:502–507

5. Watanabe K, Sasaki O, Hamano S, Kishihara K, Nomoto K, Tada I, Aoki Y (2003) *Strongyloides ratti*: the role of interleukin-5 in protection against tissue migrating larvae and intestinal adult worms. J Helminth 77:355–361

6. Bruschi F, Korenaga M, Watanabe N (2008) Eosinophils and *Trichinella* infection: toxic for the parasite and the host? Trends Parasitol 24:462–467

7. Bruschi F, Korenaga M (2012) Eosinophils and eosinophilia in parasitic infections. In: Walsh GM (ed) Eosinophils – structure. Biological properties and role in disease. Nova Biomedical, New York, p 175

8. Del Prete G, Chiumiento L, Amedei A, Piazza M, D'Elios MM, Codolo G, De Bernard M, Masetti M, Bruschi F (2008) Immunosuppression of TH2 responses in *Trichinella spiralis* infection by *Helicobacter pylori* neutrophil-activating protein. J Allergy Clin Immunol 122:908–913

9. Beckstead JH, Halverson PS, Ries CA, Bainton DF (1981) Enzyme histochemistry and immunohistochemistry on biopsy specimens of pathologic human bone marrow. Blood 57:1088–1098

10. Grouls V, Helpap B (1981) Selective staining of eosinophils and the immature precursors in tissue sections and autoradiographs with Congo Red. Stain Technol 56:323–325

11. Tomasi VH, Pérez MA, Itoiz ME (2008) Modification of Luna's technique for staining eosinophils in the hamster check pouch. Biotech Histochem 83:147–151

12. Gentilini MV, Nuñez GG, Roux ME, Venturiello SM (2011) *Trichinella spiralis* infection rapidly induces lung inflammatory response: the lung as the site of helminthocytotoxic activity. Immunobiol 216:1054–1063

13. Friend DS, Gurish MF, Austen KF, Hunt J, Stevens RL (2000) Senescent jejunal mast cells and eosinophils in the mouse preferentially translocate to the spleen and draining lymph node, respectively, during the recovery phase of helminth infection. J Immunol 165:344–352

14. Chiumiento L, Del Prete G, Codolo G, De Bernard M, Amedei A, Della Bella C, Piazza M, D'Elios S, Caponi L, D'Elios MM, Bruschi F (2011) Stimulation of TH1 response by *Helicobacter pylori* neutrophil activating protein decreases the protective role of IgE and eosinophils in experimental trichinellosis. Int J Immunopathol Pharmacol 24:895–903

15. Gansmüller A, Anteunis A, Venturiello SM, Bruschi F, Binaghi RA (1987) Antibody-dependent in-vitro cytotoxicity of newborn *Trichinella spiralis* larvae: nature of the cells involved. Parasite Immunol 9:281–292

16. Gon S, Saito S, Takeda Y, Miyata H, Takatsu K, Sendo F (1997) Apoptosis and in vivo distribution and clearance of eosinophils in normal and *Trichinella spiralis*-infected rats. J Leukoc Biol 62:309–317

Chapter 19

Interactions of Eosinophils with Nerves

Quinn R. Roth-Carter, David B. Jacoby, and Zhenying Nie

Abstract

Coculture of eosinophils and nerves is a powerful tool in determining the interactions between the two cell types. We have developed methods for culture of parasympathetic ganglia and dorsal root ganglia from humans, and we have further refined the technique to coculture with eosinophils. Here we describe methods for coculturing primary parasympathetic ganglia or dorsal root ganglia with eosinophils.

Key words Eosinophil, Parasympathetic ganglia, Dorsal root ganglia, Coculture, Nerves, Primary cell culture

1 Introduction

Interactions between eosinophils and nerves play a key role in physiology and pathology of many diseases [1]. In fact, eosinophils can be found next to and in nerves in individuals with inflammatory diseases [2–4]. Nerves recruit eosinophils to tissue using chemotactic signals, such as eotaxin [5]. Also, nerves express adhesion molecules for eosinophils, allowing direct interaction between eosinophils and nerves in tissue [6]. Conversely, eosinophils modulate neuronal phenotype and function. Eosinophils can stimulate growth of sensory nerves [7], and major basic protein released from eosinophils inhibits neuronal M2 receptor function on parasympathetic nerve [8].

The basic protocol for primary culture of airway parasympathetic neurons was developed by Dr. Allison Fryer using guinea pigs [9] and has since been modified to allow culture of parasympathetic neurons from other species, including human. We have also successfully modified protocols for culturing adult mouse sensory nerves [10] to culture human dorsal root ganglia. Using coculture of parasympathetic ganglia and eosinophils we have found that binding of eosinophils to nerves is mediated by the expression of adhesion molecules on nerves and that binding of eosinophils to nerves can stimulate degranulation of eosinophils [11].

Garry M. Walsh (ed.), *Eosinophils: Methods and Protocols*, Methods in Molecular Biology, vol. 1178, DOI 10.1007/978-1-4939-1016-8_19, © Springer Science+Business Media New York 2014

By combining coculture of eosinophils and nerves with nerve modeling techniques, we have found that eosinophils can stimulate sensory nerve growth [7]. The following protocols are currently used in our lab.

2 Materials

2.1 Tools

Small surgical scissors (2) and forceps (2), autoclaved. Store at room temperature.

1. 10 ml Beakers (2).
2. Cotton-tipped applicator (3).
3. Sterile 75 cm² rectangular cell culture flask.
4. Tissue culture-treated culture Petri dishes (100 mm × 20 mm).
5. 100 mm Culture dish.
6. 50 ml Conical tube.
7. 4 Well Chamber Slides (Lab-Tek).
8. Hemocytometer.
9. Cell culture incubator (37 °C 95 % air and 5 % CO_2).
10. Capillary tubes.
11. Surgical tools: Scissors and forceps, autoclaved. Store at room temperature.
12. ImmEdge Pen (Vector Laboratories).

2.2 Reagents (See Note 1)

1. Matrigel: Thaw on ice at 4 °C fridge overnight. Aliquot into 0.5 ml aliquots using chilled pipettes and into chilled tubes. Store aliquots at –80 °C.
2. Sodium pentobarbital (Nembutal, 50 mg/ml).
3. Dulbecco's modified Eagle's medium (DMEM), with L-glutamine.
4. Ham's F12, with L-glutamine (F12).
5. 1× Hanks' balanced salt solution (HBSS) with calcium and magnesium.
6. Guinea pig transferrin 3.7 mg/ml (ICN Biomedicals 152154).
7. 100× Penicillin–streptomycin.
8. Wash buffer: Add 1 ml of 100× penicillin–streptomycin solution into 20 ml of sterile 1× HBSS. Do not filter.
9. Fetal bovine serum (FBS): Aliquot into 5 ml aliquots, and store at –80 °C.
10. 100× Stock L-glut in DMEM: Add 7.3 mg L-glutamine in 1 ml sterile water, add 49 ml DMEM, and filter sterilize. Aliquot into 2 ml aliquots, and store at –20 °C.

11. 0.05 % Collagenase: Weigh 5 mg collagenase powder (crude type XI cell culture, Sigma C9407) and add to 10 ml of 1× HBSS. Mix well, and filter sterilize. Add 100 μl of 100× penicillin–streptomycin solution, and keep at room temperature.

12. 2 % BSA: Add 500 mg bovine serum albumin into 25 ml of DMEM.

13. 5 % FBS in DMEM: Add 2.5 ml of FBS into 47.5 ml of DMEM. Mix well, and filter sterilize.

14. Preplate media (10 % FBS in DMEM/F12): Mix 50 % Ham's F12 and 50 % DMEM. Then add 5 ml of FBS into 45 ml of DMEM/F12, and mix well.

15. 2.5S nerve growth factor (NGF, 20 μg/ml): Add 200 μg of 2.5S NGF into 10 ml of 0.1% BSA in PBS. Store aliquots at –80 °C and thaw on ice before use.

16. 5 mM Cytosine arabinoside: Add 13.98 mg of cytosine arabinoside into 10 ml of DMEM, and mix well. Keep aliquots at –20 °C.

17. Insulin–transferrin–selenium (ITS) (Mediatech 25-800-CR).

18. Serum-free media (*see* **Note 2**): Combine the components in the following order: 470 ml DMEM, 25 ml 2 % BSA, 10 ml 100× insulin–transferrin–selenium (ITS), 3.92 ml guinea pig transferrin, and 495 ml Ham's F12. The media should be immediately aliquoted and frozen at –80 °C. Freeze–thaw cycles should be limited to two. Before use, aliquot should be thawed on ice and supplemented with penicillin–streptomycin, NGF, and cytosine arabinoside to final concentration as 1× penicillin–streptomycin, 100 ng/ml of NGF, and 1 μM of cytosine arabinoside.

19. DMEM/FBS: Add 5 ml FBS to 45 ml DMEM to make 10 % FBS in DMEM. Add 500 μl 100× pen/strep.

20. RNAse-free phosphate-buffered saline (PBS).

2.3 Coculture of Eosinophils and Nerve Cells

1. Serum-free media: Combine in the following order: 95 ml DMEM, 5 ml 2 % BSA in DMEM, 2 ml 100× stock L-glut in DMEM, 2 ml 100× ITS, and 100 ml F12 medium. Divide into 10 ml aliquots, and store at –80 °C.

2. Eosinophils isolated from peripheral blood from same species as prepared parasympathetic nerves.

2.4 Mouse Dorsal Root Ganglia Preparation

1. 0.05 % Collagenase in Hanks' buffered saline solution with calcium and magnesium (HBSS). Add 5 mg collagenase (crude type XI cell culture: Sigma) in 10 ml HBSS, and filter sterilize. Use immediately after making.

2. 0.25 % Trypsin.

3. Pen/strep 100×: Aliquot into 500 µl aliquots, and store at −20 °C.

4. Sodium Pentobarbital 50 mg/ml (Nembutal).

2.5 Coculture of Peripheral Sensory Nerves with Eosinophils and Analysis of Nerve Morphology

1. Serum-free media: Combine in the following order: 95 ml DMEM, 5 ml 2 % BSA in DMEM, 2 ml 100× stock L-glut in DMEM, 2 ml 100× ITS, and 100 ml F12 medium. Aliquot into 10 ml aliquots, and store at −80 °C.

2. Eosinophils isolated from peripheral blood from same species as prepared sensory nerves.

3. Zamboni's fixative (American Mastertech).

4. PBS.

5. Blocking buffer: Add 400 µl normal goat serum (NGS) to 3.6 ml PBS. Add 4 µl Triton X-100 to make 10 % NGS and 0.1 % Triton X-100 in PBS.

6. Primary antibody solution: Add 1 µl of rabbit anti-PGP antibody to 1 ml of blocking solution.

7. Secondary antibody solution: Add 2 µl of goat anti-rabbit Alexa Flour 488 to 1 ml of blocking solution. Keep in the dark.

8. Vectasheild Mounting Medium for Fluorescence With DAPI (Vector Laboratories).

9. Cytoseal 60 (Richard Allan Scientific).

10. 22×60-1.5 Microscope Cover Glass (Fisherbrand).

---

3   Methods

3.1 Culture of Guinea Pig Parasympathetic Nerves

3.1.1 Preparation of Tracheal Smooth Muscle Strips from Guinea Pigs

1. Euthanize guinea pig by i.p. injection of a lethal dose of sodium pentobarbital (Nembutol, 2.5 ml/kg).

2. Wipe the skin of the neck with 70 % ethanol, and make a midline incision in the skin from chin to chest with sterile small surgical scissors.

3. Expose trachea by separating surrounding muscles and connective tissue.

4. Remove trachea from below the larynx to the top of the bifurcating bronchi.

5. Rinse trachea in small beaker (10 ml) with sterile wash buffer.

6. All further steps should be done in a laminar flow hood using sterile technique.

7. Transfer the beaker with trachea in laminar flow hood, and place trachea into a sterile Petri dish containing wash buffer.

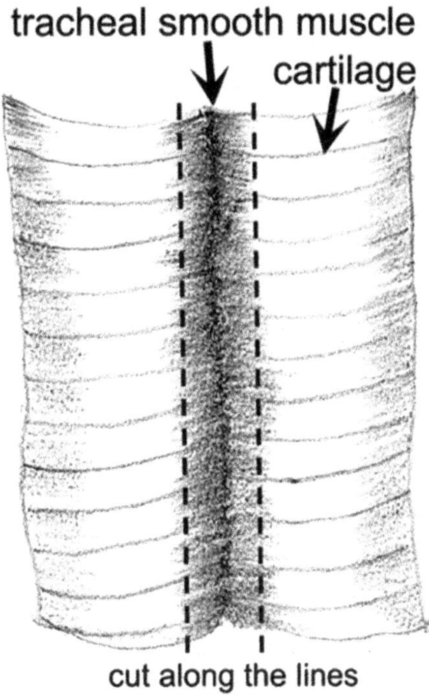

Fig. 1 Open trachea longitudinally, and remove most of the lateral portions of tracheal cartilage along the *dashed lines*, leaving a small fringe along each side of the tracheal muscle

8. Open trachea longitudinally to expose the lumen by cutting through cartilage rings with a new set of sterile small scissors and spread open so that the lumen side is face up.

9. Dip sterile cotton-tipped applicators in wash buffer, and use it to swab the lumen side of opened trachea to remove epithelial cells. Repeat three times.

10. Remove most of the lateral portions of tracheal cartilage (along the dashed line in Fig. 1), leaving a small fringe along each side of the tracheal muscle.

3.1.2 Digestion with Collagenase

1. Transfer the de-epithelialized tracheal muscle strip to a new small beaker (10 ml) with 0.5–1 ml of 0.05 % collagenase.

2. Chop and then mince the tracheal muscle strip into small homogenous pieces with scissors.

3. Transfer minced tissue into P25 tissue culture flask containing 5 ml collagenase (0.05 %) with 1× penicillin/streptomycin.

4. Incubate flask in water bath at 37 °C for 3–4 h with gentle agitation.

3.1.3 Preplate

1. Remove flask from water bath, and transfer contents to 50 ml conical centrifuge tube.

2. Inactive collagenase by adding equal volume of 5 % FBS in DMEM.

3. Centrifuge at $300 \times g$ for 10 min at room temperature.

4. Carefully remove supernatant with pipette; resuspend pellet in 5–10 ml preplate media, and centrifuge it again at $300 \times g$ for 10 min at room temperature.

5. Following the last wash, remove the supernatant carefully and resuspend cells with 4 ml of preplate media containing 1× penicillin/streptomycin.

6. Option: Small clumps of cells can be dispersed by 2–3 passages through a 20 gauge needle attached to a sterile syringe.

7. Plate cells on 100 mm × 10 mm polystyrene cell culture dish and incubate at 37 °C in 5 % CO_2 for at least 2 h and up to 18 h.

3.1.4 Coating Dishes/ Slides with Matrigel

1. Remove 0.5 ml aliquot of matrigel from –80 °C freezer and thaw on ice at 4 °C.

2. Dilute 0.5 ml matrigel aliquot with 8–12 ml 4 °C DMEM and mix thoroughly using precooled pipette.

3. Add 1 ml matrigel/DMEM per well of 6-well plate, and evenly distribute matrigel/DMEM to completely cover the bottom surface of each well.

4. Allow plate to sit at room temperature for 1 h or overnight at 4 °C.

5. Plate may either be used immediately or stored at 4 °C for up to 1 week.

6. When ready to use the plate(s), remove the excess liquid. Wash once with serum-free medium.

3.1.5 Plate Cells on Matrigel-Coated Wells

1. After 2 h of incubation, collect all nonadherent cells in the supernatant of polystyrene cell culture dish into 50 ml conical tube. Discard the dish, which contain fibroblasts, fragments of cartilage, and cellular debris that adhere to the bottom surface.

2. Centrifuge at $300 \times g$ for 10 min at room temperature.

3. Carefully aspirate supernatant, and resuspend pellet with serum-free media. Mix cell suspension thoroughly to resuspend cells.

4. Slowly remove DMEM from matrigel-coated wells, and quickly plate cells into the wells, being careful not to let the matrigel dry out.

5. Twenty-four hours after plating, remove no more than 80 % supernatant with pipette from each well and add serum-free media containing cytosine arabinoside (1.0 µM) to inhibit growth of any dividing cells. Continue to incubate cells at 37 °C for 72 h without changing media.

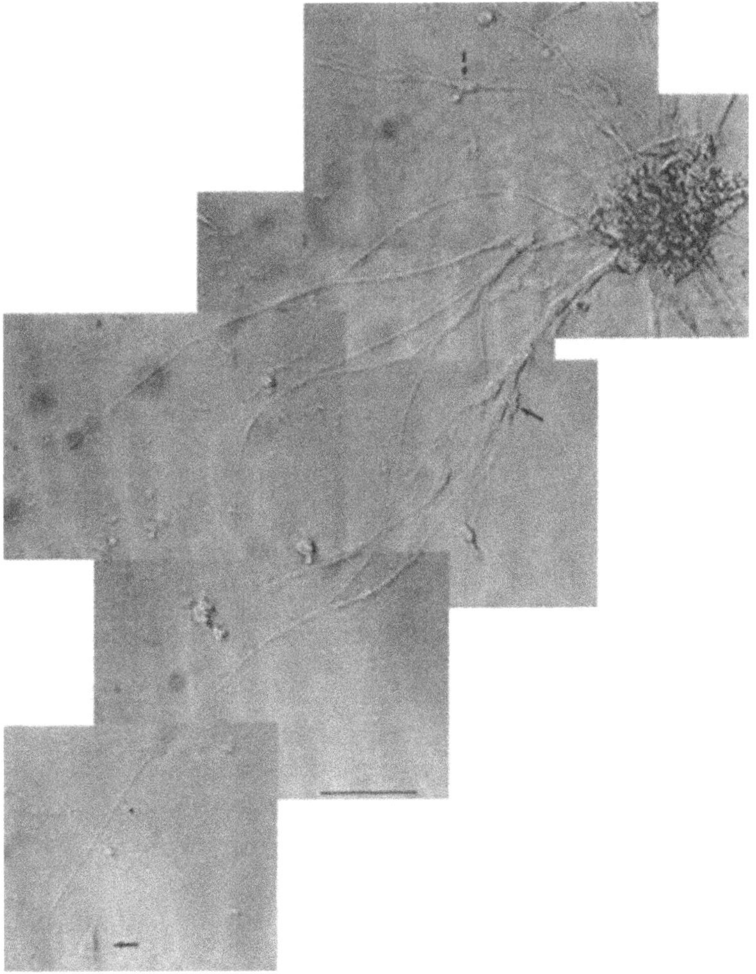

Fig. 2 Phase-contrast photomicrographs of nerve cells after 7 days in culture. A photomontage of a clump of nerve cells (*upper right*) with intertwining neuritis and cell bodies (examples of cell bodies shown by *thick arrows*) radiating outward (bar = 120 μM. There is one non-neuronal cell at the bottom of the photograph (*thin arrow*)

6. After treating with cytosine arabinoside, continue to culture cells with serum-free media at 37 °C in 5 % CO_2. Maintain the cell culture by replacing media every other day.

7. Cells are generally used for experiments in 7–10 days after plating (Fig. 2).

3.2 Culture of Human Parasympathetic Nerves

3.2.1 Preparation of Tracheal Smooth Muscle Strips from Human Trachea

1. Place the fragment of human trachea from the organ donor on a sterile Petri dish containing wash buffer in a laminar flow hood using sterile techniques.

2. Trim away the excess connective tissue outside the trachea, and cut off the smooth muscle longitudinally along the edge of cartilage.

3. Rinse the smooth muscle strip with wash buffer, and place it in a new Petri dish with the epithelial side face up.

4. Peel off the epithelium with small tweezers.

5. Transfer the de-epithelialized tracheal muscle strip to a new small beaker with 1–5 ml of 0.05 % collagenase.

6. Chop and then mince the tracheal muscle strip into small homogenous pieces with scissors.

7. Transfer minced tissue into tissue culture flask containing 25–50 ml collagenase (0.05 %) with 1× pen/strep/fungizone.

8. Incubate flask at 4 °C overnight, and then in water bath at 37 °C for at least 2 h on the next day, with gentle agitation.

9. Remove flask from water bath and inactive collagenase by adding equal volume 5 % FBS in DMEM.

10. Transfer the mixture to 50 ml conical centrifuge tubes and centrifuge at $300 \times g$ for 10 min at room temperature.

11. Carefully remove supernatant; resuspend pellet in 10–20 ml preplate media and centrifuge it again at $300 \times g$ for 10 min at room temperature.

12. Following the last wash, remove the supernatant carefully and resuspend cells with 10 ml of preplate media containing 1× pen/strep/fungizone.

13. Plate suspension on one or more 100 mm × 10 mm polystyrene cell culture dish and incubate at 37 °C in 5 % CO_2 for at least 4 h and up to 18 h.

3.2.2 Coating Dishes/ Slides with Matrigel (See Note 3)

1. Remove 0.5 ml aliquot of matrigel from −80 °C freezer and thaw on ice in fridge.

2. Dilute 0.5 ml matrigel aliquot with 8–12 ml 4 °C DMEM and mix thoroughly using precooled pipette.

3. Add 1 ml matrigel/DMEM per well of 6-well plate, and evenly distribute matrigel/DMEM to completely cover the bottom surface of each well.

4. Allow plate to sit at room temperature for 1 h or overnight at 4 °C.

5. Plate may either be used immediately or stored at 4 °C for up to 1 week.

6. When ready to use the plate(s), remove the excess liquid and wash once with serum-free media.

7. After incubation, collect all nonadherent cells in the supernatant of polystyrene cell culture dish into 50 ml conical tube. Discard the dish, which contains fibroblasts, fragments of cartilage, and cellular debris that adhere to the surface of the bottom.

8. Centrifuge at $300 \times g$ for 10 min at room temperature.

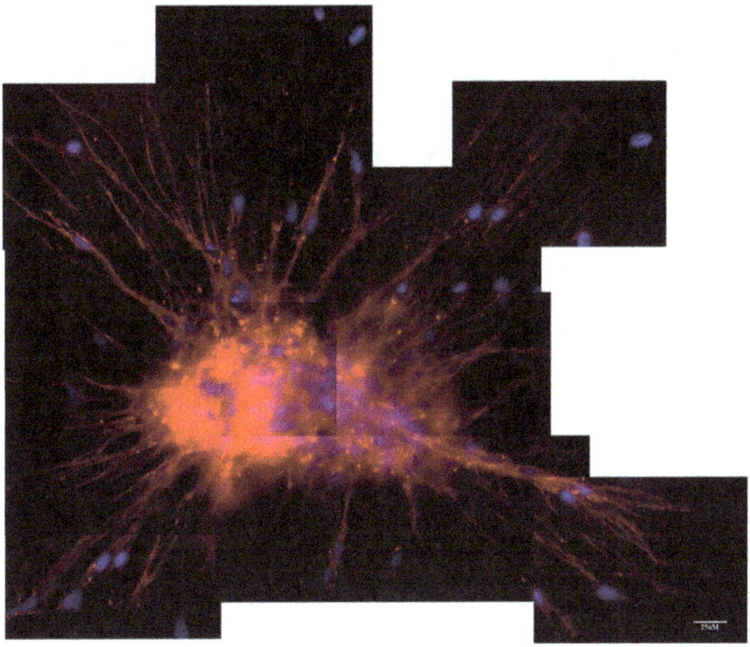

Fig. 3 A fluorescence photomontage of a human parasympathetic nerve clump after 7 days in culture. Parasympathetic neurons are stained with pan-neuronal marker PGP9.5, and all nuclei are labelled with DAPI. Bar = 25 μm

9. Carefully aspirate supernatant, and resuspend pellet with serum-free media.

10. Mix cell suspension thoroughly, plate the mixture on matrigel-coated plate, and incubate at 37 °C for 24 h.

11. Twenty-four hours after plating, remove no more than 80 % supernatant with pipette from each well and add serum-free media containing cytosine arabinoside (1.0 μM) to inhibit growth of any dividing cells. Continue to incubate cells at 37 °C for 72 h without changing medium.

12. After treatment with cytosine arabinoside, maintain cells in serum-free media at 37 °C in 5 % CO_2 and replace medium every other day with serum-free media.

13. Cells are generally used for experiments in 7–10 days after plating (Fig. 3).

3.3 Coculture of Parasympathetic Nerves with Eosinophils and RNA Harvest from Parasympathetic Ganglia (See Note 4)

1. Bring eosinophils to a concentration of 3×10^5 cells/ml with serum-free media.

2. Carefully remove the media on the nerves, replace with 1.5 ml of serum-free media with eosinophils, and incubate for 24 h at 35.5 °C.

3. Prepare glass pipette: Hold both ends of a thin wall glass capillary tube and place the middle part in a Bunsen burner

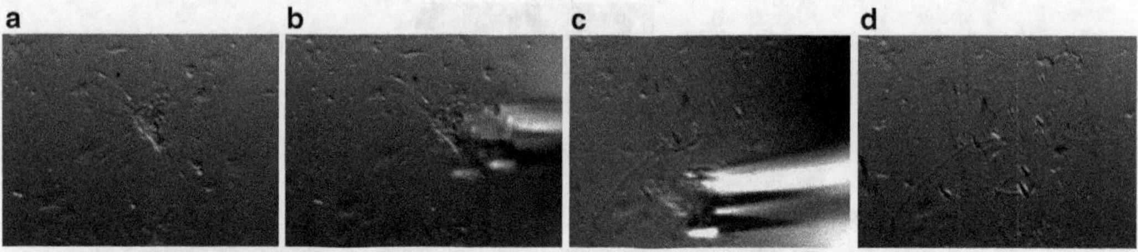

Fig. 4 Guinea pig parasympathetic nerves grow in clusters with their neuritis extending out. (**a**) Loosen the cluster from matrigel by cutting the neuritis around the cell cluster with the tip of the glass pipette, and isolate bodies. (**b**) Suck up the cell bodies by applying suction with the attached syringe (**c**) leaving the non-neuron cells behind (**d**)

flame. Pull both ends until the glass capillary tube divides into two parts. Break the tip off with a fine forceps, leaving a sterile opening finer than the original opening. Use connective tubing to attach the untouched end of the glass capillary to a syringe filled with ice-cold RNAse-free PBS.

4. Place the cell culture plate under an inverted microscope, and replace cell culture media with ice-cold RNAse-free PBS.

5. Identify nerve clusters using the inverted microscope.

6. Cut the extended neurites around the cell cluster with the tip of glass pipette, and isolate cell bodies by detaching neurites from matrigel (Fig. 4).

7. Suck up the cell bodies by applying suction with the attached syringe. Suck up as little as possible of the PBS. Eject the cells into an RNAse-free Eppendorf tube. All nerve clusters from the same dish or treatment are combined in one tube and stored on ice.

8. Change to a new glass pipette for each dish.

9. Expression of mRNA for the gene of interests is measured by real-time RT-PCR using power SYBRGreen Cells-to-CT kit (Ambion by Life Technology).

3.4 Culture of Mouse Sensory Neurons

3.4.1 Dissection and Enzymatic Dissociation of Mouse Dorsal Root Ganglia

1. Euthanize the mouse with a lethal dose of pentobarbital, 200 μl of 50 mg/ml nembutal.

2. Place mouse on its stomach, and spray the back with 70 % ethanol.

3. Using large scissors make a midline incision from the base of the skull to the tail.

4. Using new sterile scissors remove tissue around spine to expose the spinal column. Cut the spinal column just below the skull, severing it from the skull.

5. Grab the proximal end of the spinal column and lift. Using scissors cut along both edges of the spinal column, down to

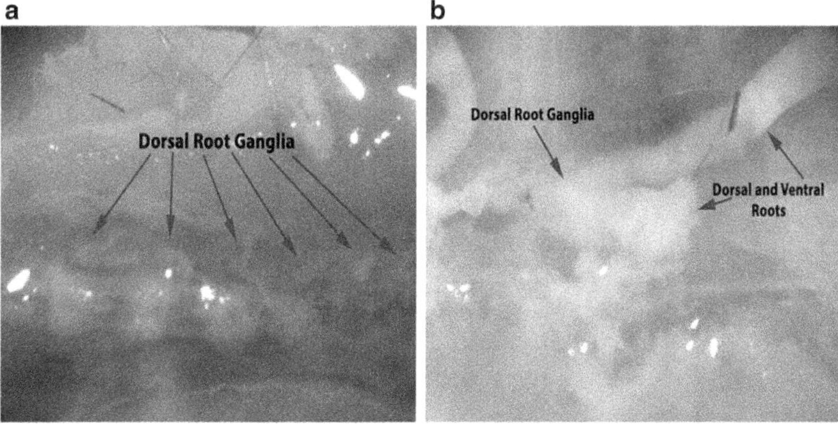

Fig. 5 There are 60 dorsal root ganglia in the mouse located in pairs at thoracic, lumbar, and sacral vertebral levels. Panel (**a**) shows the spinal canal after removal of the spinal cord. The dorsal and ventral roots can be seen and are identified by *arrows* in the image. DRGs will be located at the base of these roots. Panel (**b**) shows a close-up of dorsal and ventral roots and the DRG in relation to them

the level of the sacral end, separating the ribs, internal organs, and all tissue from the spine.

6. Cut the spine at the sacral end and place into DMEM/FBS.

7. Move the spine to 100 mm plate with DMEM/FBS under a dissecting microscope.

8. Cut the spine into two segments for ease of use. Cut the ventral side of the vertebrae, and then cut the dorsal side of the vertebrae to expose the spinal cord. Remove the spinal cord. DRGs can be identified by finding the dorsal and ventral roots, which will be present after removing the spinal cord (Fig. 5a). The DRG will be located at the base of the dorsal root (Fig. 5b). To harvest the DRGs you will have to cut away some of the spinal canal.

9. Using dissection microscope dissect DRGs and place them into fresh DMEM/FBS in a 50 ml conical tube.

10. After the dissection, spin the ganglia at $300 \times g$ for 10 min at room temperature to pellet the ganglia.

11. All further steps should be done in a laminar flow hood using sterile technique.

12. Remove DMEM/FBS. Resuspend pellet in 10 ml 0.05 % collagenase. Add 100 µl 100× pen/strep. Incubate in water bath at 37 °C with gentle shaking for 4 h.

13. After incubating, spin at $300 \times g$ for 10 min at room temperature, and remove supernatant.

14. Add 1 ml 0.25 % trypsin–EDTA, and aspirate to break up the pellet. Incubate in water bath at 37 °C with gentle shaking for 15 min.

15. Pipette cells up and down in trypsin with P1000 until DRGs are in single-cell suspension, add 10 ml DMEM/FBS, and spin at $300 \times g$ for 10 min at room temperature.

3.4.2 Preplating Cells and Coating Slides

1. Remove supernatant after spin, and resuspend the cells in 10 ml DMEM/FBS. Transfer cells to 100 mm plate and incubate overnight at 35.5 °C. This step allows adherent cells to adhere to the plate, leaving neurons in supernatant.

2. Coat slides with matrigel: This should be done on the same day the cells are preplated to allow the matrigel to coat the slides overnight.

3. To coat slides put 100 µl aliquot of matrigel on ice to thaw. Mix 10 ml chilled DMEM with matrigel using precooled pipette. Aliquot 500 µl into each well of a 4-well chamber slide. Incubate overnight at 35.5 °C.

3.4.3 Plating Cells

1. Remove supernatant from plate with 10 ml pipette, place into 50 ml conical, and spin at $300 \times g$ for 10 min at room temperature.

2. Thaw aliquots of serum-free media. Add 100 µl 100× pen/strep to each aliquot.

3. Resuspend DRGs in 1 ml serum-free media with pen/strep. Count the cells using a hemocytometer.

4. Bring the cells to a concentration of 60,000 cells/ml using serum-free media with pen/strep.

5. Carefully remove the supernatant from the 4-well chamber slides coated overnight with matrigel. Add 500 µl of cell mixture to each well. Be quick so as not to allow the matrigel to dry, and be careful not to disturb the gel on the bottom of the well.

6. Incubate 4-well chamber slides at 35.5 °C, and the nerves will be ready for experiments after incubation overnight.

3.5 Culture of Human Sensory Neurons

3.5.1 Dissect and Digest Human Dorsal Root Ganglia (See Note 5)

1. Place tissue sample onto 100 mm tissue culture plate, and add a small amount of 0.05 % collagenase to keep tissue from drying out.

2. Remove dorsal and ventral roots as well as the spinal nerve (Fig. 6).

3. Cut DRG into small, roughly 1 mm sized, pieces.

4. Move DRG pieces into 50 ml conical with remaining of 0.05 % collagenase and incubate overnight in 37 °C water bath with gentle shaking.

3.5.2 Preplate to Remove Adherent Cells and Coat Slides

1. Mix DRG in 0.05 % collagenase with 10 ml, and pipette four times to break up the remaining tissue.

2. Spin tube at $300 \times g$ for 10 min at room temperature to pellet cells. Remove supernatant.

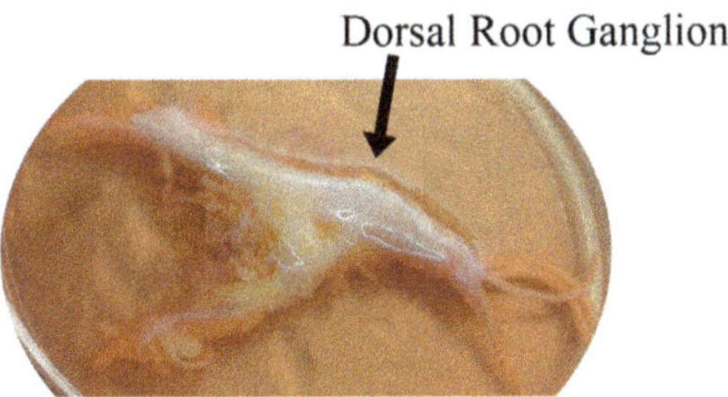

Fig. 6 Location of the dorsal root ganglion. Tissue samples from a tissue bank will come with the spinal nerve and dorsal and ventral roots still attached. The dorsal root ganglion is identified in the figure, and the spinal nerve and dorsal and ventral roots are dissected away before manually dissociating

3. Option: Incubating with 1 ml 0.25 % trypsin for 15 min in shaking water bath at 37 °C will help to break down the undigested tissue. Add 10 ml DMEM/FBS to inhibit the trypsin, and spin at $300 \times g$ for 10 min at room temperature to pellet the cells. Remove supernatant.

4. Resuspend pellet in 20 ml DMEM/FBS. Mix with 10 ml pipette to break up the pellet into a single-cell suspension.

5. Plate 10 ml/each onto two 100 mm culture plates, and incubate overnight at 35.5 °C at 5 % CO_2. This allows all adherent cells to adhere to the bottom of the plate, leaving the neurons in the supernatant.

6. Coat slides with matrigel: Thaw 100 µl aliquot of matrigel on ice. Mix 10 ml chilled DMEM with matrigel using chilled pipette. Aliquot 500 µl into each well of a 4-well chamber slide. Incubate overnight at 35.5 °C.

3.5.3 Plate Neurons

1. Thaw aliquots of serum-free media, and add 100 µl 100× pen/strep/fungizone to each aliquot.

2. Remove supernatant from preplates and place into a 50 ml conical tube. Spin tube at $300 \times g$ for 10 min at room temperature to pellet cells.

3. Resuspend cells in 1 ml of serum-free media with pen/strep/fungizone. Count cells using a hemocytometer.

4. Bring cells to a concentration of 60,000 cells/ml using serum-free media with pen/strep/fungizone.

5. Carefully remove DMEM from 4-well chamber slides, and add 500 µl of cell mixture to the wells. Be quick so as not to allow the matrigel to dry, and be careful not to disturb the gel on the bottom of the well.

6. Culture cells at 35.5 °C, and the nerves will be ready for experiments after culturing overnight.

3.5.4 Interaction Assay

1. Bring eosinophils to a concentration of 60,000 cells/ml with serum-free media.

2. Carefully remove the media from the 4-well chamber slides, replace with 500 µl of serum-free media with eosinophils, and incubate at 35.5 °C for 18 h.

3. All further steps may be done on the bench.

4. Fix cells by carefully removing media and adding 500 µl Zamboni's fixative and incubate for 15 min at room temperature.

5. Wash three times with PBS for 5 min; samples can be stored at 4 °C in PBS.

6. Remove chamber from chamber slides, following the instruction.

7. Draw barrier ring around each well using the ImmEdge pen.

8. Permeabilize and block using 100 µl blocking buffer. Incubate for 30 min on ice.

9. Remove blocking buffer, add 100 µl primary antibody solution, and incubate for 4 h at 4 °C.

10. Wash three times with PBS for 5 min.

11. Add 100 µl secondary antibody solution. Incubate for 2 h at 4 °C in the dark.

12. Wash three times with PBS for 5 min.

13. Add Vectashield to each well, and cover with cover slip. Seal the edge of the cover slip using cytoseal. Keep slide at 4 °C in the dark.

14. Image using fluorescent microscope.

15. Make nerve models using Imaris (Bitplane) software.

4 Notes

1. Prepare and store all reagents at 4 °C unless indicated otherwise.

2. Use plastic tips, pipette, tubes, or flasks to prepare the media in order to reduce contact of components, particularly of NGF, to the wall of containers. BSA should be added before insulin to reduce insulin's adsorption to the plastic. Ham's F12 should be added last because its high concentration of cysteine may reduce the activity of insulin.

3. The same as that in preparation of parasympathetic neurons from guinea pigs.

4. Because the cell density may differ among cell culture dishes and some non-neuronal cells can survive the treatment of

cytosine arabinoside, it is difficult to measure the changes of parasympathetic neuron's mRNA in response to treatment. However, we have developed a unique method to harvest parasympathetic nerve cell bodies for RNA isolation. This method takes advantage of the observation that guinea pig parasympathetic nerves grow in clusters with their neuritis extending out.

5. All steps should be done in a laminar flow hood using sterile technique.

References

1. Leiferman KM, Gleich GJ, Peters MS (2007) Dermatologic manifestations of the hypereosinophilic syndromes. Immunol Allergy Clin North Am 27(3):415–441

2. Smyth CM et al (2013) Activated eosinophils in association with enteric nerves in inflammatory bowel disease. PLoS One 8(5):e64216

3. Thornton MA et al (2013) Eosinophil recruitment to nasal nerves after allergen challenge in allergic rhinitis. Clin Immunol 147(1):50–57

4. Costello RW et al (1997) Localization of eosinophils to airway nerves and effect on neuronal M2 muscarinic receptor function. Am J Physiol Lung Cell Mol Physiol 273(1):L93–L103

5. Fryer AD et al (2006) Neuronal eotaxin and the effects of CCR3 antagonist on airway hyperreactivity and M2 receptor dysfunction. J Clin Invest 116(1):228–236

6. Nie Z, Nelson CS, Jacoby DB, Fryer AD (2007) Expression and regulation of intercellular adhesion molecule-1 on airway parasympathetic nerves. J Allergy Clin Immunol 119(6):1415–1422

7. Foster EL et al (2011) Eosinophils increase neuron branching in human and murine skin and in vitro. PLoS One 6(7):e22029

8. Jacoby DB, Gleich GJ, Fryer AD (1993) Human eosinophil major basic protein is an endogenous allosteric antagonist at the inhibitory muscarinic M2 receptor. J Clin Invest 91(4):1314–1318

9. Fryer AD et al (1996) Cultures of airway parasympathetic nerves express functional M2 muscarinic receptors. Am J Respir Cell Mol Biol 15(6):716–725

10. Malin SA, Davis BM, Molliver DC (2007) Production of dissociated sensory neuron cultures and considerations for their use in studying neuronal function and plasticity. Nat Protoc 2(1):152–160

11. Sawatzky DA et al (2002) Eosinophil adhesion to cholinergic nerves via ICAM-1 and VCAM-1 and associated eosinophil degranulation. Am J Physiol Lung Cell Mol Physiol 282(6):L1279–L1288

Chapter 20

Eosinophils Interaction with Mast Cells: The Allergic Effector Unit

Roopesh Singh Gangwar and Francesca Levi-Schaffer

Abstract

Mast cells (MC) and eosinophils are the key effector cells of allergy (Minai-Fleminger and Levi-Schaffer, Inflamm Res 58:631–638, 2009). In general, allergic reactions have two phases, namely, an early phase and a late phase. MC and eosinophils abundantly coexist in the inflamed tissue in the late and chronic phases and cross talk in a bidirectional manner. This bidirectional interaction between MC and eosinophils is mediated by both physical cell–cell contacts through cell surface receptors such as CD48, 2B4 and soluble mediators through various specific granular mediators, arachidonic acid metabolites, cytokines, and chemokines, collectively termed the "Allergic Effector Unit" (AEU) (Elishmereni et al., Allergy 66:376–385, 2011; Minai-Fleminger et al., Cell Tissue Res 341:405–415, 2010). These bidirectional interactions can be studied in vitro in a customized coculture system of MC and eosinophils derived from either mouse or human source.

Key words Allergic Effector Unit, Murine AEU, Coculture, Mast cell–eosinophil interactions, BMMC, BMEos

1 Introduction

MC are highly granulated, Fc epsilon RI (FcεRI) bearing, tissue-dwelling cells, essentially found in all tissues [1, 2]. Tissue MC express different phenotypic characteristics and are named by the tissue type in which they reside, for example connective tissue and mucosal MC. Besides their fundamental role in allergic reactions, MC also participate in various conditions such as fibrosis, responses to neoplasms, autoimmune diseases, and in host defense against bacterial or parasitic infections [3–5]. MC granules contain and release various preformed mediators such as histamine, tryptase, chymase, proteoglycans, and arachidonic acid metabolites and an array of cytokines/chemokines [6]. MC function can be regulated by their FcεRI expression which is directly affected by the IgE concentration. Additionally to FcεRI, MC also express membrane receptors, including CD48, CD300a, Fcγ RIIb, CD13, CD34,

Garry M. Walsh (ed.), *Eosinophils: Methods and Protocols*, Methods in Molecular Biology, vol. 1178, DOI 10.1007/978-1-4939-1016-8_20, © Springer Science+Business Media New York 2014

CD117 (c-kit) and various receptors from different families such as for chemokines, purinergic types, etc., which regulate their different functions, and can either positively or negatively modulate the activity of MC.

Eosinophils are multifunctional granulocytes [7, 8] that migrate into tissues in some physiological and pathological conditions where they survive for several days. Eosinophils consist of a characteristic bilobed nucleus and a cytoplasm full of secondary granules. Eosinophil granules contain the cationic proteins major basic protein (MBP), eosinophil peroxidase (EPO), eosinophil cationic protein (ECP), and eosinophil-derived neurotoxin (EDN) which are released upon cell degranulation in response to diverse stimuli along with lipid mediators, cytokines, chemokines, and neuromodulators [9] that play an important role in inflammation, allergy, parasitic infection, tissue injury and tumors. Eosinophils express various cell surface markers, such as Fc receptors, CCR3, PAF receptors, CD48, 2B4, Siglec-F, histamine receptors, etc., which are responsible for cell–cell communication via various pathways [10].

MC and eosinophils, the key effector cells of allergic inflammation [11], abundantly coexist in the inflamed tissue in the late and chronic phases and cross talk in a bidirectional manner, mediated by both the physical contacts (through cell surface receptors such as CD48, 2B4) and soluble released compounds (that is, specific mediators, various cytokines and chemokines). This bidirectional interaction between MC and eosinophils is termed as the "Allergic Effector Unit" (AEU) [12, 13]. AEU could affect the effector activities of MC and eosinophils by facilitating bidirectional exchange of regulatory information and transfer of signals. Early studies have reported that mediators of MC affect eosinophils and vice versa [2, 13, 14]. Moreover, cell surface molecules implicated in the MC–eosinophil contact mechanism (i.e., the CD2-family molecule CD48 and its high-affinity ligand 2B4 or DNAM-1 and Nectin-2) convey stimulatory signals in these cells [12, 15, 16]. Whether such MC–eosinophil interactions can indeed enforce meaningful changes on cellular functionality, and participate in shaping the allergic response in which they occur, still needs to be studied in detail and especially in vivo. Although in vivo experiments could provide relevant information, the feasibility of such studies is limited and time consuming. Therefore, the use of in vitro systems, which mimic the AEU in vivo is of great value. Indeed such MC–eosinophil interactions can be studied in vitro in a customized whole-cell coculture system employing human/murine-derived MC and eosinophils.

In this chapter, we will provide the protocols to produce the murine cell AEU by first describing the MC and eosinophils preparation and thereafter the actual AEU and its culture. We also offer some directions for producing the human AEU.

2   Materials

Prepare all the buffers/solutions with sterile deionized water (DD H$_2$O), adjust the pH with a minimum amount of acid or base, sterilize by filtration through a 0.22 μm filter, and store at 4 °C (unless indicated otherwise).

2.1   Culture Medium for BMMC and BMEos

See Tables 1 and 2.

Table 1
Medium composition for bone marrow-derived mast cells (BMMC)

BMMC culture medium components	1 l	Final concentration
RPMI 1640 medium with L-glutamine	870 ml	
Heat-inactivated fetal bovine serum/Fetal calf serum	100 ml	10 %
Pen–Strep solution (Penicillin 100,000 U/ml, Streptomycin 100 mg/ml)	10 ml	1×
Nonessential amino acids solution (100×)	10 ml	1×
BMMC cytokines (*see* Subheading 2.2)	Stock concentration	Final concentration
Recombinant murine stem cell factor (r-mSCF)	50 μg/ml	20 ng/ml
Recombinant murine IL-3 (r-mIL-3)	50 μg/ml	20 ng/ml

Table 2
Medium composition for culturing bone marrow-derived eosinophils (BMEos)

BMEos culture medium	1 l	Final concentration
RPMI 1640 medium with L-glutamine	734 ml	
Heat-inactivated fetal bovine serum/Fetal calf serum	200 ml	20 %
Pen–Strep solution (Penicillin 100,000 U/ml, Streptomycin 100 mg/ml)	10 ml	1×
L-Glutamine (200 mM)	10 ml	2 mM
Nonessential amino acids solution (100×)	10 ml	1×
HEPES (1 M)	25 ml	25 mM
Sodium pyruvate (100 mM)	10 ml	1 mM
β-mercaptoethanol (50 mM)	1 ml	50 μM
BMEos cytokines (*see* Subheading 2.3)	Stock concentration	Final concentration
(r-mSCF)	50 μg/ml	100 ng/ml
Recombinant murine Flt3-Ligand	50 μg/ml	100 ng/ml
Recombinant murine IL-5 (r-mIL-5)	5 μg/ml	10 ng/ml

2.2 BMMC Cytokines

1. Recombinant murine stem cell factor (PeproTech cat # 250-03). Prepare a stock solution of 50 µg/ml in sterile PBS, make aliquots of 32 µl each and store at –80 °C. Thaw the stock just before use and add 16 µl of this to 40 ml of BMMC culture medium.

2. Recombinant murine IL-3 (PeproTech cat # 213-13). Prepare and use same as recombinant murine SCF.

3. Once thawed, do not freeze the aliquot again, instead keep at 4 °C and this can be used up to 1 week. Do not store any cytokine at 4 °C for longer than 1 week.

2.3 BMEos Cytokines

1. Recombinant murine stem cell factor: Prepare a stock solution of 50 µg/ml as in Subheading 2.2, **item 1**. Thaw the stock just before use and add 100 µl of this to 50 ml of BMEos culture medium.

2. Recombinant murine Flt3-Ligand (PeproTech cat# 250-31). Prepare and use in same way as recombinant murine SCF for BMEos

3. Recombinant Mouse IL-5 (R&D Systems cat# 405-ML). Prepare a stock solution of 5 µg/ml in sterile PBS + 0.1 % BSA, make aliquots of 100 µl and store at –80 °C. Use 100 µl/50 ml of BMEos medium.

4. Once thawed, do not freeze the aliquot again, instead keep at 4 °C and this can be used up to 1 week. Do not store any cytokine at 4 °C for longer than 1 week.

2.4 Buffers and Solutions (See Note 1)

1. Tyrode's buffer [17] (pH 7.3) (Table 3).
   Dissolve all the components except BSA in DD H_2O (slightly less than the final volume), adjust the pH 7.3 with NaOH and make up the final volume with DD H_2O. Sterilize by filtration through 0.22 µm filter. The buffer can be stored aseptically up to 6 months at 4 °C without BSA. Add BSA 0.5 mg/ml prior to use.

2. Carbonate buffer (0.1 M, pH 9.0) (Table 4) for β-hex stop solution. Dissolve all the components in DD H_2O, adjust the pH if required, filter-sterilize through 0.22 µm filter. The buffer can be stored aseptically up to 6 months at 4 °C.

3. Toluidine blue stain: Toluidine blue 0.07 % w/v in 60 % ethanol, pH 3.5.

4. Tryptase substrate (25 mM): N-(p-Tosyl)-Gly-Pro-Lys 4-nitroanilide acetate. Dissolve 10 mg of this substrate in 630 µl of dimethyl sulfoxide (DMSO). Prepare aliquots and store at –20 °C, protect from light.

5. β-Hexosaminidase (β-hex) substrate (8 mM): 4-Nitrophenyl N-acetyl-β-D-glucosaminide. *Substrate buffer:* Citric acid (0.12 M) and Na_2HPO_4 (0.14 M) adjust the pH to 4.5 and filter-sterilize. Dissolve 20 mg of substrate in 4.5 ml of DD

Table 3
Composition of Tyrode's buffer

Buffer components	Final concentration
NaCl	135 mM
KCl	5 mM
$MgCl_2$	1 mM
$CaCl_2$	1.8 mM
Glucose	5.6 mM
HEPES	20 mM
pH	7.3 (adjust with NaOH) (*see* **Note 1**)
BSA (Fraction V)	0.5 mg/ml

Table 4
Composition of carbonate buffer

Buffer components	Final concentration
Na_2CO_3	100 mM
$NaHCO_3$	100 mM
pH	9.0 (*see* **Note 1**)

H_2O and 3 ml of substrate buffer and mix well. Prepare aliquots and store at –20 °C, protect from light.

6. OPD substrate solution for EPO (Sigma cat # P9187): Dissolve one urea hydrogen peroxide tablet (gold foil) in 20 ml of DD H_2O (mark this as *Tube A*) and dissolve one OPD tablet (silver foil) in 14.7 ml of urea hydrogen peroxide buffer from *Tube A*, cover the tube with aluminum foil to protect from light (OPD substrate, mark this as *Tube B*). Take 5.2 ml DD H_2O in a new tube (*Tube C*), cover with aluminum foil, add 4 ml Tris buffer (1 M, pH 8) and 800 µl of OPD substrate from *Tube B*, add 1.25 µl of 30 % hydrogen peroxide to this just before adding the substrate and mix well.

2.5 Other Requirements

1. Mice 6–8-week-old females (C57BL or BALB/c).
2. Sterile PBS (10× and 1×, 0.22 µm filtered).
3. DD H_2O (0.22 µm filtered).
4. Scissors and Forceps.
5. 70 % ethanol.
6. Syringes (5 or 10 ml) with needles (25 gauge).

7. Tissue culture plates, sterile (6 well, 96 well flat bottom and 96 well "U" bottom).

8. 75 cm² culture flask (sterile).

9. Temperature controlled centrifuge with swing bucket rotor.

10. Microplate Reader (spectrophotometer).

11. Microscope.

12. Centrifuge tubes (50 ml), FACS tube (5 ml polystyrene round-bottom tubes).

13. Anti-Mouse FcεRI FITC and matched isotype control antibodies.

14. Anti-Mouse CD117 (c-Kit) APC and matched isotype control antibodies.

3   Methods

The focus of the chapter is MC interactions with eosinophils. It is therefore, important to describe the protocols for the purification of MC and eosinophils. The maintenance of a coculture system greatly depends upon the source of both of these cells. There are several sources from which MC and can be obtained (*see* **Note 2**). Here we describe the differentiation of MC and eosinophils in culture from progenitors of bone marrow derived from mouse, step by step.

3.1 *Ex Vivo Differentiation and Culture of MC from Adult Mouse Bone Marrow*

Functionally competent MC [18, 19] and eosinophils [20] can be differentiated ex vivo from the bone marrow of normal mice. Mature MC differentiate from bone marrow in culture in the presence of appropriate growth factors in about 4 weeks. However, it takes only 10–14 days in culture to differentiate fully functional eosinophils from bone marrow. Therefore, culture of BMMC should be started first and 2 weeks later start the BMEos cultures.

1. Prepare 500 ml BMMC medium before harvesting the mice bone marrow and maintain at 4 °C. Aliquot 50 ml medium, warm at 37 °C water bath, and add cytokines (r-mSCF and r-mIL-3).

2. Sterilize scissors and forceps with 70 % ethanol. Euthanize mice by long exposure (2–3 min) of isoflurane and cervical dislocation and bathe in 70 % ethanol to surface-sterilize and let it dry. Remove the skin from the lower portion of the body and legs; remove hind legs from the acetabulum (joint of pubic bone with femur) and place them in 6-well plate with 10 ml RPMI 1640 medium or sterile PBS. Care should be taken not to break or cut the femurs.

3. Remove most of the flesh from the bones and separate the tibia from the femur and ankle (*see* **Note 3**).

4. Transfer the clean bones to new well/plate containing fresh medium. Add 5–10 ml culture medium to another well and fill a syringe with medium. With a sharp scalpel or scissors cut off tips of femur and tibia (stay as distal as possible). Attach a 25 gauge needle to the syringe and flush marrow from bones (*see* **Note 4**). Unify all marrow from bones of one mouse in 1 tube ≈15–20 ml, determine the cell count.

5. Centrifuge the marrow to collect the cells, 300×g, 4 °C, 7 min in swing bucket rotor. After centrifugation, discard the supernatant. Suspend the cell pellet in BMMC culture medium supplemented with BMMC cytokines (*see* Subheading 2.2) in such a way that final cell concentration should be 10^6 cells/ml, transfer to 75 cm^2 tissue culture flask and keep in 37 °C CO$_2$ (5 %) incubator.

6. Change the medium starting at day 3 two times every week by transferring the cell suspension to a sterile conical tube (50 ml) and centrifuging for 7 min at 300×g at room temperature (20 °C). Remove the supernatant and resuspend the cell pellet in fresh BMMC culture medium (maintain the cell density as 10^6 cells/ml) supplemented with cytokines and transfer to a new 75 cm^2 tissue culture flask (*see* **Note 5**).

7. After 4 weeks, the culture consists of mature BMMC. The purity is evaluated by toluidine blue staining (*see* **Note 6**). If the cells are mature, they can be utilized for experiments.

8. The BMMC should not be used after 7 weeks in culture when their reactivity begins to decrease.

3.2 Ex Vivo Differentiation and Culture of Eosinophils from Adult Mouse Bone Marrow

1. For culture of BMEos follow **steps 1–4** as described above for BMMC. The only difference is the medium composition.

2. Centrifuge the marrow cell suspension to collect the cells, 300g, 4 °C, 7 min in swing bucket rotor. By the time cells are in the centrifuge, prepare the sterile DD H$_2$O and 10× PBS. After centrifugation, discard the supernatant (medium).

3. Lyse red blood cells by resuspending the cell pellet in 9 ml DD H$_2$O (gently pipetting up and down 2–3 times, 30 s) and then immediately add 1 ml 10× PBS to make the solution isotonic.

4. Centrifuge again and repeat the previous step if necessary.

5. Resuspend the cell pellet in BMEos medium and count the cells.

6. Calculate and take the desired cell number, centrifuge, remove medium and resuspend (at a cell concentration of 10^6 cells/ml) in BMEos medium supplemented with BMEos cytokines (r-mSCF and r-mFLT3-L, *see* Subheading 2.3), transfer to 75 cm^2 tissue culture flask, and keep in 37 °C CO$_2$ incubator.

7. At Day 2 replace half of the medium. Warm the BMEos medium at 37 °C water bath. Take out the aliquots of cytokines (r-mSCF and r-mFLT3-L) from –80 °C freezer.

8. Take out the culture flask from incubator; mix by gentle shaking and transfer half of the cell suspension from each culture flask to sterile 50 ml conical tube (use separate tube for each flask).

9. Take sample for cell count (should have approximately same number of cells as started with) and centrifuge the tubes at 30 °C, $300 \times g$ for 7 min.

10. Add cytokines (r-mSCF and r-mFLT3-L) to the required amount of BMEos culture medium. Suspend cell pellet in amount of volume removed or more if necessary to adjust concentration to 10^6 cell/ml.

11. Transfer the cell suspension (with new medium) back to the respective flask and keep in 37 °C CO_2 incubator.

12. At day 4 replace the medium and cytokines (r-mSCF and r-mFLT3-L with r-mIL-5). Pre-warm the BMEos culture medium at 37 °C water bath. Thaw aliquot of r-mIL-5 and add to medium at a final concentration of 10 ng/ml (*see* Subheading 2.3, usually prepare 50–100 ml medium and use as required).

13. Transfer all the cells from culture flask to sterile 50 ml conical tube, take sample for counting and centrifuge the cells $300 \times g$, 30 °C, 7 min.

14. Remove old medium, resuspend the cell pellet (10^6 cells/ml) in medium containing r-mIL-5, transfer back to the same flask, and keep the flask in 37 °C CO_2 incubator.

15. At day 6, transfer half of the medium (cell suspension) from each culture flask to a sterile conical centrifuge tube and count the cells.

16. Centrifuge the cells at $300 \times g$, 30 °C , 7 min, and remove the old medium.

17. Resuspend the cells pellet in fresh medium containing r-mIL-5 and adjust the cell concentration to 10^6 cells/ml.

18. Transfer the cell suspension to the same flask and keep in 37 °C CO_2 incubator.

19. At day 8, transfer all the medium containing cells from the flask to a sterile conical 50 ml centrifuge tube, determine cell count and make slides for differential count.

20. Prepare fresh medium, add r-mIL-5 at a final concentration of 10 ng/ml.

21. Centrifuge the cells at $300 \times g$, 30 °C for 7 min, remove half of the medium and resuspend the cells in remaining medium.

22. Add fresh medium (containing r-mIL-5) equal to the volume removed or more if necessary to adjust the concentration to 10^6 cells/ml. Transfer the cell suspension to a new sterile flask and keep in 37 °C CO_2 incubator.

23. At day 10 replace half of the medium with fresh medium containing r-mIL-5.

24. Count and determine BMEos purity/maturity (should be >90 % eosinophils, **Notes 7** and **8**).

25. Use as desired.

26. If continuing culture, the cells will need medium replacement and cytokine supplement every 2 days (*see* **Note 9**).

3.3 The Murine AEU: Coculture of BMMC and BMEos

Before starting the actual experiment, it is mandatory to check that both the MC and eosinophils are mature and functional. Experiments can be performed on these cells only when both the BMMC and BMEos are mature. A simple FACS staining should be done to check the expression of MC and eosinophil specific surface markers (FcεR1 & c-Kit for MC and Siglec-F & CCR3 for eosinophils) (*see* **Note 7**), and functional assays for example release of β-hex, Tryptase from activated BMMC and release of EPO from activated BMEos (*see* Subheadings 3.5 to 3.7 and **Notes 10** and **11**).

There are two types of coculture: (1) short term coculture, which is usually 1 h or a few hours, (2) long term coculture, which can be from 24 h to up to several days, depending on experimental requirements. MC–Eosinophil cocultures can be set up at various cell–cell ratios (1:1, 1:0.1, 0.1:1, etc.) depending on what will be examined [21]. Here, we describe an equal MC–eosinophils (1:1) ratio.

1. Determine the cell number and take the BMMC according to your experimental requirement. Centrifuge the cells and resuspend in fresh BMMC culture medium supplemented with cytokines.

2. Sensitize BMMC by αDNP-IgE (0.5 μg/ml) in 25-cm^2 culture flask or 6-well plate in 37 °C CO$_2$ incubator overnight (It is always better to sensitize all the required cells together *see* **Note 12**).

3. The following morning, prepare/aliquot 50 ml (as required) of Tyrode's buffer (*see* **Note 13**), adjust the pH if required, add BSA (0.5 mg/ml). Count and put the required amount of cells in separate tubes, wash the cells (BMMC (sensitized) and BMEos) with Tyrode's buffer, and resuspend each of them at a cell concentration of 2×10^6 cells/ml separately.

4. Seed BMMC (2×10^5 cells/100 μl/well) in a "U shaped-bottom" 96-well tissue culture plate; add BMEos (2×10^5 cells/100 μl/well) to the BMMC wells and mix well. Control monocultures should be included in the plate as 2×10^5 BMMC and/or BMEos/100 μl/well (*see* **Note 14**). Each treatment for coculture and monoculture should be in triplicate. Keep the plate at 4 °C on ice while adding the cells.

3.4 Activation of the AEU (BMMC/ BMEos)

MCs constitutively express significant numbers of FcεRI, the high-affinity receptor for IgE, that is positively regulated by IgE concentration [22]. Usually in baseline condition, a substantial amount of IgE remains bound to the FcεRI receptor on MC. When a bivalent or multivalent antigen binds to the MC surface-FcεRI-bound IgE, cross-linking of FcεRI receptors take place, which leads to the activation of MC. Aggregation of even a small fraction of the surface FcεRI on the MC is enough to induce activation [22].

BMMC can be activated by this classical IgE-mediated mechanism. The FcεRI dependent activated MC immediately (few minutes) release amino acid metabolites such as PGD2, LTC4, etc., degranulate and release granule-associated mediators such as histamine, heparin, several proteases, proteoglycans, and certain cytokines, which lead to the induction of immediate allergic inflammation [22–24]. A few hours post activation MC synthesize and secrete cytokines, chemokines, and growth factors, which lead to chronic inflammation [2, 25, 26]: this contributes to the late phase of allergic inflammation.

The success of any experiment performed in coculture systems depends on the specific cell associated readout. In this way, one can measure the effect of each cell type on the other cell and also the combined effect of both the cell types. For example, if we want to determine the effect of MC on eosinophils in coculture then we can measure the released EPO in the culture supernatants, which will be specific for eosinophils. For MC it is possible to measure the released tryptase, histamine and β-hex (even though beta hex is also produced by eosinophils, the levels are extremely low in comparison to the BMMC and therefore it can be measured in coculture and considered as specific for BMMC) (*see* Subheadings 3.5 to 3.7 and **Note 10**). Both the BMMC and BMEos can be activated by different activators (*see* **Notes 12** and **15**) here we describe the simplest one, PAF activation (*see* **Note 16**) for BMEos and IgE mediated activation for BMMC.

1. Add activator or treatment (*see* **Note 17**) and controls (medium/buffer/vehicle) to the cells and incubate the plate (mark as *plate A*) in a CO_2 (5 %) incubator, 37 °C for 1 h. A simple experiment can be planned based on the following plate design (Fig. 1).

2. Take out the plate from incubator and immediately put it on ice for 5 min. Centrifuge the plate at $500 \times g$ for 7 min at 4 °C and collect 80 μl supernatants in a new sterile plate (mark it as *plate B*) and keep the cells in original plate (*plate A*).

3. Centrifuge both the plates again and discard the supernatants from *plate A* (which contains cells) by inverting quickly. Transfer 60 μl supernatants from the *plate B* (which contains 80 μl supernatants) to the new plate (*plate C*, this will reduce the chance of aspirating cells in the supernatant).

	1	2	3	4	5	6	7	8	9	10	11	12
A	Sensitized (Sens)-Non activated (NA) BMMC + NA - BMEos			Sens-Activated (Act) BMMC + NA-BMEos			Sens-NA-BMMC + Act-BMEos			Sens-Act BMMC + Act-BMEos		
B	BMMC Treatment			BMMC Treatment			BMMC Treatment			BMMC Treatment		
C	BMEOS Treatment			BMEOS Treatment			BMEOS Treatment			BMEOS Treatment		
D												
E												
F	NA-BMEos			Act-BMEos.			Sens-NA-BMMC			Sens-Act-BMMC		
G	NA-BMEos + BMEos Treatment			Act-BMEos + BMEos Treatment			Sens-NA-BMMC + BMEos Treatment			Sens-Act-BMMC + BMEos Treatment		
H	NA-BMEos + BMMC Treatment			Act-BMEos + BMMC Treatment			Sens-NA-BMMC + BMMC Treatment			Sens-Act-BMMC + BMMC Treatment		

Fig. 1 Schematic design of a simple coculture experiment

4. Stain the cells for FcεR1 & c-kit (for MC) and Siglec-F & CCR3 (for eosinophils) and specific marker for cell activation (Lamp-1).

5. Examine the supernatants for mediator release and cytokines by the appropriate assay (*see* Subheadings 3.5 to 3.8). In short time cocultures, granule associated preformed mediators for MC should be measured such as release of tryptase, histamine, β-hex, and amino acid metabolites like PGD_2 and for long term cocultures release of specific cytokines and chemokines

such as IL-6, TNF-α, IL-8, etc., can be measured. Also expression/up-regulation of MC and eosinophil surface markers (for example Lamp-1 and other markers of particular interest and importance) can be analyzed by FACS in any coculture experiment. One can also consider the formation of MC–eosinophils pair/couple in coculture and this can be measured by electron microscopy [12].

3.5 Tryptase Assay

1. The tryptase assay should be performed in triplicate. Take a flat bottom 96-well plate; add 2 μl of tryptase substrate and 48 μl of supernatant.

2. Cover the plate with aluminum foil to protect from direct light and incubate at 37 °C incubator for approximately 1–2 h or until a yellow color develops (*see* **Note 18**).

3. Read the absorbance at 410 nm.

3.6 Assay for Measuring β-Hex (See Also Note 10)

1. Take a flat bottom 96-well plate, add 20 μl of substrate and 20 μl of supernatant and or cell lysate.

2. Incubate for at least 2 h at 37 °C, gently mix the plate every 20 min (*see* **Note 19**). Stop the reaction by adding ice-cold stop solution 200 μl/well.

3. As soon as the stop solution is added, a yellow color will develop based on the β-hex amount present in the test wells.

4. Immediately read the absorbance at 410 nm. Calculate the percent release of β-hex or percent net specific release (*see* **Note 10**).

3.7 Assay for Measuring Released EPO from Eos (See Note 11)

1. EPO is very sticky and may stick to the wall of the culture wells and on the cells' surface itself. Block a flat bottom 96-well plate with 2.5 % BSA in PBS (300 μl/well) and incubate for a minimum of 2 h at 37 °C and thereafter rinse once with PBS.

2. Seed the cells in plate and perform the experiment in this plate.

3. Take out the plate from the incubator after completion of the experiment.

4. Add freshly prepared OPD substrate solution 100 μl/well and wait for color development (usually 5–15 min depending upon the cell number and released EPO).

5. Stop the reaction by adding 100 μl/well 2 M H_2SO_4 and read the OD at 492 nm by microplate reader.

6. The results can be represented in percent release of EPO or percent net specific release as described above for β-hex (*see* **Note 10**).

3.8 Cytokines and Chemokines

1. ELISA systems are commercially available for almost every cytokine or chemokine secreted by MC/eosinophils.

2. The manufacturer's instructions should be followed.

3.9 The Human AEU: Coculture of pbEos and CBMC

The human AEU can also be set up and studied in a similar way to the murine AEU described above. Human peripheral blood eosinophils can be purified (*see* Chapter 2) [27, 28] and cord blood derived MC can be obtained as described [29] (for other sources of MC and eosinophils of human origin *see* **Note 2**). BMMC are a more immature/mucosal type of MC and CBMC are a good human counterpart of BMMC.

3.10 Transwell Coculture

The bidirectional cross talk, which takes place between MC and eosinophils in coculture, is mediated by soluble mediators as well as physical contact. The net outcome is the cumulative effect of both of these interactions together. Distinguishing between the two might help to define the mechanism underlying a phenomenon. This can be studied in transwell coculture. In transwells, cocultures of eosinophils and MC are grown/cultured together in the same well, however, separated by a polycarbonate membrane allowing unrestricted movement of medium between the two compartments but at the same time no physical contact occurs at all. This coculture setup makes it possible to study MC–eosinophils interaction mediated exclusively by soluble mediators or secretory signals. As MC release factors that may induce eosinophil chemotaxis, which can be examined in this coculture system by a transmigration assays [21].

3.11 Blocking Receptors on the Cells

Another possibility to study the specific cell–cell contact is by preventing them to mediate the contact. The cell surface receptors (for example CD48 and or 2B4) can be blocked by antibodies (*see* **Note 20**) and then the cells cocultured to study the effect of these impaired cell–cell contact by examining the mediator release.

3.12 Knock Out Cell Coculture

Although cell surface receptors can be blocked on MC and/or eosinophils to prevent the physical contact between these cells in coculture, however, sometimes binding of antibody to a receptor can lead to activatory/inhibitory signals, which can alter the results of the experiments. Therefore, another alternative is to use the cells that are knockout for specific receptors one wants to study. The cells can be obtained from knockout mice. Availability of knockout mice may be a limitation for some researchers.

4 Notes

1. Always measure the pH before use and adjust if required. It is advisable to measure/adjust pH of any buffer at room temperature. If the buffer is cold, use the advanced pH meter with temperature probe.

2. MC can be obtained/purified from a variety of sources such as: Rat peritoneum (RPMC) [30], mouse peritoneum, mouse liver [31], mouse skin [32, 33], mouse spleen [34], mouse bone

marrow (BMMC) [35]; human mast cell leukemia HMC-1 cell line [36] and LAD 2 cell line [37], human cord blood [29], human peripheral blood [38], human lung [39], human skin [40], human intestines [41], human heart [42] human uterus [43], nasal polyps [44], etc. Similarly eosinophils can be obtained from rat peritoneum [45]. Mouse eosinophils can be isolated at high purity from peripheral blood [46] of IL-5 transgenic mice [47–49], mouse bone marrow (BMEos) [20], human peripheral blood [27, 28], and a recently described method of obtaining eosinophils from human bone marrow [50].

3. Place the bones in separate wells from different mice, and all the bones of one mouse in the same well. Clean the bone as much as possible by cutting off the attached muscle with scissors carefully not to cut/break any bone. This makes it easier to flush the marrow from bones.

4. Some workers grind the bones in mortar and pestle, but it is better to flush with needle and syringe to avoid the cross-contamination of cells from different genotypes. The bone becomes clear white when the red marrow is removed.

5. Replace the culture flasks every time the medium is changed, to remove contaminating adherent cells (usually fibroblasts). This is especially important in the beginning of the culture when many adherent cells are present. Adjust the cell density to 10^6 cells/ml after 2 weeks when the bone marrow cells start to proliferate.

6. Take a sample of cell suspension (20 μl) and add 180 μl of Toluidine blue dye. Incubate for 5 min and examine under microscope. Cells should appear dense and dark blue/purple.

7. BMMC and BMEos purity/maturity can also be determined by surface staining of FcεR1 & c-Kit (for BMMC) and Siglec-F & CCR3 (for BMEos) using flow cytometry analysis. In brief, take 10^5 cells per sample in a 96-well "U" bottom plate, centrifuge for 5 min, $450 \times g$ at 4 °C and discard the supernatant. Resuspend cells with PBS+0.1 % BSA+5 % goat serum for blocking and incubate on ice. Add fluorochrome labeled Abs [α-FcεR1 & α-c-Kit for BMMC, and α-Siglec-F & α-CCR3 (for BMEos) and respective isotype matched Ab to separate wells] and incubate for 30 min on ice in the dark. Wash off excess antibodies with PBS+0.1 % BSA (200 μl/well). Resuspend cell pellet in PBS+0.1 % BSA (200–300 μl/well) and acquire the cells on a flow cytometer. Strong expressions of these markers on the surface of respective cell indicate the maturity.

8. Balb/c bone marrow cells increases in total cell number from Day 4 to Day 10 and continues to increase thereafter. However, C57BL/6 total cell number does not increase to the same

extent and lags 1–2 days behind in % eosinophils (80 % eosinophils at Day 10, 95–100 % at Day 12). Maturity of eosinophils can be determined by the surface expression of Siglec-F and CCR3 by FACS (as described in **Note 6**).

9. The viability of eosinophils in culture decrease beyond 21 day, and therefore, it is advisable not to keep the eosinophils beyond 21st day and perform the experiment as early as possible.

10. *Assay for measuring released β-hex*: A small assay should be carried out separately on MC and eosinophils to check that the cells are functional and responding well to activators. Sensitize BMMC with IgE (for example αDNP IgE 0.5 μg/ml) overnight in CO_2 incubator (37 °C) and next day wash the cells with Ty-BSA buffer (Tyrode's buffer containing 0.5 mg/ml BSA) and seed the cells in "U" bottom 96-well plate. Control wells should be included as sensitized-non activated BMMC. Activate the cells by adding allergen (for example DNP, 10 ng/ml) and incubate for 1 h at 37 °C in CO_2 incubator. Centrifuge the plate at 1,500–2,000×*g* and transfer 80 μl of supernatant from the assay plate (*plate A*) to the new plate (*plate B*). Centrifuge both the plates and discard the supernatants from the *plate A* and from *plate B*, transfer 60 μl of supernatants to the new plate (*plate C*). Wash the cell pellet (*plate A*) once with Ty-BSA, resuspend the pellet in 100 μl Ty-BSA, lyse the cells with repeated freeze (–80 °C)–thaw cycle (minimum 3 times) or by resuspending the cells pellet in Ty-BSA+1 % Triton X-100 (100 μl/well) and incubate for 15 min at RT or until the suspension becomes clear. Aliquot 20 μl/well β-hex substrate in a flat bottom 96-well plate. To this add the 20 μl of supernatant from *plate-C* and/or 20 μl of cell lysate from *plate-A* (to each of the separate wells containing β-hex substrate). Incubate for 2 h at 37 °C and then add 200 μl/well stop solution. A yellow color will develop as soon as you add the stop solution. Read the OD at 405 nm in an ELISA microplate reader. Calculate the percent release of β-hex by the following formula.

$$\% \, release = \frac{OD \, sup.}{OD \, sup. + OD \, cell \, lysate} \times 100$$

Alternatively percent net specific release [17] can be calculated with the following formula

$$\% \, Net \, specific \, release = \frac{OD \, sup._{act.} - OD \, sup._{non \, act.}}{\left(OD \, sup. + OD \, cell \, lysate\right)_{act.} - OD \, sup._{non \, act.}} \times 100$$

OD sup.: absorbance of test supernatants [released soluble mediator content in activated (act.) or non-activated (non act.) cells]

OD cell lysate: absorbance of cell lysate [intracellular mediator content that is not released from the cells].

11. *Assay for measuring released EPO*: Block a flat bottom 96-well plate with 2.5 % BSA in PBS (300 μl/well), incubate for minimum 2 h at 37 °C, rinse once with PBS. Wash the required amount of BMEos with Ty-BSA and seed BMEos 2×10^5 cells/well/100 μl. Add PAF at a final concentration of 10^{-6} M. Control wells should be included as non-activated cells, incubate for 45 min to 1 h at 37 °C. Add freshly prepared OPD substrate solution 100 μl/well and wait for color development (usually 5–15 min depending upon the cell number and released EPO). Stop the reaction by adding 100 μl/well 4 M H_2SO_4 and read the OD at 492 nm by ELISA plate reader. The results can be represented in percent release of EPO or percent net specific release as described above for β-hex (*see* **Note 10**).

12. The BMMC can be sensitized with another kind of IgE and then can be activated by the specific allergen or by anti-igE. It is advisable to first optimize the concentration of IgE for your set of experiments by performing an experiment involving at least three different concentrations of IgE, and thereafter use the one which works best.

13. Although MC can be activated in culture medium, a stronger response is usually achieved in buffers. The use of buffer also allows for spectrometric assay such as release of β-hex without color interference, as medium often contains phenol red that can interfere with such assays and actual absorbance.

14. Setting up of monoculture is achieved in two ways and can also depend upon the design of the experiment: (a) It can be equal to the number of each contributing cell type in the same final volume. For example in our case we are establishing coculture at 1:1 cell ratio (2×10^5 cells of each type/well in 200 μl). (b) It can be equal to the total number of the cells in the coculture; that means coculture of same type of cells. Then it will be 4×10^5 cells/well/200 μl, or equal to the number of each contributing cell type in coculture and keeping the cell concentration the same as in coculture that is 2×10^5 cells/100 μl. However, in both settings the results will be different so it is good if the monoculture be established both ways and the data analyzed accordingly.

15. BMEos in vitro cultures can be activated by different activators, for example, Platelet activating factor (PAF), toxins derived from *Staphylococcus aureus* bacteria (SEB, PGN, SEA, protein A).

16. Human MC are reported to express PAF receptors and can be activated with PAF [51], but BMMC may not express PAF

receptors. In addition, using our experimental conditions for stimulation of BMMC with PAF does not result in release of tryptase or β-hex.

17. Seed BMMC first then add activator keep on ice and then add BMEos, add any other desired treatment, mix well, and keep in incubator.

18. If the released tryptase levels are very low, it takes longer than 2 h to develop the color. If there is no color after 2 h, plate can be incubated again for 2 h and read the OD after that or it may be left overnight.

19. The incubation time is directly dependent on the number of cells present in the culture. The 2 h time is sufficient to quantify β-hex from approximately 10^5 cells/100 μl. The incubation time can be adjusted accordingly depending upon the number of cells present in the culture.

20. On occasions Ab binding can activate the cells, and therefore, it must be checked beforehand whether the Ab is indeed a blocking Ab and not an activating one.

Acknowledgements

The authors would like to thank to Laila Karra for her valuable comments and critical evaluation in writing this chapter. This work was supported by the Israel Science Foundation (grant 213/05), the MAARS EU 7th framework (grant no. HEALTH-F2-2011-261366), the Aimwell Charitable Trust (London, UK). F. Levi-Schaffer is affiliated with The Dr. Adolph and Klara Brettler Center for Research in Molecular Pharmacology and Therapeutics, School of Pharmacy and the Alex Grass Center for Drug Design and Synthesis of Novel Therapeutics, School of Pharmacy of The Hebrew University of Jerusalem.

References

1. Galli SJ, Grimbaldeston M, Tsai M (2008) Immunomodulatory mast cells: negative, as well as positive, regulators of immunity. Nat Rev Immunol 8:478–486

2. Bachelet I, Levi-Schaffer F, Mekori YA (2006) Mast cells: not only in allergy. Immunol Allergy Clin North Am 26:407–425

3. Bischoff SC (2007) Role of mast cells in allergic and non-allergic immune responses: comparison of human and murine data. Nat Rev Immunol 7:93–104

4. Puxeddu I, Piliponsky AM, Bachelet I et al (2003) Mast cells in allergy and beyond. Int J Biochem Cell Biol 35:1601–1607

5. Theoharides TC, Kalogeromitros D (2006) The critical role of mast cells in allergy and inflammation. Ann N Y Acad Sci 1088: 78–99

6. Galli SJ, Tsai M, Piliponsky AM (2008) The development of allergic inflammation. Nature 454:445–454

7. Kita H (2013) Eosinophils: multifunctional and distinctive properties. Int Arch Allergy Immunol 161(Suppl 2):3–9

8. Fulkerson PC, Rothenberg ME (2013) Targeting eosinophils in allergy, inflammation and beyond. Nat Rev Drug Discov 12: 117–129

9. Gleich GJ, Adolphson CR (1986) The eosinophilic leukocyte: structure and function. Adv Immunol 39:177–253

10. Rothenberg ME, Hogan SP (2006) The eosinophil. Annu Rev Immunol 24:147–174

11. Minai-Fleminger Y, Levi-Schaffer F (2009) Mast cells and eosinophils: the two key effector cells in allergic inflammation. Inflamm Res 58:631–638

12. Elishmereni M, Alenius HT, Bradding P et al (2011) Physical interactions between mast cells and eosinophils: a novel mechanism enhancing eosinophil survival in vitro. Allergy 66:376–385

13. Minai-Fleminger Y, Elishmereni M, Vita F et al (2010) Ultrastructural evidence for human mast cell-eosinophil interactions in vitro. Cell Tissue Res 341:405–415

14. Shakoory B, Fitzgerald SM, Lee SA et al (2004) The role of human mast cell-derived cytokines in eosinophil biology. J Interferon Cytokine Res 24:271–281

15. Bachelet I, Munitz A, Mankutad D et al (2006) Mast cell costimulation by CD226/CD112 (DNAM-1/Nectin-2): a novel interface in the allergic process. J Biol Chem 281:27190–27196

16. Munitz A, Bachelet I, Fraenkel S et al (2005) 2B4 (CD244) is expressed and functional on human eosinophils. J Immunol 174:110–118

17. Blank U, Rivera J (2006) Assays for regulated exocytosis of mast cell granules. Curr Protoc Cell Biol Chapter 15, Unit 15 11

18. Berent-Maoz B, Gur C, Vita F et al (2011) Influence of FAS on murine mast cell maturation. Ann Allergy Asthma Immunol 106:239–244

19. Jensen BM, Swindle EJ, Iwaki S et al (2006) Generation, isolation, and maintenance of rodent mast cells and mast cell lines. Curr Protoc Immunol Chapter 3, Unit 3 23

20. Dyer KD, Moser JM, Czapiga M et al (2008) Functionally competent eosinophils differentiated ex vivo in high purity from normal mouse bone marrow. J Immunol 181:4004–4009

21. Elishmereni M, Bachelet I, Nissim Ben-Efraim AH et al (2013) Interacting mast cells and eosinophils acquire an enhanced activation state in vitro. Allergy 68:171–179

22. Kawakami T, Galli SJ (2002) Regulation of mast-cell and basophil function and survival by IgE. Nat Rev Immunol 2:773–786

23. Galli SJ, Kalesnikoff J, Grimbaldeston MA et al (2005) Mast cells as "tunable" effector and immunoregulatory cells: recent advances. Annu Rev Immunol 23:749–786

24. Kalesnikoff J, Galli SJ (2008) New developments in mast cell biology. Nat Immunol 9:1215–1223

25. Bloemen K, Verstraelen S, Van Den Heuvel R et al (2007) The allergic cascade: review of the most important molecules in the asthmatic lung. Immunol Lett 113:6–18

26. Prussin C, Metcalfe DD (2006) 5. IgE, mast cells, basophils, and eosinophils. J Allergy Clin Immunol 117:S450–S456

27. Pretlow TP, Wilk AI, Davis LA et al (1988) Comparison of different methods for the purification of eosinophils from human peripheral blood. Anal Biochem 175:334–341

28. Hansel TT, De Vries IJ, Iff T et al (1991) An improved immunomagnetic procedure for the isolation of highly purified human blood eosinophils. J Immunol Methods 145:105–110

29. Saito H, Ebisawa M, Sakaguchi N et al (1995) Characterization of cord-blood-derived human mast cells cultured in the presence of Steel factor and interleukin-6. Int Arch Allergy Immunol 107:63–65

30. Yurt RW, Leid RW Jr, Austen KF (1977) Native heparin from rat peritoneal mast cells. J Biol Chem 252:518–521

31. Kovarova M (2013) Isolation and characterization of mast cells in mouse models of allergic diseases. Methods Mol Biol 1032:109–119

32. Yamada N, Matsushima H, Tagaya Y et al (2003) Generation of a large number of connective tissue type mast cells by culture of murine fetal skin cells. J Invest Dermatol 121:1425–1432

33. Matsue H, Kambe N, Shimada S (2009) Murine fetal skin-derived cultured mast cells: a useful tool for discovering functions of skin mast cells. J Invest Dermatol 129:1120–1125

34. Konno S, Adachi M, Asano K et al (1993) Inhibitory effect of interferon-beta on mouse spleen-derived mast cells. Mediators Inflamm 2:243–246

35. Levi-Schaffer F, Dayton ET, Austen KF et al (1987) Mouse bone marrow-derived mast cells cocultured with fibroblasts. Morphology and stimulation-induced release of histamine, leukotriene B4, leukotriene C4, and prostaglandin D2. J Immunol 139:3431–3441

36. Nilsson G, Blom T, Kusche-Gullberg M et al (1994) Phenotypic characterization of the human mast-cell line HMC-1. Scand J Immunol 39:489–498

37. Kirshenbaum AS, Akin C, Wu Y et al (2003) Characterization of novel stem cell factor responsive human mast cell lines LAD 1 and 2 established from a patient with mast cell sarcoma/leukemia; activation following aggregation of FcepsilonRI or FcgammaRI. Leuk Res 27:677–682

38. Rottem M, Okada T, Goff JP et al (1994) Mast cells cultured from the peripheral blood of

normal donors and patients with mastocytosis originate from a CD34+/Fc epsilon RI- cell population. Blood 84:2489–2496

39. Salari H, Takei F, Miller R et al (1987) Novel technique for isolation of human lung mast cells. J Immunol Methods 100:91–97

40. Church MK, Clough GF (1999) Human skin mast cells: in vitro and in vivo studies. Ann Allergy Asthma Immunol 83:471–475

41. Fox CC, Dvorak AM, Peters SP et al (1985) Isolation and characterization of human intestinal mucosal mast cells. J Immunol 135:483–491

42. Sperr WR, Bankl HC, Mundigler G et al (1994) The human cardiac mast cell: localization, isolation, phenotype, and functional characterization. Blood 84:3876–3884

43. Massey WA, Guo CB, Dvorak AM et al (1991) Human uterine mast cells. Isolation, purification, characterization, ultrastructure, and pharmacology. J Immunol 147:1621–1627

44. Finotto S, Dolovich J, Denburg JA et al (1994) Functional heterogeneity of mast cells isolated from different microenvironments within nasal polyp tissue. Clin Exp Immunol 95:343–350

45. Cypcar D, Sorkness R, Sedgwick J et al (1996) Rat eosinophils: isolation and characterization of superoxide production. J Leukoc Biol 60:101–105

46. Penttila IA, O'Keefe DE, Jenkin CR (1982) A single-step method for the enrichment of murine peripheral blood eosinophils. J Immunol Methods 51:119–123

47. Dent LA, Daly CM, Mayrhofer G et al (1999) Interleukin-5 transgenic mice show enhanced resistance to primary infections with *Nippostrongylus brasiliensis* but not primary infections with *Toxocara canis*. Infect Immun 67:989–993

48. Dent LA, Munro GH, Piper KP et al (1997) Eosinophilic interleukin 5 (IL-5) transgenic mice: eosinophil activity and impaired clearance of *Schistosoma mansoni*. Parasite Immunol 19:291–300

49. Mishra A, Hogan SP, Brandt EB et al (2002) IL-5 promotes eosinophil trafficking to the esophagus. J Immunol 168:2464–2469

50. Wong TW, Jelinek DF (2013) Purification of functional eosinophils from human bone marrow. J Immunol Methods 387:130–139

51. Kajiwara N, Sasaki T, Bradding P et al (2010) Activation of human mast cells through the platelet-activating factor receptor. J Allergy Clin Immunol 125:1137–1145 e1136

Chapter 21

Eosinophil Interactions: Antigen Presentation

Praveen Akuthota

Abstract

Eosinophils have been demonstrated in a variety of experimental models to express MHC Class II and co-stimulatory molecules necessary to act as antigen presenting cells (APCs). They also have been experimentally observed to use these expressed proteins to function as APCs. This chapter reviews basic techniques to allow for in vitro and ex vivo experimentation of human and murine eosinophil APC function.

Key words Eosinophils, Antigen presentation, Class II major histocompatibility antigens, Granulocytes, Humans

1   Introduction

The potential for eosinophils, both human and murine, to act as MHC Class II-restricted antigen presenting cells has been recognized based on their ability to express both MHC Class II and requisite co-stimulatory molecules under the proper stimulatory conditions. Lucey and colleagues made the observation that while circulating peripheral blood eosinophils in humans do not in general express MHC Class II, they could be induced to do so ex vivo when stimulated with GM-CSF [1]. Ex vivo GM-CSF stimulation also induces upregulation of MHC Class II in murine eosinophils [2]. While GM-CSF is the most potent inducer of MHC Class II and is used in this protocol, multiple other cytokines, including IL-3, can stimulate MHC Class II expression [3].

In both humans and mice, MHC Class II expression has been observed on eosinophils in a variety of activated physiologic states. In murine systems, this phenomenon is present in models of allergic airways inflammation and intraperitoneal parasitic infection [4, 5]. Human diseases that demonstrate upregulation of MHC Class II on eosinophils include asthma, chronic eosinophilic pneumonia, and

Garry M. Walsh (ed.), *Eosinophils: Methods and Protocols*, Methods in Molecular Biology, vol. 1178,
DOI 10.1007/978-1-4939-1016-8_21, © Springer Science+Business Media New York 2014

eosinophilic esophagitis [6–8]. Similarly, under proper stimulatory conditions, both human and murine eosinophils can be induced to express requisite co-stimulatory molecules such as CD40, CD80, and CD86 [2, 4, 9].

Leveraging these observations of the ability of eosinophils to express the necessary machinery to act as APCs, a robust literature investigating the functional aspects of eosinophil-mediated antigen presentation has emerged [10]. For example, the author and colleagues utilized GM-CSF-stimulated human eosinophils to demonstrate the necessity of aggregation of MHC Class II into lipid rafts for eosinophil APC function [11]. GM-CSF-stimulated murine eosinophils were a central component of a study Wang and others that showed that eosinophils can function as true APCs in a murine model of allergic airways inflammation [8]. This protocol describes GM-CSF stimulation of human and murine eosinophils to induce the expression of MHC Class II for the purpose of studying eosinophil APC function.

2   Materials

2.1   Induction of MHC Class II Expression by Eosinophils

1. Purified human eosinophils (*see* Chapter 2).

2. Hemocytometer.

3. RPMI 1640 (with 300 mg/L L-glutamine and 25 mM HEPES) for culture medium (*see* **Note 1**).

4. Fetal bovine serum for culture medium.

5. Penicillin–Streptomycin (10,000 units–10,000 µg per ml).

6. Cell culture dishes.

7. Recombinant human GM-CSF.

8. Recombinant murine GM-CSF.

2.2   Measurement of MHC Class II Expression of Human Eosinophils by Flow Cytometry

9. 1.5-ml Eppendorf tubes.

10. Hanks' Buffered Salt Solution, without calcium or magnesium (HBSS) for flow cytometry buffer (*see* **Note 2**).

11. Bovine serum albumin (BSA) for flow cytometry buffer.

12. Anti HLA-DR (MHC Class II) antibody, FITC-conjugated (*see* **Note 3**).

13. Isotype control antibody, FITC-conjugated.

3   Methods

All steps should be performed under sterile conditions using a tissue culture hood as necessary.

3.1 Induction of MHC Class II Expression by Human Eosinophils

1. Purify human eosinophils from the peripheral blood of a volunteer donor as described in Chapter 2.

2. Count eosinophils using a hemocytometer

3. Centrifuge eosinophils at $300 \times g$ for 5 min at 4 °C. Discard supernatant and resuspend in 860 µl culture medium per 1×10^6 eosinophils and transfer to a cell culture dish of appropriate size.

4. Dilute human GM-CSF stock (10 µg/ml, *see* **Note 4**) 1:1,000 in culture medium. The resulting solution will have a GM-CSF concentration of 10 ng/ml in culture medium. Add 140 µl of this solution per 1×10^6 eosinophils in the cell suspension created in the previous step. The eosinophils will now be in a cell culture dish (or multiple cell culture dishes) with a cell concentration of 1×10^6 cells per ml of medium. The final GM-CSF concentration will be 1.4 ng/ml (100 pM).

5. Incubate at 37 °C for 2 days. MHC Class II expression should now be assayed by flow cytometry (*see* **Note 5**).

3.2 Measurement of MHC Class II Expression of Human Eosinophils by Flow Cytometry

1. Transfer 2 aliquots of 2×10^5 eosinophils to 1.5-ml Eppendorf tubes (200 µl of cell suspension per tube).

2. Centrifuge eosinophils at $300 \times g$ for 5 min at 4 °C. Discard supernatant and resuspend each sample in 50 µl of flow cytometry buffer.

3. Add 2 µl of anti-HLA-DR antibody to one sample and 2 µl of isotype control antibody to the other sample.

4. Incubate on ice for 25 min.

5. Add 1 ml of flow cytometry buffer to each sample.

6. Centrifuge eosinophils at $300 \times g$ for 5 min at 4 °C. Discard supernatant and resuspend in 500 µl of flow cytometry buffer. Transfer samples to flow cytometry tubes.

7. Measure HLA-DR versus isotype control signal by flow cytometry. Human eosinophils should express MHC Class II at this point, allowing for functional studies of antigen presenting cell function (*see* **Note 6**).

3.3 Induction of MHC Class II Expression by Murine Eosinophils

1. Purify murine eosinophils by negative selection (*see* **Note 7**).

2. Count eosinophils using a hemocytometer.

3. Centrifuge eosinophils at $300 \times g$ for 5 min at 4 °C. Discard supernatant and resuspend in 1 ml culture medium per 1×10^6 eosinophils and transfer to a cell culture dish (or multiple cell culture dishes) of appropriate size.

4. Add 1 µl of murine GM-CSF stock (10 µg/ml, *see* **Note 1**) per 1×10^6 eosinophils. The resulting final GM-CSF concentration will be 10 ng/ml (714 pM).

5. Incubate at 37 °C for 1 day (*see* **Note 8**). MHC Class II expression can now be assayed by flow cytometry if desired (*see* **Note 9** and Chapter 13).

4 Notes

1. Culture medium consists of RPMI 1640 with 10 % fetal bovine serum and 1 % penicillin–streptomycin.

2. Flow cytometry buffer consists of HBSS (calcium and magnesium free) with 0.5 % (w/v) BSA.

3. There are many commercially available antibodies against human HLA-DR available. The author has used clone TU36 from BD Pharmingen for this specific application, along with the corresponding mouse IgG_{2bK} isotype control antibody.

4. Commercially available lyophilized human and murine GM-CSF is reconstituted in sterile PBS with 0.1 % bovine serum albumin (filtered with 0.2 μm filter prior to addition to GM-CSF).

5. Because there may be donor to donor variability when working with human eosinophils, incubating with GM-CSF for 2 days rather than only 1 day is recommended to best ensure optimal expression of MHC Class II. This inherent variability between human donors is also the reason confirmation of MHC Class II expression by flow cytometry is recommended. The presence of GM-CSF in the culture medium also maintains the viability of eosinophils by inhibition of apoptosis.

6. For example, we have used a superantigen-mediated approach to study APC interactions between human eosinophils and lymphocytes [11].

7. IL-5 transgenic mice, which have an abundance of eosinophils, are an attractive option for obtaining murine eosinophils. Negative selection of peritoneal lavage fluid [12] or single cell suspensions prepared from spleens [8] can both be employed to obtain eosinophils from IL-5 transgenic mice.

8. GM-CSF incubation for 1 day has been adequate for inducing MHC Class II expression in splenic eosinophils from IL-5 transgenic mice [8].

9. Unlike the case with human eosinophils, variability does not pose as much of a challenge in murine experiments. However, assessing for MHC Class II expression is still useful as a confirmatory measure.

Acknowledgments

This work was supported by a HOPE Pilot Grant from the American Partnership for Eosinophilic Disorders to P.A.

References

1. Lucey D, Nicholson-Weller A, Weller P (1989) Mature human eosinophils have the capacity to express HLA-DR. Proc Natl Acad Sci U S A 86:1348–1351

2. Wang H, Ghiran I, Matthaei K et al (2007) Airway eosinophils: allergic inflammation recruited professional antigen-presenting cells. J Immunol 179:7585–7592

3. Weller P, Rand T, Barrett T et al (1993) Accessory cell function of human eosinophils. HLA-DR-dependent, MHC-restricted antigen-presentation and IL-1 alpha expression. J Immunol 150:2554–2562

4. MacKenzie J, Mattes J, Dent L et al (2001) Eosinophils promote allergic disease of the lung by regulating CD4(+) Th2 lymphocyte function. J Immunol 167:3146–3155

5. Mawhorter S, Pearlman E, Kazura J et al (1993) Class II major histocompatibility complex molecule expression on murine eosinophils activated in vivo by Brugia malayi. Infect Immun 61:5410–5412

6. Hansel T, Braunstein J, Walker C et al (1991) Sputum eosinophils from asthmatics express ICAM-1 and HLA-DR. Clin Exp Immunol 86:271–277

7. Beninati W, Derdak S, Dixon P et al (1993) Pulmonary eosinophils express HLA-DR in chronic eosinophilic pneumonia. J Allergy Clin Immunol 92:442–449

8. Patel A, Fuentebella J, Gernez Y et al (2010) Increased HLA-DR expression on tissue eosinophils in eosinophilic esophagitis. J Pediatr Gastroenterol Nutr 51:290–294

9. Celestin J, Rotschke O, Falk K et al (2001) IL-3 induces B7.2 (CD86) expression and costimulatory activity in human eosinophils. J Immunol 167:6097–6104

10. Akuthota P, Wang H, Spencer L et al (2008) Immunoregulatory roles of eosinophils: a new look at a familiar cell. Clin Exp Allergy 38:1254–1263

11. Akuthota P, Spencer L, Melo R et al (2012) MHC Class II and CD9 in human eosinophils localize to detergent-resistant membrane microdomains. Am J Respir Cell Mol Biol 46:188–195

12. Shi H, Humbles A, Gerard C et al (2000) Lymph node trafficking and antigen presentation by endobronchial eosinophils. J Clin Invest 105:945–953

Chapter 22

Eosinophils and Respiratory Virus Infection: A Dual-Standard Curve qRT-PCR-Based Method for Determining Virus Recovery from Mouse Lung Tissue

Caroline M. Percopo, Kimberly D. Dyer, Kendal A. Karpe, Joseph B. Domachowske, and Helene F. Rosenberg

Abstract

Several lines of investigation have indicated a role for eosinophilic leukocytes in limiting virus infectivity and promoting virion clearance. We have established a respiratory virus infection model with pneumonia virus of mice (PVM; family *Paramyxoviridae*), a natural mouse pathogen that replicates the more severe forms of human disease elicited by the phylogenetically related respiratory syncytial virus (RSV). In this chapter, we present a rapid and highly reproducible dual-standard curve qRT-PCR based method for quantitative detection of PVM replication in mouse lung tissue. We have used this assay to evaluate eosinophil-mediated antiviral host defense in mouse models of cytokine and antigen-driven eosinophilic inflammation.

Key words Inflammation, Leukocyte, Eosinophil, Pneumonia virus of mice, Polymerase chain reaction

1   Introduction

Asthma is a chronic inflammatory disease of the respiratory tract characterized by reversible airway hyperresponsiveness of uncertain etiology [1]. Although the disease is heterogeneous in nature [2, 3], eosinophils are frequently identified as components of airway infiltrates and are particularly numerous in the recently defined eosinophilic asthma phenotype [4, 5]. Mouse models of allergic airways inflammation suggest that eosinophils promote pulmonary pathology, which also includes mucus accumulation and tissue remodeling [6, 7]. Respiratory viruses play a major part in promoting asthma exacerbations, while at the same time, studies carried out in vitro and in mouse models document a role for eosinophils in limiting virus infectivity and promoting virion clearance, respectively [8–10].

Garry M. Walsh (ed.), *Eosinophils: Methods and Protocols*, Methods in Molecular Biology, vol. 1178, DOI 10.1007/978-1-4939-1016-8_22, © Springer Science+Business Media New York 2014

In our laboratory, we are exploring antiviral responses in mouse models of cytokine and antigen-driven eosinophilic airway inflammation [11]. We have established respiratory virus infections with pneumonia virus of mice (PVM; family *Paramyxoviridae*), a natural mouse pathogen that is closely related to the human respiratory syncytial virus (RSV). However, unlike RSV challenge in mice, PVM undergoes robust replication in mouse lung tissue in vivo and can elicit severe morbidity and mortality in a rodent host [12]. To facilitate these and related studies [13–15] we have developed a rapid and reproducible assay for quantitative detection of PVM replication. This assay utilizes two standard curves—one that permits determination of absolute copies of virus small hydrophobic (SH) protein nucleic acid, and the other, the cellular housekeeping GAPDH gene. This permits us to present our findings as the unitless and highly reproducible ratio of absolute copies of virus PVM_{SH} to absolute copies of cellular GAPDH. This ratio of absolute values controls for small variations in amounts of input RNA. We have shown that the results of this assay run in parallel to more traditional measurements of virus infectivity, such as tissue-culture infectious dose ($TCID_{50}$) when using lung homogenates from PVM-infected mice (Fig. 1).

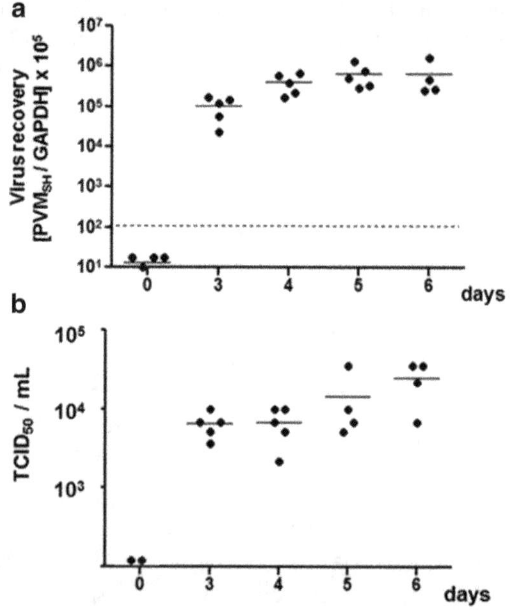

Fig. 1 Comparison of quantitative (q)RT-PCR and $TCID_{50}$ assays for detection of PVM in infected mouse lung samples. One lung from each PVM-infected mouse was used to prepare RNA for (**a**) the qRT-PCR assay and the other lung was used to prepare tissue homogenates for (**b**) the $TCID_{50}$ assay. Although each assay measures a different property of the virus—the qRT-PCR assay is designed to detect increasing levels virus nucleic acid via targeting the PVM SH gene, while the $TCID_{50}$ assay detects infectious virions—as shown here, either assay can be used to document log-fold increases in virus recovery observed during replication in lung tissue in vivo. Reprinted with permission from [15]

2   Materials

<table>
<tr><td valign="top">2.1   Storage of Tissue
and Isolation of RNA
from Tissue</td><td>

1. RNA-later (Life Technologies, catalog no. AM7020).

2. RNA-Bee (Tel-test, catalog no. Cs-104B).

3. Diethyl-pyrocarbonate (DEPC)-treated water (can be purchased, or distilled water treated with DEPC overnight at 37 °C and then autoclaved).

4. 2-Propanol.

5. Chloroform.

6. 100 % Ethanol.

7. Falcon 2059 polypropylene tubes.

8. Autoclaved pipet tips and microfuge tubes.

9. Glass transfer pipets.

10. Blade homogenizer.

11. 15 mL polypropylene screw-top tubes.

</td></tr>
<tr><td valign="top">2.2   DNase
I Digestion of Genomic
DNA Contaminants</td><td>

1. DNase I (Invitrogen catalog no. 18068-015) with 10× Reaction Buffer and 25 mM EDTA, pH 8.0 stop solution.

</td></tr>
<tr><td valign="top">2.3   First Strand
cDNA Synthesis</td><td>

1. First strand cDNA synthesis kit for RT-PCR (Roche Applied Science catalog no. 11483188001) which includes (relevant to this protocol) AMV reverse transcriptase with 10 mM dNTPs, 10× Reaction Buffer, 25 mM $MgCl_2$, 1.6 µg/µL Random primer solution, 50 U/µL RNase inhibitor and sterile water.

</td></tr>
<tr><td valign="top">2.4   Quantitative PCR
Reaction</td><td>

1. ABI TaqMan 2× Reagent (Applied Biosystems, catalog no. 4304437).

2. Primers/Probe (Mouse GAPDH; Applied Biosystems catalog no. 4352339E.

3. Primers/Probe (PVM small hydrophobic SH gene; custom design).

   Primer 1 5′-GCCGTC ATC AAC ACA GTG TGT-3′.

   Primer 2 5′-GCC TGA TGT GGC AGT GCT T-3′.

   Probe 6FAM -CGC TGA TAA TGG CCT GCA GCA-TAMRA.

Primers are reconstituted in distilled H_2O to 20 µM and probe is diluted to 7.7 µM. Primers and probe are mixed in a 1:1 ratio, divided into aliquots, and stored at −80 °C; *see* **Note 1**.

</td></tr>
<tr><td valign="top">2.5   Calibration
Standards</td><td>

1. Mouse GAPDH (mGAPDH) in pCMV Sport 6 (American Type Culture Collection catalog no. 10539385).

2. Pneumonia virus of mice (PVM) small hydrophobic (SH) gene open reading frame (GenBank accession no. AY573815) in pBacPAK8 available from authors (e-mail: hrosenberg@niaid.nih.gov).

</td></tr>
</table>

3   Methods

3.1 Extraction and Storage of Lung Tissue from Virus-Infected Mice

1. Mice are sacrificed under approved humane conditions, and lungs dissected from body cavity under aseptic conditions.

2. Lungs from each mouse are cut into multiple (3–4) pieces to increase surface to volume ratio and immersed in 4–5 mL pre-chilled RNAlater in a Falcon 2059 tube, which is kept on ice until all samples are collected. Lung tissue is stored overnight at 4 °C in RNAlater and then frozen in RNAlater at –80 °C until one is ready to isolate RNA from tissue (*see* **Note 2**).

3.2 Isolation of RNA from Lung Tissue

It is important to remember that RNA is fragile and easily hydrolyzed by trace amounts of ribonucleases, which are present in the environment and on fingertips. Gloves should be worn when handling tubes containing RNA. All pipet tips and microfuge tubes should be autoclaved or documented as RNase-free. Some labs set aside a dedicated set of Pipetman for RNA work.

1. Tissue samples are removed from the –80 °C freezer and thawed slowly on ice.

2. Lung tissue samples are removed from the RNAlater, rinsed thoroughly in DEPC-treated water and then immersed in 4 mL RNA-Bee (*see* **Note 3**) in a fresh Falcon 2059 tube. When working with RNA-Bee, which contains caustic phenol, one must wear gloves, eye-protection and a lab coat; RNA-Bee is transferred to tubes with glass transfer pipets only.

3. Tissue is blade-homogenized in RNA-Bee at a moderate setting (50–60).

4. Add 1/10 volume (400 µL) chloroform to each tube; attach top tightly, agitate to mix thoroughly and place tube on ice for 10 min.

5. Centrifuge at 4 °C, $1{,}800 \times g$ in a swinging bucket rotor in a Thermo Scientific table top centrifuge for 15 min; this promotes separation of aqueous and organic layers. The top layer (aqueous) contains the RNA; carefully remove this layer (~1 mL) with a sterile barrier tip staying clear of the dense protein layer separating the aqueous from the organic layer below.

6. Transfer aqueous phase to a 15 mL polypropylene screw-top tube. Add an equal volume of 2-propanol. Place in –20 °C freezer for 1 h to overnight to precipitate RNA.

7. Collect precipitate by centrifugation as above, $1{,}800 \times g$, 4 °C for 10–15 min. A tiny precipitate should be visible at the bottom of each tube. To remove supernatant, use a sterile 2 mL pipet with the cotton plug removed attached to vacuum suction; carefully aspirate supernatant while not disturbing the pellet.

8. Wash the pellet with 5 mL ice-cold 80 % ethanol prepared in DEPC-treated water. Centrifuge and aspirate supernatant as above. Invert tube and blot on bench paper; keep tube inverted for 5–10 min with continuous blotting.

9. Resuspend pellet in 50–100 μL DEPC-treated water, and transfer to an autoclaved microfuge tube. Determine amount of RNA and purity spectrophotometrically (A_{260}/A_{280}; **Note 4**). Remember that all RNA samples are fragile and should be handled carefully with gloves and maintained on ice. Store samples at –80 °C or use directly to generate cDNA as below.

3.3 DNase I Treatment of RNA

It is crucial to remove any contaminating DNA from the RNA preparations. Even if the PCR primers are designed so that they will not amplify genomic targets, DNA contaminants can bind to primers and interfere with quantitative reactions.

1. Combine in an autoclaved microfuge tube: 2 μL 10× DNase I reaction buffer, 2 μg RNA isolated as described in Subheading 3.1, and DEPC-treated water to 18 μL. Add 2 μL DNase I. Incubate at room temperature for 15 min.

2. After incubation, add 2 μL 25 mM EDTA to stop the reaction and incubate at 65 °C for 10 min to inactivate the DNase I enzyme.

3.4 Synthesis of First-Strand cDNA

This is accomplished with the method and reagents in the cDNA First strand synthesis kit using the DNase I-treated RNA generated in Subheading 3.2 above.

1. Combine in an autoclaved microfuge tube 2 μL of 10× Reaction Buffer, 4 μL of 25 mM $MgCl_2$, 2 μL 10 mM dNTP mix, 2 μL of random primer, 1 μL of RNase Inhibitor, 0.8 μL AMV-RT, and 8.2 μL DNase I-treated RNA. Create a duplicate control reaction with 0.8 μL DEPC-treated water in place of AMV-RT that will be included in the qPCR reactions as a (–)RT control.

2. In a thermocycler, set the following incubation times: 25 °C for 10 min to permit primer hybridization, 42 °C for 60 min to permit primed-DNA synthesis, and 99 °C for 5 min to deactivate the AMV-RT enzyme, followed by cessation of the reaction at 4 °C for 5 min. The samples can then be removed and stored at –80 °C or used immediately.

3.5 Quantitative Polymerase Chain Reaction (qPCR)

Each cDNA generated above will be evaluated in the dual standard curve assay, with assays run in duplicate to assess the C_t, or cycle threshold, using primers and probe for the virus SH gene as well as those targeting the cellular housekeeping gene (GAPDH). The no reverse transcriptase (–RT) controls can be run in single wells. At the same time, qPCR is performed in duplicate on tenfold serial dilutions of known copy numbers of plasmids that encode either the virus SH gene or mouse GAPDH to generate standard curves (i.e., C_t vs. gene copy; Fig. 2). A comprehensive review of absolute quantitation using qRT-PCR can be found from Invitrogen—Applied Biosciences at http://tools.invitrogen.com/content/sfs/manuals/cms_041436.pdf.

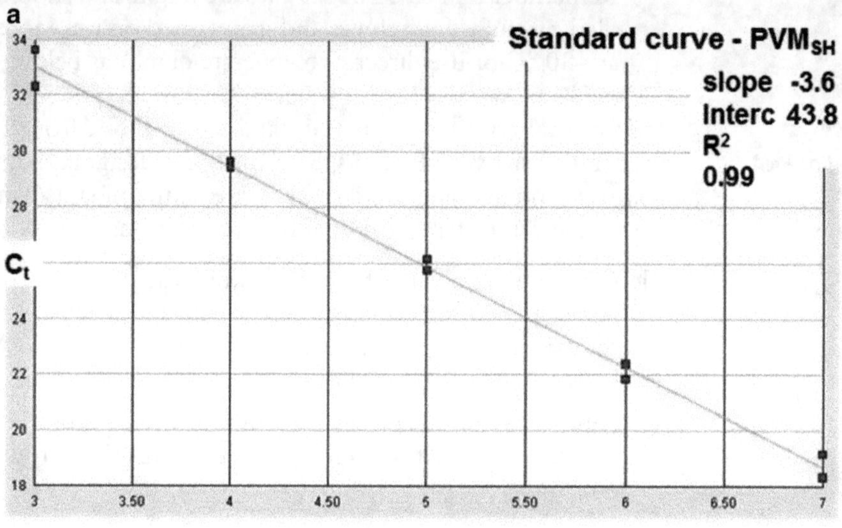

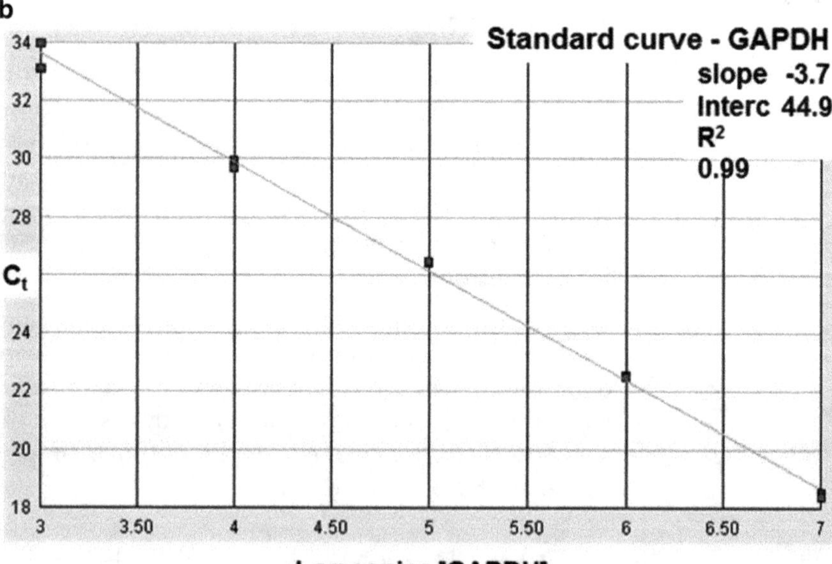

Fig. 2 Standard curves for determination of virus recovery (PVM_SH/GAPDH). Shown are the results of qPCR using serial tenfold dilutions of plasmids encoding target (**a**) virus SH gene (PVM_SH-pBACpaK8) and (**b**) mouse GAPDH (mGAPDH-pCMVSport6). Copy numbers from unknowns—both PVM_SH and GAPDH—can be determined by interpolating graphs of C_t versus copy number as shown

1. A single qPCR test primer reaction (25 μL total) includes 12.5 μL 2× ABI TaqMan 2× Reagent, 10.5 μL distilled water, 1.0 μL PVM SH Custom Primers/Probe, and 1.0 μL cDNA template prepared as in Subheading 3.3. This reaction is run in duplicate for each cDNA template. A mastermix can be created and distributed (24 μL/well) with cDNA added as the final step.

2. On the same plate, serial dilutions of known quantities of the PVM_{SH} pBacPAK8 plasmid are included in duplicate 25 μL reactions prepared as above. Suggested quantities include 10^2–10^9 molecules per reaction, added in 1.0 μL volumes. See support protocol (Subheading 3.5) for information on calculating quantities of molecules from plasmid preparations.

3. A single qPCR control reaction (also 25 μL total) is prepared as described in **step 1**, save for the use of 1.0 μL mGAPDH commercial primers/probe; as above, this reaction is to be run in duplicate for each cDNA template, and a mastermix can be created and distributed (24 μL/well) with cDNAs added as a final step. These reactions can be run on a separate plate from the test reactions.

4. As in **step 2**, serial dilutions of known quantities of mGAPDH-pCMV Sport 6 plasmid are included in duplicate 25 μL reactions. Suggested quantities include 10^6–10^9 molecules added in 1.0 μL volumes. The GAPDH reactions can be run on a separate plate from the PVM_{SH} reactions, but each standard curve should be on the same plate with its own test samples.

5. Thermocycling parameters for the ABI 7500 thermocycler using the Absolute Quantitation Program can be set at 50 °C for 2 min, 95 °C for 10 min, followed by 40 cycles of alternating 95 °C for 15 s and 60 °C for 1 min (*see* also **Note 5**).

3.6 Support Protocol: Calculating Molecules per μL for Standard Curves

These calculations assume that the reader can perform a standard plasmid isolation. We typically isolate plasmids using the PowerPrep HP plasmid isolation kit following the package insert instructions, which can also be found online at http://www.origene.com/other/Plasmid_Purification/more.aspx. The following is a calculation used to determine the number of molecules at a given concentration.

1. The PVM SH gene has been introduced into the pBacPAK8 plasmid; the vector plus insert together represent 5,778 base pairs. With the average molecular mass of a nucleotide base pair at 660 Da, the estimated plasmid molecular mass is 3.8×10^6.

2. The concentration of plasmid in solution is determined by measuring the absorbance at 260 nm (i.e., OD_{260} of $1.0 = 50$ μg/mL double-stranded DNA). If the concentration of the plasmid

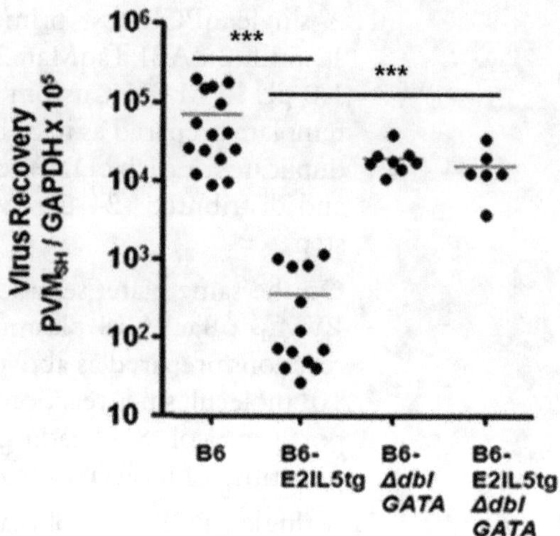

Fig. 3 Eosinophils limit virus infectivity in vivo. Virus recovery at 4 days after inoculation with pneumonia virus of mice (PVM), determined as absolute copy number of virus SH gene per absolute copy number cellular GAPDH (PVM$_{SH}$/GAPDH) in samples of total lung RNA; ***$p < 0.005$ (Mann–Whitney, two-tailed), mouse strains include wild-type C57BL/6 (B6), pulmonary eosinophil-enriched B6-E2IL5tg [16] and eosinophil-deficient strains B6-ΔdblGATA and B6-E2IL5tg-ΔdblGATA. Reprinted with permission from [11]

preparation of 1.0 μg/μL, or 10^{-6} g/μL, this represents $10^{-6}/3.8 \times 10^6 = 0.26 \times 10^{-12}$ or 2.6^{-13} mol/μL at this concentration.

3. With Avogadro's number (1 mol contains 6.023×10^{23} molecules), this converts to 15.7 or 16×10^{10} molecules/μL at this concentration.

4. As the plasmid contains 2 copies of the SH gene per molecule, we divide this in half, so at a concentration of 1.0 μg/μL, the value becomes 8×10^{10} SH gene copies/μL.

5. From here, one prepares serial tenfold dilutions as appropriate to generate multiple points as for a standard curve. The same calculations can be done for the mGAPDH pCMV-Sport 6 plasmid, which includes 5,651 base pairs and calculates to an estimated molecular mass of 3.73×10^6.

We have used this method to examine the impact of degranulating eosinophils on virus recovery from mouse lung tissue (Fig. 3).

4   Notes

1. *Virus sequences.* It is always worthwhile amplifying and sequencing the virus target and confirming 100 % match before ordering primers and probe.

2. *Stabilizing tissue in RNAlater.* We do this routinely, as isolating RNA is very time-consuming and needs one's full attention. The tubes containing RNAlater should be chilled on ice prior to adding tissue, an important step particularly when planning to store eosinophil-enriched tissue. While many protocols suggest that tissue should be removed from RNAlater prior to freezing, we have had no difficulty with isolating high quality RNA from lung tissue that was frozen in RNAlater, although one must be diligent about washing the samples off in DEPC-treated water prior to immersing them in RNA-Bee. There are recipes for RNAlater substitutes available on the Internet; we have not had the opportunity to examine them.

3. *Use of RNA-Bee.* RNA-Bee is a phenol-based RNA isolation reagent with blue dye that marks the organic solvent layer. This is helpful but probably not absolutely necessary; other RNAzol-type reagents may be substituted. Note that this reagent is caustic and protective gear (eye protection, lab coat, gloves) should be worn at all times.

4. *Quality control.* If the GAPDH C_ts are greater than 25, the RNA may be degraded (not fixable) or may simply need further cleaning (fixable). A post-isolation RNA cleanup kit may be used; RNAeasy mini kit, Qiagen catalog no. 74104. Start by targeting the samples with high GAPDH values; if successful in reducing the GAPDH values to a useful range ($C_t = 18$–22), use the kit on all samples in a set for overall consistency.

5. *ABI 7500 use and maintenance.* This machine should be used carefully and calibrated at least once a year according to the manufacturer's directions. This includes yearly maintenance by an ABI service representative and additional calibration as necessary using Spectral calibration kits I and II (ABI catalog numbers 4349180 and 4351151, respectively).

Acknowledgements

Support provided by NIAID Division of Intramural Research (AI000941 and AI000943) to HFR and Children's Miracle Network of New York to JBD.

References

1. Edwards MR, Bartlett NW, Hussell T, Openshaw P, Johnston SL (2012) The microbiology of asthma. Nat Rev Microbiol 10:459–471

2. Gibson PG (2009) Inflammatory phenotypes in adult asthma: clinical applications. Clin Respir J 3:198–206

3. Lin TY, Poon AH, Hamid Q (2013) Asthma phenotypes and endotypes. Curr Opin Pulm Med 19:18–23

4. Walsh GM (2013) Profile of reslizumab in eosinophilic disease and its potential in the treatment of poorly controlled eosinophilic asthma. Biologics 7:7–11

5. Castro M, Mathur S, Hargreave F, Boulet LP, Xie F, Young J, Wilkins HJ, Henkel T, Nair P, Res-5-0010 Study Group (2010) Reslizumab for poorly controlled, eosinophilic asthma: a randomized, placebo controlled study. Am J Respir Crit Care Med 184:1125–1132

6. Thomas A, Busse W (2012) The evolving role of eosinophils in asthma. In: Lee JJ, Rosenberg HF (eds) Eosinophils in health and disease. Elsevier, Inc., Waltham, MA, pp 448–461

7. Rosenberg HF, Dyer KD, Foster PS (2013) Eosinophils: changing perspectives in health and disease. Nat Rev Immunol 13:9–22

8. Domachowske JB, Dyer KD, Bonville CA, Rosenberg HF (1998) Recombinant human eosinophil-derived neurotoxin/RNase 2 functions as an effective antiviral agent against respiratory syncytial virus. J Infect Dis 177:1458–1464

9. Adamko DJ, Yost BL, Gleich GJ, Fryer AD, Jacoby DB (1999) Ovalbumin sensitization changes the inflammatory response to subsequent parainfluenza infection. Eosinophils mediate airway hyperresponsiveness, m(2) muscarinic receptor dysfunction and antiviral effects. J Exp Med 190:1465–1478

10. Phipps S, Lam CE, Mahalingam S, Newhouse M, Ramirez R, Rosenberg HF, Foster PS, Matthaei KI (2007) Eosinophils contribute to innate antiviral immunity and promote clearance of respiratory syncytial virus. Blood 110:1578–1586

11. Percopo CM, Dyer KD, Ochkur SI, Luo JL, Fischer ER, Lee JJ, Lee NA, Domachowske JB, Rosenberg HF (2014) Activated mouse eosinophils protect against lethal respiratory virus infection. Blood. 123:743–752

12. Bem RA, Domachowske JB, Rosenberg HF (2011) Animal models of human respiratory syncytial virus disease. Am J Physiol Lung Cell Mol Physiol 301:L148–L156

13. Gabryszewski SJ, Bachar O, Dyer KD, Percopo CM, Killoran KE, Domachowske JB, Rosenberg HF (2011) Lactobacilllus-mediated priming of the respiratory mucosa protects against lethal pneumovirus infection. J Immunol 186:1151–1161

14. Garcia-Crespo KE, Chan CC, Gabryszewski SJ, Percopo CM, Rigaux P, Dyer KD, Domachowske JB, Rosenberg HF (2013) Lactobacillus priming of the respiratory tract: heterologous immunity and protection against lethal pneumovirus infection. Antiviral Res 97:270–279

15. Glineur SF, Renshaw RW, Percopo CM, Dyer KD, Dubovi EJ, Domachowske JB, Rosenberg HF (2013) Novel pneumoviruses (PnVs): evolution and inflammatory pathology. Virology 443:257–264

16. Ochkur SI, Jacobsen EA, Protheroe CA, Biechele TL, Pero RS, McGarry MP, Wang H, O'Neill KR, Colbert DC, Colby TV, Shen H, Blackburn MR, Irvin CC, Lee JJ, Lee NA (2007) Co-expression of IL-5 and eotaxin-2 in mice creates an eosinophil-dependent model of respiratory inflammation with characteristics of severe asthma. J Immunol 178:7879–7889

Chapter 23

Antimicrobial Activity of Human Eosinophil Granule Proteins

Anu Chopra and Janendra K. Batra

Abstract

Eosinophils secrete a number of proinflammatory mediators, like cytokines, chemokines, and granule proteins which are responsible for the initiation and sustenance of inflammatory response caused by them. The eosinophil granule proteins, ECP, EDN, MBP, and EPO possess antimicrobial activity against bacteria, helminths, protozoa, and viruses. In this chapter, we describe various assays used to detect and quantitate the antimicrobial activities of eosinophil granule proteins, particularly ECP and EDN. We have taken a model organism for each assay and described the method for antiviral, antihelminthic, antiprotozoan, and antibacterial activity of purified eosinophil granule proteins.

Key words Eosinophil granule protein, Antiviral, Antibacterial, Antihelminthic, Antiprotozoan

1 Introduction

Eosinophils are non-dividing, terminally differentiated leukocytes having a bilobed nucleus with highly condensed chromatin and densely granulated cytoplasm [1]. These granules have a crystalloid core that contains major basic protein (MBP), while the matrix of the granule is composed of highly charged eosinophil cationic protein (ECP), eosinophil derived neurotoxin (EDN), and eosinophil peroxidase (EPO) along with lysosomal hydrolases and a number of cytokines [2].

MBP is the most predominant protein in eosinophil granules and gets its name because of its relative abundance and highly basic character [3]. MBP has been strongly implicated in the pathogenesis of asthma and other allergic disorders characterized by eosinophilia [4]. EDN derives its name as a neurotoxin by virtue of its ability to cause neurotoxicity in animal models [5, 6]. ECP is a highly basic granule protein which acts as a clinical marker for monitoring various inflammatory diseases [7, 8]. Both ECP and EDN are weak ribonucleases and have been classified under the RNase A superfamily. EPO is a heme-containing haloperoxidase [9].

Garry M. Walsh (ed.), *Eosinophils: Methods and Protocols*, Methods in Molecular Biology, vol. 1178,
DOI 10.1007/978-1-4939-1016-8_23, © Springer Science+Business Media New York 2014

267

It is an important constituent of the innate immune system and is a mediator for various hypersensitivity mechanisms [10, 11].

The beneficial function of eosinophils has been primarily attributed to their ability to defend the host against parasitic helminths. Upon infection, the eosinophils aggregate and degranulate to secrete their granule proteins in the local vicinity of damaged parasites [12]. MBP and ECP are potent helminthotoxins [13, 14], while EDN is marginally toxic to schistosomula of *Schistosoma mansoni* [15], newborn larvae of *Trichinella spiralis* [16], and microfilariae of *Brugia pahangi* and *Brugia malayi*, the parasite nematodes that trigger filariasis and tropical pulmonary eosinophilia [17]. ECP also exhibits toxicity on protozoans like *Trypanosoma cruzi* [18–20], *Plasmodium falciparum* [21], and *Leishmania donovani* [22]. EPO is potent toxin for bacteria and parasites like *Mycobacterium tuberculosis* [23], *S. mansoni* [24], *T. spiralis* [25], *and Brugia* species [17]. ECP and MBP are bactericidal and reported to be active against both gram-positive and gram-negative bacteria [22, 26]. *E. coli* and *H. pylori* infections induce the release of ECP in serum and gastric juice of the affected individuals [27, 28] while increased degranulation of MBP is observed in the intestinal eosinophils of patients infected with *Vibrio cholerae* and *Shigella* [29, 30]. EDN, and to a lesser extent ECP possesses antiviral activity against single stranded RNA viruses like RSV [31]. Recombinant EDN is also reported to possess inhibitory activity against HIV and hepatitis B virus [32, 33].

The eosinophil granule proteins can be purified from patients with hypersensitivity and eosinophilia [34] or prepared using recombinant technology. In our lab, we have cloned and expressed recombinant ECP and EDN in *E. coli* BL21 RIL, and purified to homogeneity from inclusion bodies ([22, 35] and as described in Chapter 10). Various assays are available for the detection of antimicrobial activity of these proteins in vitro. The antihelminthic activity of the granule proteins is measured on *Schistosoma mansoni* by incubating the *schistosomula* with varying concentrations of the purified granule protein and fluorochrome DAPI, and then scoring the dead microorganisms [15, 36, 37]. *S. mansoni* is maintained in *Blomphalaria glabrata* snails, and golden hamsters or mice [37]. The antibacterial activity of the eosinophil granule proteins, ECP and MBP is measured by the bactericidal assay described by Lehrer et al. [26]. The stationary phase bacterial cultures are incubated with the eosinophil proteins and plated onto broth plates. The bactericidal activity is assessed by counting the number of colony forming units as a function of protein concentration. The antiprotozoan activity of ECP is measured by taking *Leishmania donovani* as a model organism [22]. Leishmania promastigotes are incubated with varying concentrations of the protein and the live cells are determined by MTT assay. The MTT cell viability assay is a colorimetric assay which measures the reduction of a tetrazolium component,

MTT into an insoluble formazan product by the mitochondria of viable cells. The antiviral activity of EDN and ECP is measured on ssRNA virus RSV by shell vial assay described by Domachowske and Bonville [31] with some modifications [38]. The Hep-2 mammalian cell line is infected with RSV-B virus, and incubated with the granule proteins. Indirect immunofluorescence staining using anti-RSV antibody is used to count the infected cells and antiviral activity expressed as ID_{50} value that represent the concentration of protein that inhibit viral infection by 50 %. A PCR based method has also been used to quantify anti-RSV activity of the eosinophil granule proteins, wherein expression of a virus-specific G protein is quantified in infected cells by real-time PCR [38].

2   Materials

Prepare all solutions using ultrapure water prepared by purifying deionized water to attain a sensitivity of 18 MΩ cm at 25 °C and use analytical grade reagents. Prepare and store all reagents at room temperature (unless indicated otherwise). All the autoclaving is done at 121 °C, 15 psi for 15 min.

2.1   Culture Media and Buffers

1. Dulbecco's MEM high glucose (DMEM) pH 7 and 7.2.

2. Fetal Calf Serum (FCS): Heat-inactivate the serum at 55 °C for 1 h in a waterbath before use. Aliquot in 50 ml tubes and store at –20 °C (*see* **Note 1**).

3. M199 medium.

4. Luria–Bertani medium (LB): Dissolve 10 g Tryptone, 5 g yeast extract, and 10 g NaCl in 950 ml water. Adjust the pH of the solution to 7.0 with NaOH and bring the volume up to 1 l and autoclave.

5. LB agar: Add 1.5 g agar in 100 ml LB medium and autoclave.

6. Phosphate buffered saline, 50 mM, pH 7.4 (PBS): Add 39 mM Na_2HPO_4, 11 mM $NaH_2PO_4·2H_2O$, and 138 mM NaCl in 950 ml water and adjust the pH with 10 N NaOH. Make up the volume to 1 l.

7. 100× antibiotic–antimycotic solution: 10,000 U/ml penicillin and 10,000 μg/ml streptomycin.

2.2   Shell Vial Assay

1. Complete DMEM with 10 % FCS: To 100 ml of DMEM add 10 ml FCS and 1 ml antibiotic–antimycotic solution.

2. DMEM with 2 % FCS: Add 2 ml heat-inactivated FCS to filter-sterilized 100 ml DMEM. No antibiotic is added to it when used to propagate RSV.

3. 10× Trypsin-EDTA (Invitrogen): Make small aliquots of the stock bottle and keep at –20 °C (*see* **Note 1**).

4. Acetone: Chill the acetone at –20 °C for at least 1 h before using for fixation.

5. Saponin solution, 0.01 % for permeabilization: Weigh 1 mg saponin and dissolve it in 10 ml autoclaved water.

6. Blocking solution: 3 % Normal goat serum (NGS). Prepare 5 ml blocking solution by adding 150 μl NGS in 4.85 ml saponin solution as prepared above.

7. Glycerol.

8. Neubauer's chamber and trypan blue dye for cell counting (*see* **Note 2**).

9. Autoclaved coverslips: clean the coverslips by keeping them overnight in acetone and wash them with autoclaved water. Put the coverslips in glass petri dishes and autoclave (*see* **Note 3**).

10. 24-well plate with lid.

2.3 Antibody and Conjugate

1. Mouse anti-RSV antibody.

2. Goat anti-mouse FITC conjugate.

2.4 RT-PCR Assay for Antiviral Activity Against RSV

1. Autoclaved DEPC treated water: Add 0.1 % DEPC in water, stir overnight in a dark bottle on a magnetic stirrer and then autoclave.

2. Trizol-LS reagent (Invitrogen).

3. Chloroform.

4. Isopropanol.

5. 75 % ethanol: Mix 75 ml ethanol with 25 ml autoclaved DEPC treated water.

6. dNTP mix: Add 5 μl of each dNTP (dATP, dGTP, dCTP and dTTP) from 10 mM stock in a microfuge tube and add 180 μl fresh autoclaved water. Store it at –20 °C.

7. Random hexamers.

8. 10× Reaction buffer.

9. M-MuLV Reverse transcriptase (200 U/μl).

10. RNase Inhibitor (40 U/μl).

11. TAE buffer: It is composed of 40 mM Tris, 20 mM acetic acid, and 1 mM EDTA (pH 8.0).

12. 2.5 % agarose gel: Weigh 2.5 g agarose and add 100 ml TAE buffer. Boil to dissolve the agarose. Allow to cool and when the solution is luke-warm, add 2.5 μl of ethidium bromide (10 mg/ml) and pour the solution in the gel casting tray of the gel apparatus. Allow it to solidify (*see* **Notes 4** and **5**). Run the gel in 1× TAE buffer and observe the gel under UV in a trans-illuminator.

13. SYBR green mix (Applied Biosystem/Invitrogen): keep at 4 °C if to be stored for a short period but for long-term storage keep at –20 °C.

14. Primers (*see* **Note 6**).

   G protein Forward primer: 5'ACTCATCCAAACAACCC ACA3'.

   G protein Reverse primer: 5'GGAACAAAATTGAACAC TTC3'.

2.5 Assay for Antihelminthic Activity Against S. mansoni	1. *B. glabrata* snails infected with *S. mansoni*. These can be obtained from NIAID Schistosomiasis Resource Centre; http://www.schisto-resource.org/. 2. Conditioned water. Pass tap water through activated charcoal filter and aerate it for 3 days. 3. Iodine solution. Dissolve 4 g potassium iodide and 2 g iodine in 100 ml water; store in a dark bottle. 4. Complete DMEM with 10 % FCS as prepared above without antibiotics. 5. DMEM with 1 % FCS: Add 1 ml heat-inactivated FCS to 100 ml DMEM. 6. Percoll solution: To prepare 40 ml of percoll gradient suspension, add 24 ml Percoll, mix 4 ml 10× Eagle's minimum essential medium (EMEM), 1.5 ml antibiotic mixture containing 10,000 U/ml penicillin and 10 mg/ml streptomycin, 1 ml 1 M HEPES in 0.85 % NaCl. Make up the volume by adding approximately 9.5 ml distilled water. 7. DAPI (4',6-diamidino-2-phenylindole). 8. 96-well round bottom microtiter plates with lid.
2.6 Assay of Antiprotozoan Activity Against L. donovani	1. M199 culture medium supplemented with 10 % FCS. 2. Formaldehyde. 3. 96-well flat bottom microtiter plates with lid. 4. MTT (3-(4,5-dimethylthiazol-2-yl)-diphenyl-tetrazolium bromide 10 mg/ml: carefully weigh 10 mg of powdered MTT and dissolve it in 1 ml of M199 culture medium. Mix by vortexing (*see* **Notes 7** and **8**). 5. Lysis solution: for 50 ml solution, weigh 10 g SDS and dissolve in 25 ml dimethyl formamide (DMF). Make up the volume to 50 ml with autoclaved water. Cover the solution with aluminum foil to avoid exposure to light.
2.7 Assay of Antibacterial Activity Against E. coli	1. LB medium. 2. LB agar plates: Pour 25 ml warm autoclaved LB agar per plate and allow to solidify in laminar hood. 3. PBS: prepare PBS, pH 7.4 as mentioned above and autoclave.

3   Methods

3.1   Assay of Antiviral Activity Against RSV

This is done by two different assays. The shell vial assay measures the effect of eosinophil protein on the infectivity of the virus, whereas the real-time PCR based assay assesses the effect of protein directly on the virus.

3.2   Propagation of RSV-B

The virus handling is strictly done in Class II cabinets. Gloves must be worn at all times while handing the virus. The discard should be disposed off carefully to avoid any contamination. The waste plasticware should be packed in separate bags, while spirit should be added in the liquid waste before disposal.

1. Grow Hep-2 cells to monolayers in T25 flasks in DMEM, pH 7.2 with 10 % FCS (*see* **Note 9**).

2. Remove the FCS by washing the Hep-2 monolayer with filter-sterilized PBS.

3. Inoculate the monolayer with RSV-B stock in 0.5 ml DMEM, pH 7.

4. Incubate the cells with the virus for 1 h at 37 °C to allow adsorption of virus. The flask must be occasionally tilted to avoid drying of the cells (*see* **Note 10**).

5. Remove the inoculum and add 4 ml of DMEM pH 7 supplemented with 2 % FCS.

6. Grow the cells till syncytia formation is observed. It may take 4–5 days, so change the growth medium every 2 days.

7. Lyse the cells by freezing at −70 °C followed by thawing at 37 °C in a water bath.

8. Aliquot and store the lysed suspension containing the RSV-B virions at −70 °C.

3.3   Shell Vial Assay for Antiviral Activity

Seeding of Hep-2 Monolayer

1. Take a fully confluent T-25 flask of Hep-2 cells and dislodge the cells using 1× trypsin-EDTA (*see* **Note 11**).

2. Place one autoclaved coverslip in each well of a 24-well plate.

3. Count the cells in Neubauer's chamber and seed 1.5×10^5 Hep-2 cells/well in 1 ml DMEM, pH 7.2 with 10 % FCS on autoclaved coverslips placed in the 24-well plate (*see* **Note 2**).

4. Allow the cells to grow for 48 h to form a monolayer.

Treatment of RSV with Eosinophil Protein

1. Filter-sterilize the purified eosinophil granule protein (ECP/EDN) using a 0.2 μm filter.

2. Add different dilutions of filtered protein in 20 μl to 0.2 ml of RSV-B suspension in DMEM, pH 7.

3. Allow the protein and viral suspension to mix for 2 h at room temperature using an end to end shaker.

Infection of Hep-2 Cells with Virus

1. Remove the culture medium and wash the Hep-2 monolayers on coverslips twice with PBS.

2. To the washed Hep-2 monolayer add 0.2 ml of the protein treated or untreated viral suspensions in different wells.

3. Centrifuge the plates at $300 \times g$ for 30 min to allow adsorption of the virus to the cells.

4. Add 1 ml of DMEM, pH 7 containing 2 % FCS to each well and incubate the plates at 37 °C in 5 % CO_2 for 48 h.

5. Gently remove the medium from each well at the end of 48 h.

6. Wash the cells twice with PBS.

7. Fix the cells by adding 0.5 ml of chilled acetone for 5 min.

8. Wash the cells with PBS (*see* **Note 12**).

Indirect Immunoflourescence

1. Add 500 µl blocking solution in each well containing a coverslip, and keep it at room temperature for 30 min.

2. Wash the cells twice with PBS.

3. Add 150 µl of 1:150 dilution of mouse anti-RSV antibody in PBS and incubate it in a humidified chamber for 45 min at room temperature.

4. Wash off the antibody from the cells by washing the cells thrice with PBS.

5. Add 150 µl of 1:50 dilution of goat anti-mouse FITC conjugate in each well and incubate for 30 min in a humidified chamber (*see* **Note 13**).

6. Wash the cells twice with PBS after incubation to remove excess unbound antibody.

7. Mount the coverslip on a glass slide and view the cells under a fluorescent microscope (*see* **Note 14**).

8. The cells infected with RSV will appear fluorescent green when viewed using a blue filter in the microscope.

9. Count the infected fluorescent cells in all the experimental sets and compare the percentage of infected cells in wells treated with proteins with untreated cells (controls). The antiviral activity is expressed as ID_{50} value that represents the concentration of protein which inhibits the viral infection by 50 %.

3.4 RT-PCR Based Assay for Antiviral Activity Against RSV

Filter-sterilize the purified eosinophil granule protein (ECP/EDN) using a 0.2 µm filter.

Incubation of Virus with Protein

1. To 1 ml of RSV suspension, add various serial dilutions of the desired eosinophil protein (EDN/ECP) in 20 µl.

2. Allow the protein and viral suspension to mix for 30 min at room temperature using an end to end shaker.

3. Isolate RNA from these protein and viral suspension mixtures using Trizol-LS (Invitrogen) reagent or RNeasy mini kit (Qiagen) as per manufacturer's instructions.

RNA Isolation Using
Trizol-LS Reagent

1. To the RSV-protein mixture add 3 ml of Trizol-LS reagent, mix well.

2. Allow it to stand for 5 min at room temperature.

3. Add 800 μl of RNA grade chloroform and shake the tube vigorously for about 15 s.

4. Allow it to stand for 10 min at room temperature and then centrifuge at 12,000×*g* for 15 min at 4 °C (*see* **Note 15**).

5. Carefully remove the top aqueous layer with a pipette and transfer to a fresh tube (*see* **Note 16**).

6. Add 2.0 ml isopropanol and mix gently. Leave it at room temperature for 10 min.

7. Centrifuge at 12,000×*g* for 10 min at 4 °C (*see* **Note 17**).

8. Place the tubes on ice. A barely visible pellet may be observed at the bottom of the tube.

9. Carefully decant the liquid and add 2.5 ml of 75 % ethanol in DEPC treated water. Mix gently.

10. Centrifuge at 12,000×*g* for 5 min at 4 °C.

11. Pour off the ethanol and air-dry the pellet (*see* **Note 18**).

12. Add 25 μl autoclaved DEPC-treated water to the RNA pellet. Leave at room temperature for 30 min to dissolve well.

13. Determine the concentration and purity of the RNA by measuring its absorbance at 260 and 280 nm. A good quality RNA has a 260/280 ratio greater than 1.8.

14. Prepare complementary DNA from each of these RNA samples.

cDNA Preparation

1. Take 10 μl of RNA from untreated and RSV samples treated with eosinophil protein and add 4 μl of dNTP mix (2.5 mM) and 2 μl of random hexamers (0.4 μg/μl).

2. Heat the mix in a thermal cycler at 70 °C for 5 min.

3. Immediately transfer the tubes containing the mix to ice.

4. Add the following to this mixture:

10× Reaction buffer	2.0 μl
M-MuLV reverse transcriptase (200 U/μl)	1.0 μl
RNase inhibitor (40 U/μl)	1.0 μl

5. Incubate the mix at 42 °C for 60 min.

6. Incubate at 95 °C for 5 min to inactivate the reverse transcriptase.

7. Dilute the reaction mixture to 50 μl using autoclaved DEPC water.

8. Quantitative analysis of viral particle is done by performing SYBR real-time PCR for expression of mRNA for G protein of RSV.

SYBR Real-Time PCR

1. Set up the PCR in triplicate for all samples. A typical reaction mixture contains

2× SYBR green mix:	10 µl
Template cDNA:	2 µl
1 µM Fwd primer:	2 µl
1 µM reverse primer:	2 µl
Nuclease-free water:	2 µl

Set up a no-template control (NTC) which contains water instead of the template.

2. The PCR cycles are set as follows

95 °C for 10 min, followed by 40 cycles of 95 °C, 15 s and 60 °C, 1 min.

3. Analyze the real-time PCR data using the *Comparative Ct method* $(2^{-[\Delta][\Delta]Ct})$ to compare the results obtained from protein treated and untreated RSV samples.

where, $[\Delta][\Delta]Ct = [\Delta]Ct\ Test - [\Delta]Ct\ Control$

Ct Test is value for viral sample treated with protein and Ct Control is for the untreated viral sample.

4. Additionally, after the PCR is over, run a 2.5 % agarose gel to visualize a 217 bp band for DNA for G protein of RSV and quantitate by densitometry (*see* **Note 4**).

3.5 Assay of Anti-helminthic Activity Against S. mansoni

In Vitro Transformation of S. mansoni Cercariae to Schistosomules (See Note 19)

1. Place the infected snails that are shedding cercariae in 100 ml beakers in conditioned water at a density of one snail per 2 ml water.

2. Put the beaker under a strong light source for 2 h (ensure that the water does not overheat during this period).

3. Remove the snails from water with a small strainer or feather-weight forceps.

4. Filter the suspension of cercariae in water with a 100 µm filter to remove any debris.

5. Gently suspend the cercariae in water and draw 3 aliquots of 200 µl each for counting.

6. Dilute the three aliquots to 2 ml with water, add a few drops of iodine solution, and count the stained intact cercariae using a dissection microscope.

7. Put the cercariae in water in a 50 ml centrifuge tube and place the tube on ice for 30 min.

8. Centrifuge at $100 \times g$ at 4 °C for 2 min.

9. Remove the supernatant leaving behind 3 ml at the top of the pellet.

10. Add 3 ml of cold DMEM and vortex at high speed for 45 s.

11. Place the tube on ice for 3 min, then vortex again for 45 s.

12. Gently layer the cercarial suspension on top of 40 ml Percoll suspension in a fresh 50 ml tube.

13. Centrifuge at $500 \times g$ at 4 °C for 15 min.

14. Discard 40 ml of the supernatant and resuspend the pellet by tapping in residual medium.

15. Add DMEM to the resuspended pellet to a final volume of 50 ml.

16. Centrifuge the tube for 5 min at $100 \times g$ at 4 °C.

17. Wash the final pellet twice with DMEM.

Effect of Eosinophil Granule Proteins on S. mansoni

1. Resuspend the schistosomule pellet in DMEM with 10 % FCS, in tissue culture flasks, at a density of approximately 500 organisms/ml, and incubate at 37 °C in a 5 % CO_2 incubator for 3 h. The schistosomules will gradually undergo morphological and physiological changes (*see* **Note 20**).

2. Wash the schistosomules twice with incomplete DMEM and resuspend them at a concentration of 1,000 schistosomules/ml in DMEM containing 1 % FCS.

3. Add 1 µg of the fluorochrome DAPI per ml.

4. Aliquot 100 µl of this suspension in each well of a 96-well microtiter plate.

5. Add the granule proteins in various serial dilutions in triplicates and make the final volume up to 200 µl in each well.

6. Place the plates in a humidified chamber at 37 °C for 18 and 36 h

7. Visualize the plate under inverted fluorescent microscope (Nikon) to determine the number of dead schistosomules in each well (*The dead schistosomules are immobile and granular, and have a deep blue fluorescence due to uptake of DAPI*).

8. The result is expressed as LD_{50} (lethal dose) for the protein, which is the concentration of the protein at which 50 % of the schistosomules are dead upon treatment with the granule protein.

3.6 Assay of Antiprotozoan Activity Against Leishmania donovani UR6 (See Note 21)

1. The *Leishmania* promastigotes are maintained in M199 medium containing 10 % FCS at 23 °C.

2. Centrifuge active promastigotes at $500 \times g$ for 10 min to pellet dead cells.

3. The supernatant containing the live cells are centrifuged at $1,200 \times g$ and pelleted cells resuspended in 1 ml of M199 medium.

4. For counting of *Leishmania* cells, take 10 μl of cells from the culture and fix them by adding 900 μl of 4 % formaldehyde. Mix them thoroughly with the help of a pipette. Put 10 μl of the fixed cells on the Neubauer's haemocytometer and leave at room temperature for 5 min to allow the cells to settle down. Count the cells in 4 squares, average the value, and multiply the number by 10^6 to determine the number of cells present in 1 ml of culture.

5. Plate *L. donovani* cells at a concentration of 2×10^6 cells/well in a 96-well flat bottom microtiter plate.

6. Filter-sterilize the granule proteins and add various concentrations to leishmania in the wells, in triplicate and maintain the final volume at 200 μl/well.

7. Incubate the plate at 23 °C for 72 h.

8. Determine the number of live cells and LD_{50} for the protein by MTT assay

MTT Assay

1. Prepare 10 mg/ml stock of MTT in M199 medium and add 20 μl of this solution to each well containing the cells to obtain a final concentration of 1 mg/ml.

2. Continue the incubation at 23 °C for 6 h to allow the uptake and oxidation of the dye by viable cells.

3. Aspirate the medium with the help of a pipette and add 100 μl of the lysis solution in each well.

4. Visually inspect to ensure complete dissolution of purple colored dye crystals and read the MTT absorption at 570 nm using an ELISA plate reader. The absorption at 650 nm was subtracted from the values obtained at 570 nm.

5. LD_{50} value for each protein, which represents the concentration of the protein that killed 50 % of parasites, is determined by plotting the percentage of live cells against concentration of protein.

3.7 Assay of Antibacterial Activity Against E. coli

1. Pick a single colony from a LB-agar plate streaked with required bacteria and inoculate in 5 ml LB medium.

2. Grow the culture overnight at 37 °C.

3. Transfer the culture to a 15 ml tube and centrifuge it at $1,000 \times g$ for 15 min.

4. Discard the supernatant and add 2 ml sterile PBS and re-centrifuge. Repeat PBS wash and resuspend the cells in PBS at a dilution of 1:100 of the original volume.

5. In separate microcentrifuge tubes, to 100 μl of this bacterial suspension add varying concentrations of granule proteins (EDN/ECP/MBP) in 100 μl, mix, and incubate at 37 °C for 6 h.

6. After incubation, plate ten-fold serial dilutions of the treated bacterial suspensions in duplicates on LB plates and grow overnight at 37 °C (*see* **Note 22**).

7. Count the colony forming units (CFU)/ml for each experiment the next day. Plot the CFU/ml versus the protein concentration to determine LD_{50}. LD_{50} is defined as the concentration of the protein required to kill 50 % of the bacterial population. Perform the experiment in triplicate and determine the standard error.

4 Notes

1. Aliquoting and storing reagents like FCS and trypsin-EDTA in small fractions prevents their loss of activity and degradation due to repeated freezing and thawing.

2. Mix 10 μl of trypan blue dye with 10 μl single cell suspension, and load 10 μl of this mix onto Neubauer's chamber and count the cells in the four large squares. Average the count to per square and multiply by 2×10^4 to obtain the number of cells per ml of cell suspension.

3. Use an autoclaved pair of forceps for handing coverslips once they are cleaned and autoclaved.

4. 2.5 % Agarose gel tends to solidify very fast. Be quick to add ethidium bromide and pour the gel in the apparatus before it starts solidifying.

5. Always wear gloves while handling ethidium bromide as it is carcinogenic.

6. We measure the RSV infection by quantitating DNA encoding G protein of RSV. The primers are designed by "Primer Express Software version 3.0" (ABI, USA).

7. MTT may not dissolve completely. Vortex it well and allow it to settle before using.

8. Cover the MTT solution with aluminum foil as it is light sensitive.

9. The pH of DMEM should be maintained carefully at 7 and 7.2. The medium should not be stored for long, as the pH tends to increase with time. The medium should be kept at 4 °C and brought to room temperature before use.

10. The cells should not be allowed to dry and the flask should be tilted every 10–15 min.

11. While dislodging, the flask should be gently tapped so that the cells separate from each other and do not form a cluster. Cells should appear as single cells because clusters hinder proper cell counting.

12. After fixation, the remaining procedures can be done outside the laminar hood. The fixed slides can be kept at 4 °C overnight and proceeded for IFA the following day.

13. Since the secondary antibody is light sensitive, use a dark colored chamber or cover the chamber with aluminum foil.

14. While mounting, it is advisable to add antifade onto the coverslip so that the fluorescence is not quenched easily.

15. Remove the tubes very carefully from the centrifuge so as not to disturb the layers.

16. While pipetting, leave some of the aqueous phase so as to prevent any DNA contamination. It is preferable to use a smaller volume pipette as it is harder to control the rate and force of fluid withdrawal with a larger volume pipette.

17. If a low yield is expected, centrifuge for 30 min.

18. RNA may aggregate and not resolubilize if the pellet is left to dry for too long. Presence of ethanol also hinders solubilization of RNA into solution. It is advisable to recentrifuge after decanting ethanol so as to remove residual ethanol.

19. Schistosomes are a biohazard, therefore investigators must wear latex gloves at all times while handling them. *S. mansoni* is maintained in *Blomphalaria glabrata* snails. The infectious stage of *Schistosoma* is the cercariae stage. The cercariae of *S. mansoni*, obtained from the snails are transformed in vitro to their next developmental stage, the schistosomules by vortexing.

20. Always use freshly prepared schistosomules for cytotoxicity assay.

21. Handling of Leishmania is done strictly in Class II cabinets in tissue culture room. Gloves should be worn at all times while working with *Leishmania*.

22. While plating the triplicates of bacterial suspensions, take care not to mix spreaders as it can lead to erroneous results.

References

1. Walsh GM (2001) Eosinophil granule proteins and their role in disease. Curr Opin Hematol 8:28–33

2. Weller PF (1991) The immunology of eosinophils. N Engl J Med 324(16):1110–1118

3. Gleich GJ, Adolphson CR, Leiferman KM (1993) The biology of the eosinophilic leukocyte. Annu Rev Med 44:85–101

4. Kita H, Adolphson, CR, Gleich, GJ (1998) Biology of eosinophils. In Allergy: principles and practice (5th ed), Middleton Jr E, Reed CE, Ellis EF, Adkinson Jr NF, Yunginger JW, Busse WW (Eds.), Mosby, St Louis, pp 242–260

5. Durack DT, Sumi SM, Klebanoff SJ (1979) Neurotoxicity of human eosinophils. Proc Natl Acad Sci U S A 76:1443–1447

6. Gordon MH (1933) Remarks on Hodgkin's disease: a pathogenic agent in the glands, and its application in diagnosis. Br Med J 1: 641–644

7. Venge P, Bystrom J, Carlson M, Hakansson L, Karawacjzyk M, Peterson C, Seveus L, Trulson

A (1999) Eosinophil cationic protein (ECP): molecular and biological properties and the use of ECP as a marker of eosinophil activation in disease. Clin Exp Allergy 29:1172–1186

8. Boix E, Carreras E, Nikolovski Z, Cuchillo CM, Nogues MV (2001) Identification and characterization of human eosinophil cationic protein by an epitope-specific antibody. J Leukoc Biol 69:1027–1035

9. Wever R, Hamers MN, Weening RS, Roos D (1980) Characterization of the peroxidase in human eosinophils. Eur J Biochem 108:491–495

10. Henderson WR, Chi EY, Klebanoff SJ (1980) Eosinophil peroxidase-induced mast cell secretion. J Exp Med 152:265–279

11. Motojima S, Frigas E, Loegering DA, Gleich GJ (1989) Toxicity of eosinophil cationic proteins for guinea pig tracheal epithelium in vitro. Am Rev Respir Dis 139:801–805

12. Butterworth AE, David JR, Franks D, Mahmoud AA, David PH, Sturrock RF, Houba V (1977) Antibody-dependent eosinophil-mediated damage to 51Cr-labeled schistosomula of *Schistosoma mansoni*: damage by purified eosinophils. J Exp Med 145:136–150

13. Gleich GJ, Adolphson CR (1986) The eosinophilic leukocyte: structure and function. Adv Immunol 39:177–253

14. Butterworth AE (1984) Cell-mediated damage to helminths. Adv Parasitol 23:143–235

15. Ackerman SJ, Gleich GJ, Loegering DA, Richardson BA, Butterworth AE (1985) Comparative toxicity of purified human eosinophil granule cationic proteins for schistosomula of *Schistosoma mansoni*. Am J Trop Med Hyg 34:735–745

16. Hamann KJ, Barker RL, Loegering DA, Gleich GJ (1987) Comparative toxicity of purified human eosinophil granule proteins for newborn larvae of Trichinella spiralis. J Parasitol 73:523–529

17. Hamann KJ, Gleich GJ, Checkel JL, Loegering DA, McCall JW, Barker RL (1990) In vitro killing of microfilariae of *Brugia pahangi* and *Brugia malayi* by eosinophil granule proteins. J Immunol 144:3166–3173

18. Villalta F, Kierszenbaum F (1984) Role of inflammatory cells in Chagas' disease. I. Uptake and mechanism of destruction of intracellular (amastigote) forms of *Trypanosoma cruzi* by human eosinophils. J Immunol 132:2053–2058

19. Kierszenbaum F, Villalta F, Tai PC (1986) Role of inflammatory cells in Chagas' disease. III. Kinetics of human eosinophil activation upon interaction with parasites (*Trypanosoma cruzi*). J Immunol 136:662–666

20. Molina HA, Kierszenbaum F, Hamann KJ, Gleich GJ (1988) Toxic effects produced or mediated by human eosinophil granule components on *Trypanosoma cruzi*. Am J Trop Med Hyg 38:327–334

21. Waters LS, Taverne J, Tai PC, Spry CJ, Targett GA, Playfair JH (1987) Killing of *Plasmodium falciparum* by eosinophil secretory products. Infect Immun 55:877–881

22. Singh A, Batra JK (2011) Role of unique basic residues in cytotoxic, antibacterial and antiparasitic activities of human eosinophil cationic protein. Biol Chem 392:337–346

23. Borelli V, Vita F, Shankar S, Soranzo MR, Banfi E, Scialino G, Brochetta C, Zabucchi G (2003) Human eosinophil peroxidase induces surface alteration, killing, and lysis of *Mycobacterium tuberculosis*. Infect Immun 71:605–613

24. Jong EC, Mahmoud AA, Klebanoff SJ (1981) Peroxidase-mediated toxicity to schistosomula of Schistosoma mansoni. J Immunol 126:468–471

25. Buys J, Wever R, Ruitenberg EJ (1984) Myeloperoxidase is more efficient than eosinophil peroxidase in the in vitro killing of newborn larvae of *Trichinella spiralis*. Immunology 51:601–607

26. Lehrer RI, Szklarek D, Barton A, Ganz T, Hamann KJ, Gleich GJ (1989) Antibacterial properties of eosinophil major basic protein and eosinophil cationic protein. J Immunol 142:4428–4434

27. Svensson L, Wenneras C (2005) Human eosinophils selectively recognize and become activated by bacteria belonging to different taxonomic groups. Microbes Infect 7:720–728

28. Aydemir SA, Tekin IO, Numanoglu G, Borazan A, Ustundag Y (2004) Eosinophil infiltration, gastric juice and serum eosinophil cationic protein levels in *Helicobacter pylori*-associated chronic gastritis and gastric ulcer. Mediators Inflamm 13:369–372

29. Qadri F, Bhuiyan TR, Dutta KK, Raqib R, Alam MS, Alam NH, Svennerholm AM, Mathan MM (2004) Acute dehydrating disease caused by *Vibrio cholerae* serogroups O1 and O139 induce increases in innate cells and inflammatory mediators at the mucosal surface of the gut. Gut 53:62–69

30. Raqib R, Moly PK, Sarker P, Qadri F, Alam NH, Mathan M, Andersson J (2003) Persistence of mucosal mast cells and eosino-

phils in Shigella-infected children. Infect Immun 71:2684–2692

31. Domachowske JB, Dyer KD, Bonville CA, Rosenberg HF (1998) Recombinant human eosinophil-derived neurotoxin/RNase 2 functions as an effective antiviral agent against respiratory syncytial virus. J Infect Dis 177: 1458–1464

32. Bedoya VI, Boasso A, Hardy AW, Rybak S, Shearer GM, Rugeles MT (2006) Ribonucleases in HIV type 1 inhibition: effect of recombinant RNases on infection of primary T cells and immune activation-induced RNase gene and protein expression. AIDS Res Hum Retroviruses 22:897–907

33. Ding J, Liu J, Xue CF, Li YH, Gong WD (2003) Construction and expression of prokaryotic expression vector for pTAT-HBV targeted ribonuclease fusion protein. Xi Bao Yu Fen Zi Mian Yi Xue Za Zhi 9: 49–51

34. Slifman NR, Loegering DA, Mckean DJ, Gleich GJ (1986) Ribonuclease activity associated with human eosinophil-derived neurotoxin and eosinophil cationic protein. J Immunol 137: 2913–2917

35. Sikriwal D, Seth D, Dey P, Batra JK (2007) Human eosinophil-derived neurotoxin: involvement of a putative non-catalytic phosphate-binding subsite in its catalysis. Mol Cell Biochem 303(1–2):175–181

36. Yazdanbakhsh M, Tai PC, Spry CJ, Gleich GJ, Roos D (1987) Synergism between eosinophil cationic protein and oxygen metabolites in killing of schistosomula of *Schistosoma mansoni*. J Immunol 138:3443–3447

37. Lewis F (1999) Schistosomiasis. In: Coico R (ed) Current protocols in immunology, vol III. Wiley, New York, pp 19.1.1–19.1.28

38. Sikriwal D, Seth D, Parveen S, Malik A, Broor S, Batra JK (2012) An insertion in loop L7 of human eosinophil-derived neurotoxin is crucial for its antiviral activity. J Cell Biochem 113(10):3104–3112

Chapter 24

Eosinophils and the Ovalbumin Mouse Model of Asthma

F. Daubeuf and Nelly Frossard

Abstract

Mouse models of asthma are essential to understand asthma pathogenesis and eosinophil recruitment in the airways, and to develop new therapeutic strategies. Animal models try to mimic features of the human disease including airway hyperresponsiveness (AHR), eosinophilic inflammation, and remodeling, which are the typical asthma-related characteristics. The mouse is now the species of choice for asthma research due to the availability of transgenic animals and a wide array of specific reagents and techniques available. Cellular responses may be studied with innovative imaging and flow cytometry methods while lung mechanics may be precisely measured by the forced oscillation technique, and airway responsiveness approached by barometric plethysmography in conscious and unconstrained animals. Here, we describe procedures to generate acute models of hypereosinophilic asthma in mice, with ovalbumin (OVA) as the allergen. The presented allergic asthma models offer a large and reproducible eosinophil recruitment, measured in the bronchoalveolar lavage (BAL), accompanied with AHR, inflammation, and remodeling, and are particularly suited to assess the activity of drug candidates. We here present the classical 21-day allergic asthma model to OVA, and adjustments for a rapid 8-day model of airway allergic hypereosinophilia, and a more chronic 57-day model suitable for C57BL/6 mice to develop AHR together with airway eosinophilic inflammation and remodeling.

Key words Allergic asthma, Mouse model, Ovalbumin, Airway eosinophilia

1 Introduction

Human allergic asthma is defined as a chronic eosinophilic inflammatory disorder of the airways and is characterized clinically by airway hyperresponsiveness (AHR) and intermittent, reversible airway obstruction [1]. Histopathological features of asthma show the presence of a large eosinophilic infiltrate in the bronchi, and structural changes grouped as "airway remodeling" including subepithelial fibrosis, goblet cell hyperplasia, airway smooth muscle thickening, and increased vascularity. It is accepted that AHR and remodeling result from repeated exposure to allergen, that lead to chronic inflammation of the airways [2]. Studies in laboratory animals have produced a large amount of knowledge on the mechanisms responsible for allergic asthma. Among animal models, the

Garry M. Walsh (ed.), *Eosinophils: Methods and Protocols*, Methods in Molecular Biology, vol. 1178,
DOI 10.1007/978-1-4939-1016-8_24, © Springer Science+Business Media New York 2014

mouse is now the most widely used species. Mice are not naturally prone to asthma, but asthma-like artificial reactions may be induced in the respiratory tract to develop inflammation and symptoms that are reflecting those of the human disease. Some differences persist however in the pathophysiology of asthma between mouse and human. AHR in mice follows allergen challenge and is transient, while it is present at any time in human even in the absence of symptoms [3]. Chronic models appear difficult to develop in mice, probably due to the absence of environmental cofactors such as pollution, lung infection, and also probably due to the employed allergen. These observations suggest that allergic asthma models in mice do not exactly replicate the human disease, but the observations made in these mouse models support most existing paradigms and are useful to develop new antiasthma strategies [4].

The most commonly used strain for allergen challenge models and eosinophil recruitment is the Th2-type BALB/c mice, but the C57BL/6 or A/J strains have also been used successfully for allergen challenge studies and development of asthma features [5]. A/J mice seem more sensitive to allergen and are suitable for development of chronic models [6]. Allergens that may have clinical relevance, such as house dust mite or cockroach extracts [7, 8], have been recently successfully developed for asthma models in the mouse. However, ovalbumin (OVA) derived from chicken egg is until now a more frequently used allergen since it induces a robust and reproducible allergic bronchial inflammation, particularly in acute allergic responses [9]. Various sensitization and challenge procedures have been developed to induce acute asthma symptoms to OVA. For priming, allergen sensitization requires multiple systemic administrations of OVA in the presence of an adjuvant via intraperitoneal route. Aluminum hydroxide $(Al(OH)_3)$ is a commonly used adjuvant to promote the development of a Th2 immune response to OVA [10]. After the sensitization period allowing IgE production (usually from 5 to 21 days), all protocols require local challenges with the allergen. OVA may be applied to the airways by nebulization, or by intratracheal (i.t.) or intranasal (i.n.) instillation [11, 12]. Following these procedures, mice develop key features of clinical asthma, including increased levels of allergen-specific IgE in serum, eosinophil and Th2 cell infiltration into the airways referred to as airway inflammation, mucus hyperproduction and collagen deposition as airway remodeling, and AHR to methacholine.

The influx of inflammatory cells in the airways, in particular eosinophil infiltration, is studied in the bronchoalveolar lavage (BAL) [20]. BAL is performed after euthanasia and differential cells are counted by optical microscopy as eosinophils, neutrophils, macrophages, and lymphocytes [15]. For more specific assessments, flow cytometric methods can be applied, e.g., to identify T cell phenotypes in the cell composition of BAL fluid in asthma models [21].

We here describe the optimized procedures to sensitize and challenge mice to OVA, in order to develop reproducible features of airway inflammation, e.g., eosinophil infiltration assessed in BAL fluid, remodeling, and hyperresponsiveness. To do so, we present the classical acute 21-day asthma model in Balb/c mice and special adjustments for a rapid 8-day model of airway allergic hypereosinophilia and a more chronic 57-day model suitable for C57BL/6 mice to develop AHR associated with inflammation and remodeling. In a following step, we describe an easy-to-perform, inexpensive, and reproducible manner to obtain BAL to measure inflammatory cell recruitment in mouse airways.

2 Materials

Prepare all solutions using sterile and pyrogen-free commercial saline (NaCl 0.9 %, B. Braun, Boulogne, France), and all reagents on ice. OVA solutions are prepared, aliquoted, and frozen ready-to-use to increase reproducibility of the experiment.

2.1 Ovalbumin Solutions and Aluminum Hydroxide Powder

1. Prepare a sterile 2 mg/ml solution of OVA as follows: weigh 80 mg OVA (Sigma-Aldrich, A5503) and dissolve it in 40 ml cold sterile saline in a 50 ml Falcon tube with a vortex (at maximal speed, *see* **Note 1**)

2. For sensitization procedures in the 8-day and 21-day models, take 25 ml of this solution and distribute as 1.1-ml aliquots into 1.5-ml microtubes. Immediately freeze and store aliquots at −80 °C.

3. For challenge procedures in the 8-day and 21-day models, take 8 ml of the remaining 2 mg/ml solution and dilute it 1/5th by adding 32 ml cold sterile saline in a 50-ml Falcon tube with a vortex (at maximal speed, *see* **Note 1**). Distribute as 1-ml aliquots in 1.5-ml microtubes. Immediately store aliquots at −80 °C.

4. For sensitization and challenge procedures in the 57-day model, take 8 ml of the 2 mg/ml solution and dilute it 1/2.5th by adding 12 ml cold sterile saline in a 50-ml Falcon tube with a vortex (at maximal speed, *see* **Note 1**). Distribute as 1-ml aliquots in 1.5-ml microtubes. Immediately store aliquots at −80 °C.

5. In addition, prepare aliquots of ready-to-use sterile saline for control experiments. Transfer 1 ml sterile saline into 1.5-ml microtubes and 4 ml saline into sterile culture tubes (BD Falcon, 352003). Immediately store the aliquots at −80 °C.

6. As soon as the aluminum hydroxide powder [$Al(OH)_3$, alum, Sigma-Aldrich, cat. no. 239186] (*see* **Note 2**) arrives at the lab, weigh aliquots of 80 mg in 5-ml sterile culture tubes. Be careful to store alum aliquots protected from light at room temperature.

***2.2 Ovalbumin
and Alum Conjugates***

Conjugation of OVA to alum is a critical step to guarantee the reproducibility of the sensitization.

1. Before use, bring an aliquot of 2 mg/ml OVA solution and an aliquot of 4-ml sterile saline to room temperature.

2. Take an aliquot of alum (80 mg), add 1 ml OVA solution (2 mg/ml) and 3 ml sterile saline. This suspension should be prepared fresh every day.

3. Gently homogenize the OVA–alum suspension for 4 h at 4 °C on a rotator mixer to allow adsorption of OVA on alum. (Alum is not entirely soluble and this will be presented as a suspension.)

4. Before administration to animals, bring the suspension to room temperature on a rotator mixer for 10 min (18–23 °C).

***2.3 Anesthetic
Solution for in
Administration***

1. In a 15 ml Falcon tube, add 1.5 ml of a 100 g/l commercial solution of ketamine, Imalgene®), 0.5 ml of a 20 g/l commercial solution of xylazine (Bayer, Rompun® 2 %) and 10 ml of sterile saline. The prepared solution contains 12.5 mg/ml ketamine base and 0.83 mg/ml xylazine base from hydrochloride. This preparation may be stored at 4 °C for 10 days.

2. Before use in animals, bring the solution to room temperature. Inject 100 µl of the anesthetic solution per mouse (25 g), i.e., 4 ml/kg. The administered dose is 50 mg/kg ketamine and 3.3 mg/kg xylazine.

***2.4 Anesthetic
Solution for
Bronchoalveolar
Lavage Procedure***

1. In a 15 ml Falcon tube, add 4.5 ml of a 100 g/l commercial solution of ketamine, 1.5 ml of a 20 g/l commercial solution of xylazine, and 6 ml of sterile saline. The prepared solution contains 37.5 mg/ml ketamine base and 24.9 mg/ml xylazine base from hydrochloride. This preparation may be stored at 4 °C for 10 days.

2. Before use in animals, bring the solution to room temperature. Inject 100 µl of the anesthetic solution per mouse (25 g), i.e., 4 ml/kg. The administered dose is 150 mg/kg ketamine and 10 mg/kg xylazine.

***2.5 Solutions
for Bronchoalveolar
Lavage Procedure***

1. Saline–EDTA 2.6 mM: in a sterile 1-l DURAN® glass bottle, add 970 mg of EDTA (ethylenediaminetetraacetic acid disodium salt dihydrate), 9 g of sodium chloride, and 1-l of ultrapure water. Add a PTFE coated stir bar in the bottle and place it on a magnetic stirrer for 30 min until dissolved. Adjust pH to 7.3 with a 2 N sodium hydroxide solution. This preparation may be stored at 4 °C for 1 week.

2. Potassium chloride 0.6 M: in a sterile 500-ml DURAN® glass bottle, add 22.36 g of potassium chloride and 500 ml of ultrapure water.

3 Methods

This procedure describes how mice sensitized and challenged to OVA will develop reproducible and robust allergic asthma features, in particular eosinophil infiltration to be recovered in the BAL. Mice should be sensitized intraperitoneally, then challenged by intranasal administration at the indicated times (Fig. 1). Repeated exposure to OVA is required to induce cytokine production and increase eosinophil recruitment (Fig. 2). Eosinophils recovered in the BAL fluid are presented in Fig 3. Control mice are sensitized with the OVA–alum suspension for the 8-day and 21-day models or with OVA in the absence of adjuvant for the 57-day model. They are challenged with solvent (saline) alone.

Asthma features will be assessed 24 h after the last OVA challenge: AHR may be measured by whole body plethysmography as described [13] or the forced oscillation technique [14] and inflammatory cell recruitment in particular eosinophils assessed in the collected BAL [15] described below and presented on Fig. 3.

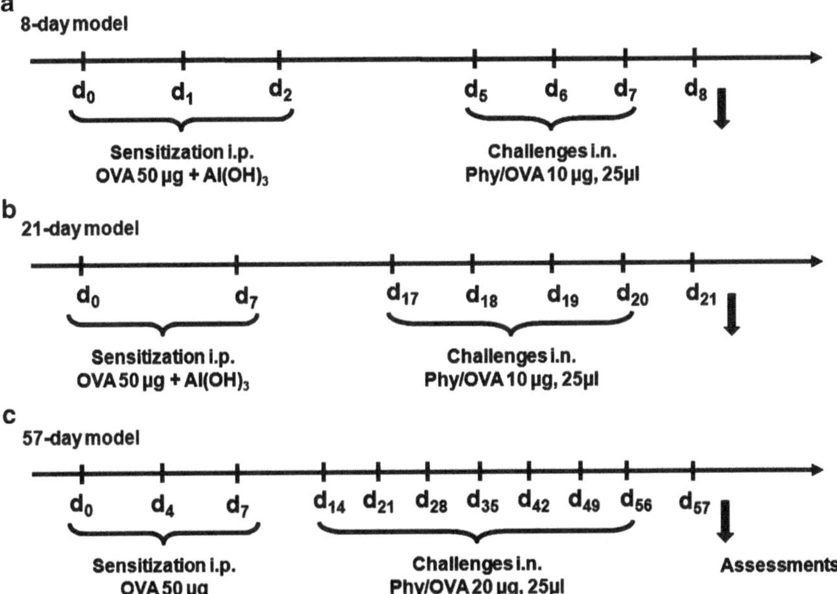

Fig. 1 Allergic asthma models to ovalbumin (OVA) in mice. (**a**) The 8-day rapid model of hypereosinophilia is composed of a sensitization step with intraperitoneal (i.p.) administrations of OVA–alum suspension on days 0, 1, and 2, followed by intranasal (i.n.) challenges with OVA or saline for control mice on days 5, 6, and 7. (**b**) The 21-day acute model of asthma is composed of a sensitization step with i.p. administrations of OVA–alum suspension on days 0 and 7, followed by i.n. challenges with OVA or saline for control mice on days 17, 18, 19, and 20. (**c**) The 57-day chronic model of asthma is composed of a sensitization step with i.p. administrations of OVA alone (no adjuvant) on days 0, 4, and 7, followed by i.n. challenges with OVA or saline for control mice weekly for 7 weeks. Assessments of AHR, OVA-specific IgE production, airway inflammatory cell recruitment, and airway remodeling are performed 24 h after the last OVA challenge

3.1 Perform Ovalbumin Sensitization with Adjuvant in the 8-day and 21-day Models

1. Take the OVA–alum suspension (*see* Subheading 2.2).

2. Hold the mouse (*see* **Note 3**) in your hand by the dorsal skin so that its head is up and its rear legs are down. Maintain its tail in a fixed position with your fingers.

3. Use 1-ml syringes and 25-G needles to inject the OVA–alum suspension and administer 4 ml/kg, i.e., 100 μl per mouse (of 25 g) by intraperitoneal injection. Gently homogenize the

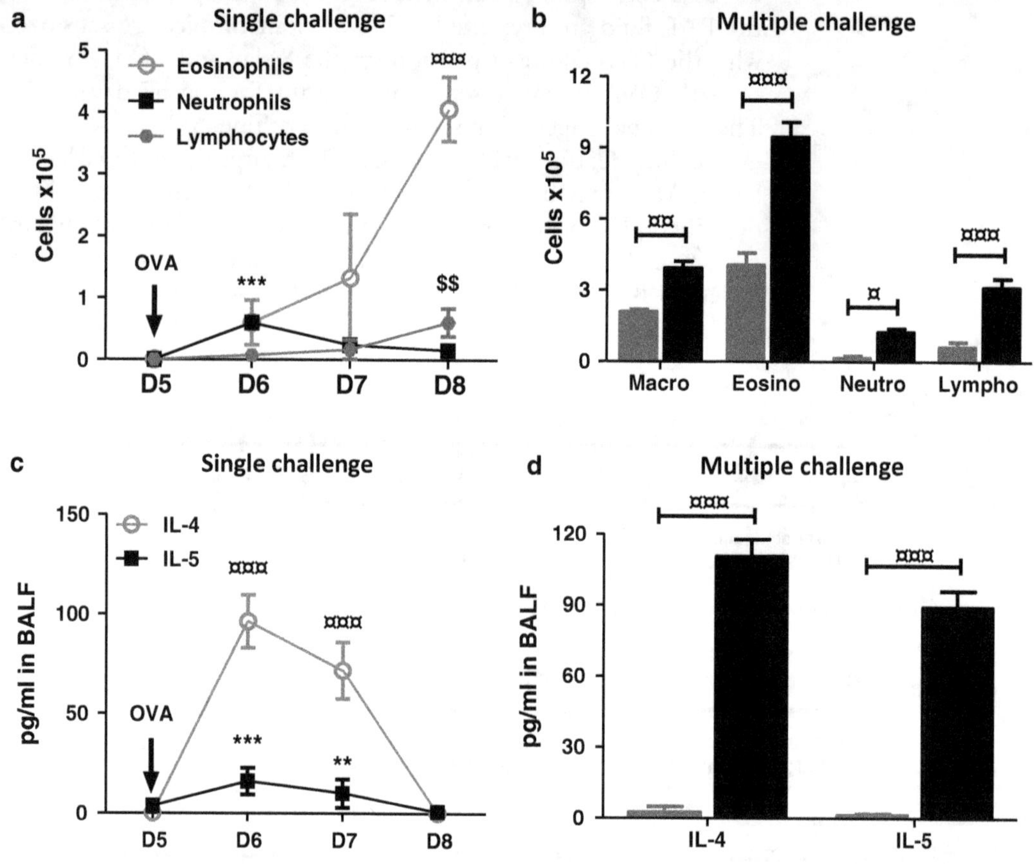

Fig. 2 Repeated exposure to OVA is required to induce both eosinophil recruitment and cytokine production. Example of the 8-day model. (**a**) Evolution of absolute numbers of eosinophils, neutrophils, and lymphocytes in the bronchoalveolar lavage fluid (BALF) 24 h (D6), 48 h (D7), and 72 h (D8) after a single challenge to OVA (performed on D5 and represented by the *arrow*) in mice sensitized to OVA. *Dots* are means and *bars* are SEM values (n=3–6 mice per group). ^{ooo} $P \leq 0.001$ versus D5 for eosinophils, *** $P \leq 0.001$ versus D5 for neutrophils, and $^{\$\$}$ $P \leq 0.01$ versus D5 for lymphocytes. (**b**) Absolute numbers of macrophages (Macro), eosinophils (Eosino), neutrophils (Neutro), and lymphocytes (Lympho) in BALF on D8 after a single challenge to OVA on D5 (*grey blocks*) or 3 challenges to OVA on 3 consecutive days (D5, D6, and D7) (*black blocks*). *Blocks* are means and *bars* are SEM values (n=6 mice per group). ^{o} $P \leq 0.05$; ^{oo} $P \leq 0.01$; ^{ooo} $P \leq 0.001$ (**c**) Evolution of IL-4 and IL-5 cytokine levels recovered in BALF 24, 48, and 72 h after a single challenge to OVA on D5 (represented by the *arrow*). *Dots* are means and *bars* are SEM values (n=3–6 mice per group). ^{ooo} $P \leq 0.001$ versus D5 for IL-5 and ** $P \leq 0.01$, *** $P \leq 0.001$ versus D5 for IL-4. (**d**) Levels of IL-4 and IL-5 recovered in BALF on D8 after a single challenge to OVA on D5 (*grey blocks*) or 3 challenges to OVA on 3 consecutive days (D5, D6, and D7) (*black blocks*). Blocks are means and *bars* are SEM values (n=6 mice per group). ^{ooo} $P \leq 0.001$

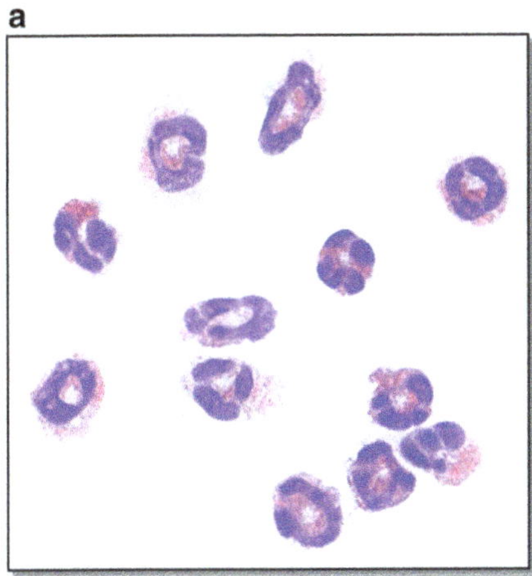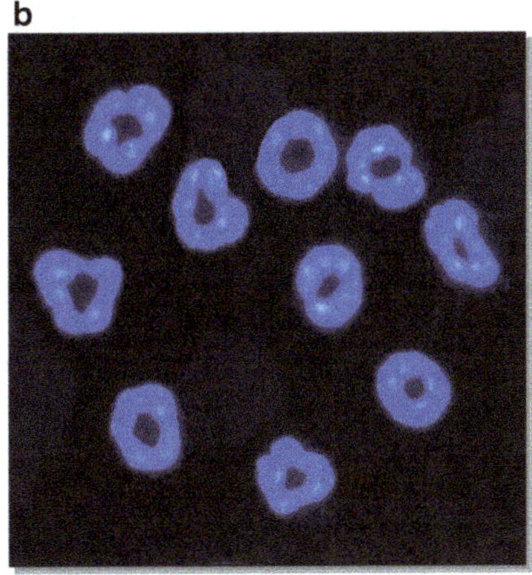

Fig. 3 Photograph of eosinophils recovered in BALF in the 21-day acute model of asthma to OVA in mice. (**a**) Bright field photograph of cytospun eosinophils stained with Diff-Quick. (**b**) Fluorescent photograph of eosinophils stained with DAPI to highlight the typical circular nucleus of murine eosinophils

suspension between each injection (*see* **Note 4**). Each mouse receives 50 μg OVA adsorbed on 2 mg alum in saline.

3.2 Perform Ovalbumin Sensitization in the 57-day Model

1. Bring an aliquot of 0.8 mg/ml OVA solution to room temperature and vortex for 5 s at maximal speed (*see* **Note 1**).

2. Hold the mouse (*see* **Note 3**) in your hand by the dorsal skin so that its head is up and its rear legs are down. Maintain its tail in a fixed position with your fingers.

3. Use 1-ml syringes and 25-G needles to inject OVA and administer 5 ml/kg, i.e., 125 μl per mouse (of 25 g) by intraperitoneal injection. Each mouse receives 50 μg OVA in saline.

3.3 Ovalbumin Challenge

1. Bring an aliquot of 0.4 mg/ml (8-day and 21-day models) or 0.8 mg/ml (57-day model) OVA solution to room temperature and vortex for 5 s at maximal speed (*see* **Note 1**).

2. Mice should be anesthetized for intranasal administration. Anesthetize mice as follows: Hold the mouse in your hand by the dorsal skin so that its head is up and its rear legs are down. Maintain its tail in a fixed position with your fingers and use 1-ml syringes and 25-G needles to inject 4 ml/kg of the anesthetic solution (*see* **Note 5**) by intraperitoneal injection.

3. Place the mouse in the cage and wait until vibrissae do not move any more.

4. Hold the mouse in your hand in a vertical position with its head up and its rear legs down. Administer drop by drop 12.5 μl OVA solution, or saline alone for controls, in each nostril using sterile tips and a 20-μl precision pipette (*see* **Note 6**). Each mouse receives 10 μg (8-day and 21-day models) or 20 μg (57-day model) of OVA.

5. Keep the mouse in your hand in a vertical position for at least 1 min so that the solution can be distributed in the airways, and check that the mouse breathes normally (*see* **Note 7**).

6. Next place the mouse in a horizontal decubitus on a heating blanket until the mouse is completely conscious.

3.4 Bronchoalveolar Lavage Procedure

1. Mice should be anesthetized for BAL procedure as follows: Hold the mouse in your hand by the dorsal skin so that its head is up and its rear legs are down. Maintain its tail with fingers and use 1-ml syringes and 25-G needles to inject 4 ml/kg of the anesthetic solution (*see* Subheading 2.4) by intraperitoneal injection.

2. Place the animal in a dorsal decubitus position until the mouse is deeply anesthetized.

3. Using scissors, make a small incision in the neck skin. Separate salivary glands, incise the sternohyoid muscle to expose the trachea, and place a cotton thread (black haberdashery cotton thread no. 40) under the trachea.

4. Make a small semi-incision of the trachea to allow a 21-G lavage tube to pass into the trachea (*see* **Note 8**). Stabilize the tube and needle by attaching them with a cotton thread.

5. Load a 1-ml syringe with 0.5 ml sterile saline–EDTA, place it in the 21-G lavage tube and inject 0.5 ml saline–EDTA into the lung. Massage the chest for 10 s, re-aspirate saline of the first lavage, and keep the recovered lavage fluid into a 5-ml tube placed on ice.

6. Repeat the procedure 10 times per animal (*see* **Note 9**).

7. Pool lavages recovered and centrifuge them for 5 min at $300 \times g$ at 4 °C to pellet the cells. Discard the supernatant and add 1500 μl ultrapure water to the cell pellet for erythrocyte hemolysis. Wait for 10 s, add 500 μl KCl (0.6 M), and homogenize by inverting.

8. Centrifuge the BAL fluid for 5 min at $300 \times g$ at 4 °C. Discard the supernatant, add 500 μl saline–EDTA to the cell pellet, and homogenize by inverting.

3.5 Inflammatory Cell Counting

1. For total cell count: place 5 μl of the cell suspension on a hemocytometer, count the cells, and calculate the total cell number in BALF.

2. For differential cell count: homogenize by inverting and dilute with saline–EDTA to obtain a final concentration of 250,000 cells/ml. In a cytofunnel place 200 μl of the cell suspension. Cytocentrifuge for 10 min at $200 \times g$, air-dry the slide, and proceed to cell staining.

3. Cell staining with Diff-Quick staining kit: immerse the slide for 15 s in Diff-Quick fixative reagent, for 30 s in Diff-Quick solution I then for 15 s in Diff-Quick solution II and rinse the slide for 5 s in tap water. Let the slide air-dry (*see* **Note 10**).

4. Count and identify 400 cells under light microscopy on each slide. Magnification 1,000×; oil immersion. Manual counting allows to identify eosinophils, neutrophils, macrophages, and lymphocytes. The percentage of each cell population is reported as the total number of cells, and the absolute number of each cell population is then calculated in BALF.

4 Notes

1. OVA is a protein that may be difficult to dissolve in saline. In our experience, it is better to use a high speed vortex, with maximal speed $\geq 3,000$ rpm to dissolve OVA rapidly and prevent the formation of a turbid suspension composed of hydrated OVA particles.

2. Be very careful while choosing the aluminum hydroxide reagent. The quality of aluminum hydroxide influences the number of eosinophils recovered in BAL in the 8-day and 21-day models. We recommend to use aluminum hydroxide from Sigma-Aldrich (cat. no. 239186).

3. These protocols are developed to be used with 9-week-old male or female Balb/c mice to study AHR, OVA-specific IgE production, airway inflammatory cell recruitment, and airway remodeling [16–19]. C57BL6 mice may be used to study eosinophilic airway inflammation in the 8-day and 21-day models, but AHR cannot be measured (Fig. 4). To measure AHR together with eosinophil assessment in C57BL6 mice, we recommend the 57-day allergic asthma model. In addition, the described steps may be used for various other asthma models. Most of asthma models are dependent on the number of sensitizations and challenges, the dose of OVA and alum used, and the time between sensitizations and/or challenges.

4. Gently homogenize the suspension by 3–4 repeated reversal of the tube/syringe between each use so that the suspension does not drop at the bottom of the tube/syringe.

5. Anesthesia is key to successful intranasal administration. Too light anesthesia reduces reproducibility of inflammatory cells recruitment, and too deep anesthesia enhances respiratory failure during and after i.n. administration. It may be necessary to adapt the dose of anesthetic to warrant the best quality of anesthesia. It is often necessary to increase the dose over time.

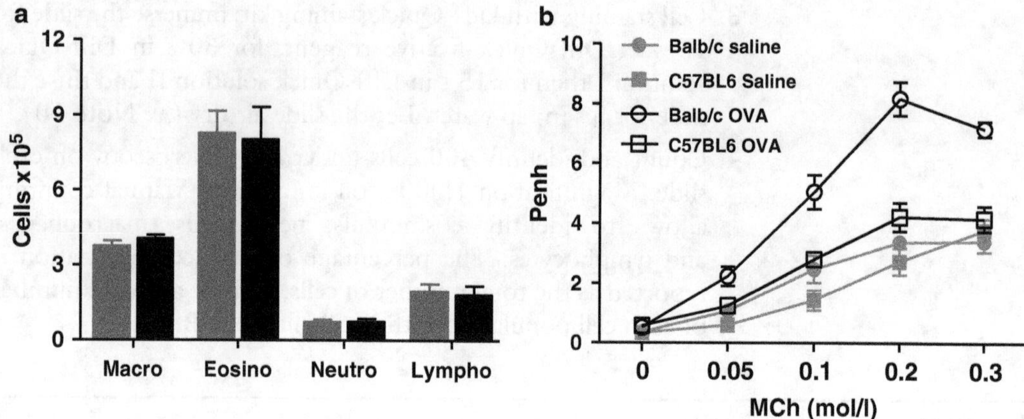

Fig. 4 Comparison of inflammatory cell recruitment and airway hyperresponsiveness between Balb/c and C57BL6 in the 21-day allergic asthma model. (**a**) Inflammatory cells in BALF on day 21 in Balb/c mice (*grey blocks*) or in C57BL6 mice (*black blocks*). *Blocks* are means and *bars* are SEM values. (**b**) Airway hyperresponsiveness to methacholine measured by plethysmography on vigil and unrestrained mice (EMKA Technologies, Paris, France) on day 21. *Dots* are means and *bars* are SEM values

6. The solution has to be administered drop by drop, slowly and very carefully, to maximize the distribution of OVA into the airways. Intranasal challenge is a simple and easy-to-perform technique, but it requires expertise to obtain reproducible responses.

7. If the mouse does not breathe normally, perform a thorax massage by pressing the rib cage several times, quickly but carefully. Please take care to identify each mouse who stops breathing, because this may affect AHR and eosinophilic inflammation of the airways.

8. While semi-incising the trachea, take care not to cut through the trachea. For tracheotomy, use a 21-G lavage tubing, carefully placed over a 21-G needle or a single-use Terumo surshield® IV catheter (Terumo, 1SR*SFA2025A).

9. Supernatant from the first two lavages should be pooled and separated from the eight following lavages for cytokine or mucus analysis, since a higher concentration is present in the 2 first lavages. In this case, centrifuge the initial two first lavages for 5 min at $300 \times g$ at 4 °C, then freeze the supernatant for further analysis, and add the cell pellet to the eight following lavages.

10. We describe the staining of cytospun cells with the commercial Diff-Quick staining : this staining requires to be performed in less than an hour of cytospinning. Other commercial staining may be useful such as RAL 555 (RAL-diagnostics) or could be advantageously replaced by a homemade staining described in [15].

Acknowledgements

This work was supported by the "Fonds de Dotation Recherche en Santé Respiratoire, Appel d'Offres Blanc 2010." FD is a recipient of a fellowship from the Laboratory of Excellence Medalis Initiative of Excellence (IdEx), Strasbourg University, France.

References

1. Global Initiative for Asthma (GINA) (2012) Pocket guide for asthma management and prevention. http://www.ginasthma.org/

2. Berend N, Salome CM, King GG (2008) Mechanisms of airway hyperresponsiveness in asthma. Respirology 13:624–631

3. Bates JH, Rincon M, Irvin CG (2009) Animal models of asthma. Am J Physiol Lung Cell Mol Physiol 297(3):L401–L410

4. Epstein MM (2006) Are mouse models of allergic asthma useful for testing novel therapeutics? Exp Toxicol Pathol 57(Suppl 2):41–44

5. Kumar RK, Herbert C, Foster PS (2008) The "classical" ovalbumin challenge model of asthma in mice. Curr Drug Targets 9(6):485–494

6. Shinagawa K, Kojima M (2003) Mouse model of airway remodeling: strain differences. Am J Respir Crit Care Med 168(8):959–967

7. Lukacs NW, John A, Berlin A, Bullard DC, Knibbs R, Stoolman LM (2002) E- and P-selectins are essential for the development of cockroach allergen-induced airway responses. J Immunol 169(4):2120–2125

8. Ulrich K, Hincks JS, Walsh R et al (2008) Anti-inflammatory modulation of chronic airway inflammation in the murine house dust mite model. Pulm Pharmacol Ther 21:637–647

9. Nials AT, Uddin S (2008) Mouse models of allergic asthma: acute and chronic allergen challenge. Dis Model Mech 1(4–5):213–220

10. McKee AS, Munks MW, MacLeod MK et al (2009) Alum induces innate immune responses through macrophage and mast cell sensors, but these sensors are not required for alum to act as an adjuvant for specific immunity. J Immunol 183:4403–4414

11. Zosky GR, Sly PD (2007) Animal models of asthma. Clin Exp Allergy 37(7):973–988

12. Daubeuf F, Frossard N (2013) Acute asthma models to ovalbumin in the mouse. Curr Protocols Mouse Biol 3:31–37

13. Daubeuf F, Reber L, Frossard N (2013) Measurement of airway responsiveness on vigil and unrestrained mouse. http://www.bio-protocol.org/wenzhang.aspx?id=328

14. Daubeuf F, Reber L, Frossard N (2013) Measurement of airway responsiveness in the anesthetized mouse. http://www.bio-protocol.org/wenzhang.aspx?id=645

15. Daubeuf F, Frossard N (2012) Performing bronchoalveolar lavage in the mouse. Curr Protoc Mouse Biol 2:167–175

16. Delayre-Orthez C, Becker J, De Blay F, Frossard N, Pons F (2004) Dose-dependent effects of endotoxins on allergen sensitization and challenge in the mouse. Clin Exp Allergy 34:1789–1795

17. Daubeuf F, Hachet-Haas M, Gizzi P, Gasparik V, Bonnet D, Utard V, Hibert M, Frossard N, Galzi JL (2013) An antedrug of the CXCL12 neutraligand blocks experimental allergic asthma without systemic effect in mice. J Biol Chem 288(17):11865–11876

18. Gasparik V, Daubeuf F, Hachet-Haas M, Rohmer F, Gizzi P, Haiech J, Galzi JL, Hibert M, Bonnet D, Frossard N (2011) Prodrugs of a CXC chemokine ligand 12, CXCL12, neutraligand active in vivo in a new asthma model. ACS Med Chem Lett 3:10–14

19. Hachet-Haas M, Balabanian K, Rohmer F et al (2008) Small neutralizing molecules to inhibit actions of the chemokine CXCL12. J Biol Chem 283:23189–23199

20. Andreasen CB (2003) Bronchoalveolar lavage. Vet Clin Small Anim 33:69–88

21. Reber LL, Daubeuf F, Plantinga M, De Cauwer L, Gerlo S, Waelput W, Van Calenbergh S, Tavernier J, Haegeman G, Lambrecht BN, Frossard N, de Bosscher K (2012) A fully dissociated glucocorticoid receptor modulator reduces airway hyperresponsiveness and inflammation in a murine model of asthma. J Immunol 188:3478–3487

Chapter 25

Mutant Mice and Animal Models of Airway Allergic Disease

Marie-Renée Blanchet, Matthew Gold, and Kelly M. McNagny

Abstract

Eosinophilia is a hallmark of allergic airway inflammation, and eosinophils represent an integral effector leukocyte through their release of various granule-stored cytokines and proteins. Numerous mouse models have been developed to mimic clinical disease and they have been instrumental in furthering our understanding of the role of eosinophils in disease. Most of these models consist of intranasal (i.n.) administration of antigenic proteases including papain and house dust mite (HDM) or the neo-antigen ovalbumin, with a resulting Th2-biased immune response and airway eosinophilia. These models have been particularly informative when combined with the numerous transgenic mice available that modulate eosinophil frequency or the mechanisms involved in their migration. Here, we describe the current models or allergic airway inflammation and outline some of the transgenic mice available to study eosinophils in disease.

Key words Asthma, Inflammation, Eosinophil, Mouse

1 Introduction

Allergic airway disease such as asthma is characterized by airway inflammation, airway hyperresponsiveness, and tissue remodelling [1]. In recent years, the vast majority of the research on asthma has focused on furthering our understanding of the development of the pulmonary allergic reaction using animal models and assessing their response to a variety of naturally occurring antigens, such as house dust mite (HDM) extract [2], papain [3] and model antigens such as ovalbumin (OVA) [4]. Inhalation of these antigens leads to a pulmonary allergic reaction, involving recruitment of granulocytes and a strong inflammatory response. Eosinophils are known to play a major role in the development of Th2-driven allergic airway inflammation in response to exposure to airborne allergens. Coincident with eosinophil and mast cell infiltration and degranulation, airway hyperresponsiveness develops and, after repeated attacks and chronic inflammation, airway remodelling ensues. These three hallmarks of asthma (eosinophil infiltration, airway hyperresponsiveness and tissue remodelling) are tightly linked and mimic the symptoms occurring in asthmatic patients.

Garry M. Walsh (ed.), *Eosinophils: Methods and Protocols*, Methods in Molecular Biology, vol. 1178,
DOI 10.1007/978-1-4939-1016-8_25, © Springer Science+Business Media New York 2014

As stated, a major contribution to the understanding of the role of eosinophils in the pathophysiology of this disease has been the development of animal models which mimic either one or all of the characteristics of human asthma [5]. This has been further enhanced through the use of genetically-modified mice including those completely lacking eosinophils [6, 7], and has led to several breakthrough findings on the role of this cell population in airway inflammation and other disease. Here we briefly describe several genetically-modified mouse strains and their relative utility in assessing eosinophil function (*PHIL, dbl-GATA, eoCRE, Cd34*$^{-/-}$, *Rora*$^{sg/sg}$) and provide in-depth protocols for three different mouse models of allergic airway inflammation (the OVA model of asthma, the HDM model of asthma, and the papain model of eosinophilia) which are widely used to study eosinophil function. Finally, we also present a non-eosinophilic model of airway inflammation, hypersensitivity pneumonitis (HP), which is a useful and important negative control for distinguishing between Th2 and Th1/17-driven disease and eosinophil function.

1.1 Mouse Strains to Study the Role of Eosinophils in Allergic Responses

The PHIL Mouse

The *PHIL* mouse [6] was one of the first genetically-modified mouse strains developed and used to study the importance of eosinophils in disease. In these mice, transgenic expression of diphtheria toxin is driven by the eosinophil peroxidase promoter, leading to ablation of all eosinophils shortly after the commitment of precursors to the eosinophil lineage. These mice therefore do not possess mature eosinophils and have been widely used to study the role of eosinophils in disease and various phenotypes [6, 8].

The dblGATA Mouse

Another eosinophil-deficient mouse which is available to study the role of the presence of eosinophils in disease is the *dblGATA* mouse [8, 9]. These mice carry a site-directed mutation of tandem GATA-1 binding sites in the eosinophil specific GATA-1 promoter. This very subtle mutation selectively ablates expression of GATA-1 in the eosinophil lineage and ablates development of eosinophils during early stages of precursor commitment while all other GATA-1-dependent lineages (erythroid and megakaryocytic) are spared. Thus, like the *PHIL* mice, the *dblGATA* mice are extremely useful for delineating general eosinophil-dependent aspects of normal development and disease.

The eos-CRE Mouse

The CRE recombinase system is widely used to target mutations to specific cell lineages. These mice provide an invaluable method for inactivating genes that would otherwise be embryonic lethal selectively in one lineage or tissue via transgenic expression of CRE. This strategy is extremely useful in determining the cell autonomous function of a particular gene in the absence of possible bystander effects in other lineages. Recently, an eosinophil lineage-specific CRE mouse was developed by expressing CRE-recombinase under the control of the eosinophil peroxidase promoter [10]. This now paves the way for evaluating the functional evaluation of a number of critical genes selectively in the eosinophil lineage. Such mice will likely quickly become widely used to study the importance of gene expression in eosinophils in disease such as allergic airway inflammation.

The Cd34$^{-/-}$ Mouse

Although several eosinophil-deficient mouse strains exist and can be used to evaluate the absolute requirement for eosinophils in disease, they do not permit the analysis of more subtle aspects of eosinophil function. Recently, we showed that eosinophils express the hematopoietic stem cell marker CD34 and that, although these mice produce normal numbers of eosinophils in the bone marrow and peripheral blood, they fail to traffic efficiently to the sites of Th2 driven inflammation [4]. Thus, CD34-deficient mice offer an interesting opportunity for distinguishing the functional significance of inflammatory eosinophil recruitment from steady state eosinophilopoiesis. However, it is also important to note that CD34 is expressed by a number of other mature hematopoietic cells in mice including mast cells and dendritic cells [4, 11, 12], and this needs to be taken into consideration when using this mouse to study cell trafficking in disease.

The Rora$^{sg/sg}$ Mouse

Group 2 innate lymphoid cells (ILC2s) are a recently described subset of the innate immune compartment identified by their unique expression of surface antigens (CD45$^+$Lineage$^-$CD127$^+$CD 25$^+$CD90$^+$ST2$^+$Sca1$^+$) [13–15]. They reside in multiple tissue sites but predominantly at mucosal surfaces and other potential portals of pathogen entry and they are potent producers of a variety of Th2 polarizing cytokines, predominantly IL-5 and IL-13. As such, these cells play a critical innate role in the initiation of Th2-driven disease and the recruitment and frequency of eosinophils [16–21]. While ILC2 development has been shown to be dependent on the transcription factors *Id2* [13], *Gata3* [17, 18], and *Tcf7* [20], two-groups independently identified the transcription factor RORα to be highly expressed in ILC2 development and mice deficient in RORα activity have a specific loss of ILC2 cells without abnormalities in most other hematopoietic compartments [22, 23]. Therefore, these mice too can be used to investigate the significance of eosinophil recruitment to specific sites of Th2-driven inflammation as well as the upstream processes that initiate Th2 inflammation.

1.2 Mouse Models to Study the Role of Eosinophils in Disease

Ovalbumin Model of Asthma

The OVA-based model of asthma has, historically, been the most widely used model and has been studied in depth. It involves a systemic priming step via intraperitoneal OVA injection, with or without aluminum hydroxide (Al(OH)$_3$), as a Th2 polarizing adjuvant. Typically, following sensitization, mice are "rested" for a minimum of 7 days to permit time for the production of

OVA-specific antibodies (predominantly IgG$_1$ and IgE), before mice are subsequently challenged either via intranasal instillation (i.n.) or aerosol exposure to OVA. Several different temporal regimens for sensitization and challenges have been published in the literature but these seem to create similar responses. Here, we present the exact timing we have used for over 10 years and with which we obtain reproducible eosinophil-driven responses [5, 24–26]. We find that when combined with intraperitoneal adjuvant priming, OVA induces a potent and robust eosinophil recruitment to the lung and thus this is a useful measure of their function in an allergic disease.

Various studies using genetically modified mice have demonstrated the importance of eosinophils in this Th2 airway inflammatory response. Interestingly, initial analyses of eosinophil-deficient *PHIL* mice [6] and *dblGATA* mice using this model, came to different conclusions on the importance of eosinophils in allergic airways disease [6, 8, 9]. With *PHIL* mice, the presence of eosinophils was fully necessary to induce airway inflammation and airway hyperresponsiveness, two major hallmarks of the disease. In stark contrast, the dbl*GATA* mice failed to show a significant defect in airway hyperresponsiveness and in mucus secretion and only exhibited protection from airway remodelling and collagen deposition. Thus, these authors argued for a relatively minor role for eosinophils in the full asthma phenotype. This discrepancy was later resolved to be an effect of the genetic backgrounds of the mice used (B6 for *PHIL* and Balb/c for *dblGATA*). These two background strains are well-known to have different predispositions to Th2 driven immune responses. Indeed, when both strains were evaluated in a B6 background, it was found that eosinophils are essential for the development of airway allergic responses [8].

The conclusions on the significance of eosinophils in OVA-induced asthma are further supported by studies in the *Cd34$^{-/-}$*, eosinophil migration-deficient mouse. Studies utilizing these mice revealed that efficient eosinophil migration to the lung is crucial for development of airway inflammation and AHR, even in the presence of normal levels of Th2 cytokines and bone marrow blood eosinophil precursors [4], thus highlighting the importance of local recruitment. Therefore, there is currently strong evidence for a role for eosinophils in the development of the allergic airway inflammation and AHR in this model, making it one of the best models to study eosinophil function and recruitment to the lung in allergy.

House Dust Mite (HDM)
Model of Asthma

While the use of the OVA model of asthma helped increase our understanding of eosinophil function in this disease, it quickly became evident that a mouse model based on naturally-occuring antigens, using the natural intranasal route of sensitization and which did not require the use of synthetic adjuvants such as

Al(OH)$_3$ was necessary. The HDM extract-based model of asthma was first described in 1996 [27] and it fulfills these criteria. Briefly, mice are sensitized i.n. for 3 consecutive days with HDM extract. The fact that HDM extract leads to a local sensitization to this antigen is likely linked to the intrinsic protease activity of several proteins in this antigen extract [28] which directly stimulate the airway epithelium to cause sensitization. Following sensitization, several i.n. challenges are used to induce allergic airway disease characterized in part by the recruitment of eosinophils to the alveolar space and lung tissue.

Although it is quickly increasing in popularity amongst the asthma basic research community, the characterization of this model and of the role of eosinophils in this model remains in its infancy. For example, no studies using eosinophil-deficient mice have been used in this model. However, as exposure to HDM causes very similar inflammation to OVA-based models (a Th2 cytokine response with high levels of IL-5 and IL-13, recruitment of eosinophils in the alveolar space and bronchi, AHR and antigen-specific IgE), this model is very likely to be dependent on the presence and recruitment of eosinophils to the lung as has previously shown with the OVA model. Likewise the dearth of antigen-specific transgenic TCR mice for HDM antigens has, until recently, impaired the ability to study downstream T cell driven responses. This has recently been remedied [29], and therefore, this model that uses a common human allergen is likely to be important for most future studies on eosinophil function in allergy.

Intriguingly, $Cd34^{-/-}$ and $Rora^{sg/sg}$ mice have been used in this model (Gold et al., unpublished and submitted data) and confirm an important role for eosinophils migration ($Cd34^{-/-}$ mice) and recruitment ($Rora^{sg/sg}$) in disease induced by HDM. Studies using $Rora^{sg/sg}$ mice in particular show that recruitment of eosinophils in response to a local antigen route of priming with HDM is solely dependent on the presence of innate lymphoid ILC2 cells, and that without ILC2 cells (and consequently, eosinophils), mice did not develop airway inflammation in response to HDM (unpublished, submitted data).

Papain Model of Eosinophilia

Although mouse models of asthma are useful tools to study eosinophil biology, they are complex and require the highly coordinated interaction of several hematopoietic cell populations. For some purposes, it would be more desirable to have a simple and acute model which consists of a relatively pure eosinophil-recruitment reaction. The papain-induced eosinophilia model is almost entirely eosinophilic, and fulfills these criteria [3].

Papain is a protease antigen that is a causative agent of occupational asthma [30]. While intradermal administration has been used to model basophil recruitment and Th2 development [31], inhalation of papain induces a robust and relatively selective recruitment of airway eosinophils. This response is independent of T and B cells as papain-induced eosinophil recruitment is not affected in $Rag2^{-/-}$ mice [31]. Papain induces release of IL-33 [32], a potent activator of group 2 innate lymphoid cells (ILC2s) that release large amounts of IL-5 and IL-13 and are responsible for papain-induced airway eosinophilia [15]. This model has become invaluable in determining early innate mediators of airway eosinophilia and is especially useful in highlighting the importance of the newly defined ILC2 subset of the innate immune cell repertoire.

Hypersensitivity Pneumonitis as a Negative Control to Study Eosinophil Function

One of the challenges of working with genetically modified mice and models to study eosinophil function is the lack of a robust Th1/Th17 allergic airway model to serve as a good negative control, i.e., in which it has been clearly shown that eosinophils do not play a role. In terms of a negative control for the eosinophilic response, the mouse model of hypersensitivity pneumonitis (HP) is the perfect candidate. HP is a Th1/Th17 allergic airway inflammatory disease characterized by an important alveolar infiltration of lymphocytes and lack of AHR. Eosinophils are not characteristic of the inflammation observed in HP, nor are any of the common eosinophil-related cytokines including IL-3, IL-5, or IL-13. Rather, HP relies on the release of Th1 and Th17 cytokines including IFN-gamma and IL-17 [33, 34]. Therefore, the mouse model of HP remains one of the few non-Th2 allergic airway inflammatory models, and it can be used to rule out the role of eosinophils in genetically modified mice phenotypes.

In mouse, HP is induced by i.n. administration of purified antigen from the bacteria *Saccharopolyspora rectivirgula* (SR), which grows in humid environments such as damp hay. The specific SR-dependent form of HP is also less formally known as "Farmer's lung" [35]. Typically, the SR antigen is obtained by bead-crushing live purified SR bacteria. The highly purified antigen preparation is complex to prepare, as contamination with other bacterial strains during preparation can easily occur and specific equipment is needed to produce efficient antigen. Indeed, in our hands, antigen produced by techniques such as sonication does not demonstrate the appropriate antigenic properties (unpublished observation). It is therefore highly recommended to get in touch with specialists in the field to obtain highly purified antigen.

The SR-induced Th-1/Th17 inflammatory response is characterized by an alveolar lymphocytosis and SR-specific IgG. In response to SR, neither humans nor mice develop AHR, which furthers separate this model from the mouse models of eosinophil-driven asthma previously described. It is therefore an appropriate and very useful negative control for the study of eosinophils or the significance of molecules on the molecules elaborated by eosinophils in disease [11].

2 Materials

2.1 Ovalbumin Model of Asthma

1. Mice (minimum of 6 weeks old at start of experiment and age and sex matched). All animal experiments must be conducted according to your institutions guidelines.
2. Albumin from chicken egg white, Grade V.
3. Injectable Alum.
4. Phosphate Buffered Saline.
5. 1 mL syringes.
6. 26–28 G needles.
7. Isoflurane.

2.2 House Dust Mite Model of Asthma

1. HDM lyophilized extract, *Dermatophagoides pteronyssinus* (Greer Labs, cat #: XPB82D3A), resuspended to 2.5 mg/mL in sterile PBS.

2.3 Papain Model of Eosinophilia

1. Papain (from *Carica papaya*, Sigma-Aldrich, supplied as a 25 mg/mL solution).

2.4 Hypersensitivity Pneumonitis: Negative Control for Eosinophilic Responses

1. SR antigen (home-grown or contact specialists in the field to obtain efficient antigen).

2.5 Assessment of Airway Inflammation

1. Ketamine/xylazine (20/1 mg/mL; 100 μl/10 g IP).
2. Surgical scissors and forceps.
3. 70 % Ethanol.
4. Catheters 22 g.
5. Suture thread.
6. 1 mL Tuberculin syringe.
7. PBS.
8. 15 mL conical tubes.
9. 10 % neutral buffered formalin.
10. Red Cell Lysis Buffer (Invitrogen, cat #: A1049201).
11. Hemacytometer.
12. Trypan Blue solution, 0.4 %.
13. Microscope slides.
14. Shandon Filter Cards.
15. Cytospin 4 Cytocentrifuge.

16. Wright-Giemsa Stain.

    (a). Fixative (Fisher Scientific, cat #: 122-929), or use methanol (Fisher Scientific, cat #: A412).

    (b). Solution I: PROTOCOL HEMA-3 (Fisher Scientific, cat #: 122-937).

    (c). Solution II: PROTOCOL HEMA-3 (Fisher Scientific, cat #: 122-952).

17. Permount Mounting Medium.

2.6 Lung Inflation and Fixation for Histology

1. 30 mL Luer-Lok syringe.

2. 18 G needle.

3. 500 mL volume Erlenmeyer Filter Flask.

4. 10 mL polystyrene serological pipette.

3 Methods

(Note that disease timelines are presented in Fig. 1 for all four models described below (Subheadings 3.1–3.4)).

3.1 Ovalbumin Model Disease Induction [4]

1. Dilute OVA in PBS to make a 4 mg/mL solution.

2. Shake the aluminum hydroxide solution well before use, then dilute the 4 mg/mL OVA solution 1:1 with the alum, for a final OVA concentration of 2 mg/mL.

3. Mix the OVA/Alum mixture for 30 min at room temperature in order for the alum to effectively adsorb the OVA antigen.

4. Immunize mice intraperitoneally on days 0 and 7 with 100 µL of the OVA/alum mixture using a 1 mL syringe and 28 G needle.

5. For intranasal challenges on days 21, 22, 23, 25, and 27, dilute OVA in PBS to make a 10 mg/mL solution.

6. Anesthetize mice until breathing rate reduces to approximately one per second (oxygen 1.5 L/min with 3.5 % isoflurane).

7. Once mice are appropriately sedated, intranasally administer 50 µL of 10 mg/mL OVA solution, adding dropwise through the nares.

8. Monitor the mice until they recover from anesthesia (approximately 5 min).

3.2 HDM-Extract Model Disease Induction [2]

1. Reconstitute lyophilized HDM extract to a stock concentration of 2.5 mg/mL in PBS.

2. Anesthetise mice with isoflurane as described in **step 6** of Subheading 3.2.

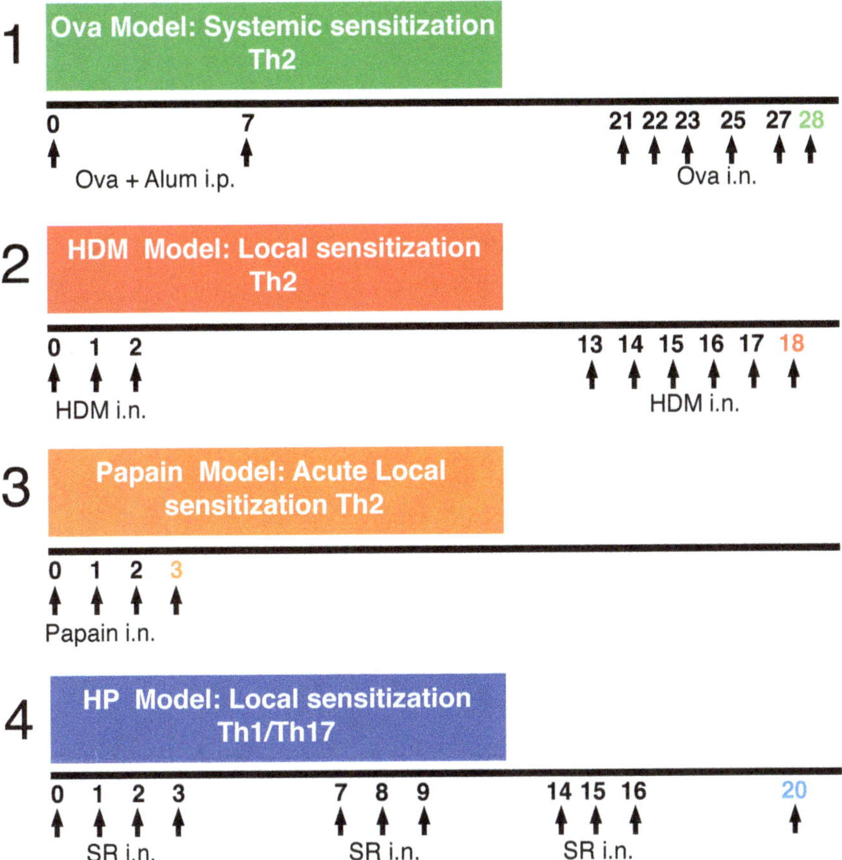

Fig. 1 Timelines for each model presented in the chapter

3. For HDM challenges on days 0, 1, and 2, dilute stock HDM solution to 2 mg/mL in PBS, intranasally administer 50 μL dropwise through the nares.

4. For HDM challenges on days 13–17, dilute stock HDM solution to 500 μg/mL in PBS and intranasally administer 50 μL dropwise through the nares.

5. Monitor the mice until they recover from anesthesia (approximately 5 min).

3.3 Papain Model Disease Induction [22]

1. Papain is supplied as a 25 mg/mL solution, dilute to 250 μg/mL with sterile PBS.

2. Anesthetise mice with isoflurane as described in **step 6** of Subheading 3.2.

3. Administer 40 μL of 250 μg/mL papain solution dropwise through the nares. Administer PBS alone or heat-inactivated papain as a negative control (*see* **Note 6**) on days 0, 1, and 2.

4. Monitor the mice until they recover from anesthesia (approximately 5 min).

3.4 HP Model Disease Induction [10]

1. Reconstitute lyophilized SR antigen to a stock concentration of 4 mg/mL in PBS.

2. Anesthetise mice with isoflurane as described in **step 6** of Subheading 3.2.

3. For challenges on all challenge days, administer 50 μl dropwise through the nares.

4. Monitor the mice until they recover from anesthesia (approximately 5 min).

3.5 Analysis of Disease Severity: Broncho-alveolar Lavage (BAL)

1. Anesthetise mice with a ketamine/xylazine overdose (20/1 mg/mL; 100 μL/10 g IP).

2. Place the mice ventral side up and pin down forepaws and hind-paws.

3. Using scissors and forceps, remove skin above the neck area. Carefully pull the parotid and submaxillary gland laterally.

4. Upon visualization of the trachea, remove the muscle layer surrounding it, then make a pinhole partial cut of the trachea just inferior of the larynx and thyroid. Carefully insert the flexible 22 G catheter into the trachea, using the suture thread to secure the catheter.

5. Prepare three 1 mL slip-tip syringes filled with 1 mL of PBS. Lavage the lungs three times with 1 mL of PBS, slowly advancing and recovering the PBS lavage liquid. Pool the collected lavages into a 15 mL conical tube and store on ice until further use.

6. After collecting the BAL, dissect open the thoracic cavity, exposing the left lung and the four lobes of the right lung (superior, middle, inferior, and post-caval).

7. Dissect out some lung specimens for histology, and place in ten volumes worth of 10 % buffered formalin. Store specimens at 4 °C for 24 h and then replace the formalin with 70 % ethanol for long term storage at 4 °C before paraffin embedding and histology.

3.6 Analysis of BAL Fluid: Enumeration and Differential Counts of BAL Leucocytes

1. Record collected BAL volume and then centrifuge at $1,200 \times g$ for 5 min.

2. Resuspend cell pellet in 1 mL of red-cell lysis buffer and incubate for 3–5 min, then dilute with PBS and centrifuge at $1,200 \times g$ for 5 min.

3. Resuspend cell pellet in 1 mL of PBS or media. Collect aliquot of cells for dilution with trypan blue and enumeration on hemocytometer.

4. Count total number of BAL cells and report it on the BAL volume (total number of BAL cells/mL BAL fluid).

5. Prepare aliquots of cells for cytospins. Dilute aliquots to 5.0–7.5 × 10^5 cells/mL, and cytospin 100 μL of cell dilutions to each slide for 3 min at 200 × g (approximately 50,000–75,000 cells/slide).

6. Allow slides to dry for 2 h to overnight, before staining.

7. Insert the slides for 30 s each into methanol, solution I and solution II of the PROTOCOL HEMA-3 staining set. Allow excess methanol/stain to drip down in-between solutions.

8. Allow the slides to air-dry and then, if desired, mount with coverslip using Permount.

9. Perform differential cell counts from a minimum of 400 cells/slide using standard morphological criteria of macrophages, lymphocytes, neutrophils, and eosinophils.

3.7 Histology and Tissue Inflammation Analysis

1. Paraffin embed lung specimens and section 3–6 μm thick, then stain with H and E.

2. Under microscopic examination, score disease severity based on the following criteria in 4–5 airway sections per mouse and average the results:

   (a) Perivascular infiltration, score of 0–4.

   - 0, no cells.
   - 1, a few cells.
   - 2, entire encirclement of vessel with infiltrate 1–2 cells deep.
   - 3, entire encirclement of vessel with infiltrate 3–5 cells deep.
   - 4, entire encirclement of vessel with infiltrate >5 cells deep.

   (b) Peribronchiolar infiltration, score of 0–4.

   - 0, no cells.
   - 1, a few cells.
   - 2, entire encirclement of bronchiole with infiltrate 1–2 cells deep, slight loss of uniformity of airway epithelium.
   - 3, entire encirclement of bronchiole with infiltrate 3–5 cells deep, with a more pronounced hyperplasia and metaplasia of the airway epithelium.
   - 4, entire encirclement of vessel with infiltrate >5 cells deep, complete loss of airway epithelial structure including tissue damage leading to rupture of the bronchiole.

(c) Parenchymal infiltration, score of 0–4.

- 0, no cells.
- 1, a few scattered cells throughout the lung.
- 2, one quadrant of the lung with a high degree of infiltration.
- 3, two quadrants of the lung with a high degree of infiltration.
- 4, more than two quadrants of the lung with a high degree of infiltration.

4 Notes

1. Most methods mentioned above are tailored for mice on the C57Bl/6 J background. Due to the increased Th2 bias of the immune response in other inbred strains (Balb/cJ or 129S1/SvImJ for example), it would be advisable to titrate down the antigen concentration for both the OVA and HDM asthma models if these Th2-skewed strains were to be used.

2. It is important to use only age and sex matched mice for all asthma experiments due to the reported sex differences in asthma susceptibility in mice [36, 37].

3. It is important to insure that the levels of LPS are as low as possible (and similar between lots) for the OVA and HDM stocks. Increased levels of LPS will lead to a neutrophilic response rather than an eosinophilic response using these antigens.

4. The protease activity in the HDM stock should be verified and kept similar between lots to insure reproducibility.

5. We also notice that the aluminum hydroxide tends to lose its potency after 4–6 months. Be sure to shake the bottle carefully before using as it tends to precipitate.

6. As a negative control, treat mice i.n. with heat-inactivated papain. This can be easily achieved by boiling the papain mixture for 10 min at 100 °C.

7. To avoid the entrance of blood in the BAL, avoid performing cardiac punctures until after the collection of the BAL. The blood obtained can then be later used for serum antibody and cytokine quantifications.

8. For intranasal administration, it is imperative to treat the mice at the optimal sedation point to insure the antigen is aspired into the lungs and not expulsed (mouse not sedated enough) or drained directly into the throat and swallowed (mouse too sedated). One good indication of the right level of sedation is to count the number of breaths per second: antigen should be administered when the mouse breathes at the rate of one breath per second.

References

1. Barnes PJ (2008) Immunology of asthma and chronic obstructive pulmonary disease. Nat Rev Immunol 8:183–192

2. Phipps S, Lam CE, Kaiko GE, Foo SY, Collison A, Mattes J, Barry J, Davidson S, Oreo K, Smith L, Mansell A, Matthaei KI, Foster PS (2009) Toll/IL-1 signaling is critical for house dust mite-specific helper T cell type 2 and type 17 [corrected] responses. Am J Respir Crit Care Med 179:883–893

3. Soto-Mera MT, Lopez-Rico MR, Filgueira JF, Villamil E, Cidras R (2000) Occupational allergy to papain. Allergy 55:983–984

4. Blanchet MR, Maltby S, Haddon DJ, Merkens H, Zbytnuik L, McNagny KM (2007) CD34 facilitates the development of allergic asthma. Blood 110:2005–2012

5. Jacobsen EA, Helmers RA, Lee JJ, Lee NA (2012) The expanding role(s) of eosinophils in health and disease. Blood 120:3882–3890

6. Lee JJ, Dimina D, Macias MP, Ochkur SI, McGarry MP, O'Neill KR, Protheroe C, Pero R, Nguyen T, Cormier SA, Lenkiewicz E, Colbert D, Rinaldi L, Ackerman SJ, Irvin CG, Lee NA (2004) Defining a link with asthma in mice congenitally deficient in eosinophils. Science 305:1773–1776

7. Humbles AA, Lloyd CM, McMillan SJ, Friend DS, Xanthou G, McKenna EE, Ghiran S, Gerard NP, Yu C, Orkin SH, Gerard C (2004) A critical role for eosinophils in allergic airways remodeling. Science 305:1776–1779

8. Blanchet MR, Gold M, Maltby S, Bennett J, Petri B, Kubes P, Lee DM, McNagny KM (2010) Loss of CD34 leads to exacerbated autoimmune arthritis through increased vascular permeability. J Immunol 184:1292–1299

9. Walsh ER, Sahu N, Kearley J, Benjamin E, Kang BH, Humbles A, August A (2008) Strain-specific requirement for eosinophils in the recruitment of T cells to the lung during the development of allergic asthma. J Exp Med 205:1285–1292

10. Doyle AD, Jacobsen EA, Ochkur SI, Willetts L, Shim K, Neely J, Kloeber J, Lesuer WE, Pero RS, Lacy P, Moqbel R, Lee NA, Lee JJ (2013) Homologous recombination into the eosinophil peroxidase locus generates a strain of mice expressing Cre recombinase exclusively in eosinophils. J Leukoc Biol 94:17–24

11. Blanchet MR, Bennett JL, Gold MJ, Levantini E, Tenen DG, Girard M, Cormier Y, McNagny KM (2011) CD34 is required for dendritic cell trafficking and pathology in murine hypersensitivity pneumonitis. Am J Respir Crit Care Med 184:687–698

12. Drew E, Merkens H, Chelliah S, Doyonnas R, McNagny KM (2002) CD34 is a specific marker of mature murine mast cells. Exp Hematol 30:1211–1218

13. Moro K, Yamada T, Tanabe M, Takeuchi T, Ikawa T, Kawamoto H, Furusawa J, Ohtani M, Fujii H, Koyasu S (2010) Innate production of T(H)2 cytokines by adipose tissue-associated c-Kit(+)Sca-1(+) lymphoid cells. Nature 463:540–544

14. Halim TY, Krauss RH, Sun AC, Takei F (2012) Lung natural helper cells are a critical source of Th2 cell-type cytokines in protease allergen-induced airway inflammation. Immunity 36:451–463

15. Neill DR, Wong SH, Bellosi A, Flynn RJ, Daly M, Langford TK, Bucks C, Kane CM, Fallon PG, Pannell R, Jolin HE, McKenzie AN (2010) Nuocytes represent a new innate effector leukocyte that mediates type-2 immunity. Nature 464:1367–1370

16. Yasuda K, Muto T, Kawagoe T, Matsumoto M, Sasaki Y, Matsushita K, Taki Y, Futatsugi-Yumikura S, Tsutsui H, Ishii KJ, Yoshimoto T, Akira S, Nakanishi K (2012) Contribution of IL-33-activated type II innate lymphoid cells to pulmonary eosinophilia in intestinal nematode-infected mice. Proc Natl Acad Sci U S A 109:3451–3456

17. Molofsky AB, Nussbaum JC, Liang HE, Van Dyken SJ, Cheng LE, Mohapatra A, Chawla A, Locksley RM (2013) Innate lymphoid type 2 cells sustain visceral adipose tissue eosinophils and alternatively activated macrophages. J Exp Med 210:535–549

18. Barlow JL, Bellosi A, Hardman CS, Drynan LF, Wong SH, Cruickshank JP, McKenzie AN (2012) Innate IL-13-producing nuocytes arise during allergic lung inflammation and contribute to airways hyperreactivity. J Allergy Clin Immunol 129(191–198): e191–e194

19. Klein Wolterink RG, Serafini N, van Nimwegen M, Vosshenrich CA, de Bruijn MJ, Fonseca Pereira D, Veiga Fernandes H, Hendriks RW, Di Santo JP (2013) Essential, dose-dependent role for the transcription factor Gata3 in the development of IL-5+ and IL-13+ type 2 innate lymphoid cells. Proc Natl Acad Sci U S A 110:10240–10245

20. Hoyler T, Klose CS, Souabni A, Turqueti-Neves A, Pfeifer D, Rawlins EL, Voehringer D, Busslinger M, Diefenbach A (2012) The transcription factor GATA-3 controls cell fate and maintenance of type 2 innate lymphoid cells. Immunity 37:634–648

21. Yang Q, Monticelli LA, Saenz SA, Chi AW, Sonnenberg GF, Tang J, De Obaldia ME, Bailis W, Bryson JL, Toscano K, Huang J, Haczku A, Pear WS, Artis D, Bhandoola A (2013) T cell factor 1 is required for group 2 innate lymphoid cell generation. Immunity 38:694–704

22. Wong SH, Walker JA, Jolin HE, Drynan LF, Hams E, Camelo A, Barlow JL, Neill DR, Panova V, Koch U, Radtke F, Hardman CS, Hwang YY, Fallon PG, McKenzie AN (2012) Transcription factor RORalpha is critical for nuocyte development. Nat Immunol 13:229–236

23. Halim TY, MacLaren A, Romanish MT, Gold MJ, McNagny KM, Takei F (2012) Retinoic-acid-receptor-related orphan nuclear receptor alpha is required for natural helper cell development and allergic inflammation. Immunity 37:463–474

24. Naus S, Blanchet MR, Gossens K, Zaph C, Bartsch JW, McNagny KM, Ziltener HJ (2010) The metalloprotease-disintegrin ADAM8 is essential for the development of experimental asthma. Am J Respir Crit Care Med 181:1318–1328

25. Blanchet MR, Israel-Assayag E, Cormier Y (2005) Modulation of airway inflammation and resistance in mice by a nicotinic receptor agonist. Eur Respir J 26:21–27

26. Haddon DJ, Antignano F, Hughes MR, Blanchet MR, Zbytnuik L, Krystal G, McNagny KM (2009) SHIP1 is a repressor of mast cell hyperplasia, cytokine production, and allergic inflammation in vivo. J Immunol 183:228–236

27. O'Brien R, Ooi MA, Clarke AH, Thomas WR (1996) Immunologic responses following respiratory sensitization to house dust mite allergens in mice. Immunol Cell Biol 74:174–179

28. Thomas WR, Smith WA, Hales BJ, Mills KL, O'Brien RM (2002) Characterization and immunobiology of house dust mite allergens. Int Arch Allergy Immunol 129:1–18

29. Jarman ER, Tan KA, Lamb JR (2005) Transgenic mice expressing the T cell antigen receptor specific for an immunodominant epitope of a major allergen of house dust mite develop an asthmatic phenotype on exposure of the airways to allergen. Clin Exp Allergy 35:960–969

30. Milne J, Brand S (1975) Occupational asthma after inhalation of dust of the proteolytic enzyme, papain. Br J Ind Med 32:302–307

31. Sokol CL, Barton GM, Farr AG, Medzhitov R (2008) A mechanism for the initiation of allergen-induced T helper type 2 responses. Nat Immunol 9:310–318

32. Oboki K, Ohno T, Kajiwara N, Arae K, Morita H, Ishii A, Nambu A, Abe T, Kiyonari H, Matsumoto K, Sudo K, Okumura K, Saito H, Nakae S (2010) IL-33 is a crucial amplifier of innate rather than acquired immunity. Proc Natl Acad Sci U S A 107:18581–18586

33. Joshi AD, Fong DJ, Oak SR, Trujillo G, Flaherty KR, Martinez FJ, Hogaboam CM (2009) Interleukin-17-mediated immunopathogenesis in experimental hypersensitivity pneumonitis. Am J Respir Crit Care Med 179:705–716

34. Gudmundsson G, Hunninghake GW (1997) Interferon-gamma is necessary for the expression of hypersensitivity pneumonitis. J Clin Invest 99:2386–2390

35. Girard M, Cormier Y (2010) Hypersensitivity pneumonitis. Curr Opin Allergy Clin Immunol 10:99–103

36. Melgert BN, Oriss TB, Qi Z, Dixon-McCarthy B, Geerlings M, Hylkema MN, Ray A (2010) Macrophages: regulators of sex differences in asthma? Am J Respir Cell Mol Biol 42:595–603

37. Melgert BN, Postma DS, Kuipers I, Geerlings M, Luinge MA, van der Strate BW, Kerstjens HA, Timens W, Hylkema MN (2005) Female mice are more susceptible to the development of allergic airway inflammation than male mice. Clin Exp Allergy 35:1496–1503

Murine Models of Eosinophilic Leukemia: A Model of FIP1L1-PDGFRα Initiated Chronic Eosinophilic Leukemia/Systemic Mastocytosis

Yoshiyuki Yamada, Jose A. Cancelas, and Marc E. Rothenberg

Abstract

Chronic eosinophilic leukemia (CEL) was distinguished from hypereosinophilic syndrome (HES) in the 2001 World Health Organization (WHO) criteria. Subsequently, the FIP1L1-PDGFRα *(F/P)* fusion tyrosine kinase was identified in patients with HES and found to be the most common clonal defect in CEL and the second most frequent mutation in systemic mastocytosis (SM). Introduction of F/P into bone marrow hematopoietic stem cells and progenitors has been used to establish murine models of F/P--myeloproliferative neoplasm and F/P–CEL. IL-5 overexpression and introduction of F/P is required to develop murine CEL. This F/P-CEL model is thought to be an accurate model of the clinical disease. Here we describe the method of F/P-CEL/SM model development and assessment.

Key words FIP1L1-PDGFRα, Chronic eosinophilic leukemia (CEL), Hypereosinophilic syndromes (HES), Systemic mastocytosis (SM), Eosinophils

1 Introduction

Chronic eosinophilic leukemia (CEL) is a rare hematological disorder with primary eosinophilia. CEL was distinguished from hypereosinophilic syndrome (HES) by the World Health Organization (WHO) in 2001 [1]. Diagnosis of CEL is based on the exclusion of reactive or secondary causes of hypereosinophilia, lymphocytic variants of hypereosinophilia, and the presence of myeloid cells with clonal cytogenetic abnormality or clonality, or blasts in the peripheral blood (higher than 2 %) or marrow (more than 5 % but less than 20 %) as well as persistent eosinophilia more than 1.5×10^9/L in blood and myeloblasts <20 % in blood or marrow. A novel fusion tyrosine kinase produced by an interstitial chromosomal deletion on 4q12, FIP1L1-PDGFRα (F/P), was identified in patients with HES and eosinophil cell line Eol-1 [2, 3]. The initially diagnosed HES patients with F/P were reclassified as having CEL according to the WHO criteria because the *F/P* fusion is

Garry M. Walsh (ed.), *Eosinophils: Methods and Protocols*, Methods in Molecular Biology, vol. 1178, DOI 10.1007/978-1-4939-1016-8_26, © Springer Science+Business Media New York 2014

a clonal cytogenetic abnormality. Since then, F/P-positive CEL has become the most frequent clonal defect demonstrated in CEL. With increasing recognition of the importance of the molecular definition, characterized eosinophilic syndromes such as F/P-positive CEL have been assembled into a new category of myeloid neoplasms known as "myeloid and lymphoid neoplasm with eosinophilia and abnormalities of PDGFRA, PDGFRB or FGFR1" in the revised 2008 WHO criteria [4].

Just after the discovery of F/P, Cools et al. attempted to develop a disease model of CEL by retroviral transduction of the *F/P* fusion gene into bone marrow hematopoietic stem cells and progenitors (HSC/P) and transplantation into recipient mice [5]; however, this induced a murine model of myeloproliferative neoplasm (MPN) similar to that found in p210-BCR/ABL-induced chronic myelogenous leukemia-like disease (F/P-MPN). Thus, in this murine model, F/P expression induced proliferation of myeloid lineages that are not eosinophil-predominant, suggesting F/P might require secondary events for the development of CEL-like disease. Candidates for these secondary events include IL-5, which is considered to be the most relevant cytokine in the pathogenesis of HES/CEL. Indeed, elevated serum IL-5 levels have been reported in imatinib-responsive HES patients including those expressing F/P [6]; anti-IL-5 responsive F/P+ patients have also been observed [7]. Therefore, we hypothesized that F/P in conjunction with IL-5 overexpression may induce murine CEL-like disease [8]. Wild-type recipient mice were transplanted with the *F/P* fusion gene via retrovirus transduction of HSC/P derived from the bone marrow of CD2-IL-5 transgenic mice, which overexpress IL-5 in a T-cell dependent fashion. The mice developed rapidly progressive disease characterized by intense leukocytosis with hypereosinophilia in peripheral blood, hepatosplenomegaly, and tissue eosinophilia in multiple organs, resembling human HES (F/P-CEL) [8]. The specificity of this combination of IL-5 overexpression and F/P has been examined. Although other MPN such as CML are occasionally associated with eosinophilia, p210-BCR/ABL in the presence of transgenic T-cell overexpression of IL-5 does not induce CEL-like disease. In addition, F/P but not p210-*BCR/ABL* increased the expression and frequency of IL-5Rα+ cells in splenocytes in comparison to vector controls. These findings suggest expression of the F/P fusion gene may specifically induce eosinophil differentiation during myeloproliferation.

Clinically, F/P-positive CEL is characterized by systemic mastocytosis (SM) as well as clonal hypereosinophilia, multiple organ dysfunctions due to eosinophil infiltration, and a dramatic response to treatment with imatinib mesylate. The murine CEL model generated by introduction of F/P and IL-5 overexpression also exhibits systemic mastocytosis [9] resembling clinical F/P-positive CEL. The molecular mechanism underlying the development of CEL/ SM by F/P has been shown in a few reports. F/P synergizes with

SCF stimulation through c-kit to promote mast cell development and activation [9] and specifically enhances eosinophil development from HSC/P via the MAPKs cascades by controlling the expression and activity of lineage-specific transcription factors, such as *C/EBPα*, *GATA-1*, and *GATA-2* in mouse [10]. In addition, F/P activates JAK2 synergistically with IL-5 resulting in cellular proliferation and infiltration of human F/P$^+$ cells [11].

Thus, the murine F/P-positive CEL model is a well-established model of human CEL. We describe the method for developing this model here.

2 Materials

2.1 Mice

Prepare donor and recipient mice for transplantation.

1. Prepare donor mice. Interleukin-5 (IL-5) transgenic (Tg) mice (7–12 weeks old, CD2$^+$ T-cell–dependent IL-5Tg BALB/c mice) (*see* **Note 1**) [12] serve as bone marrow (BM) donors. As a control, BALB/c (wild type) female mice (7–12 weeks old) should be used (National Cancer Institute Frederick, MD or Taconic Farms Germantown, NY, USA.).

2. Use BALB/c (wild type) female mice as recipients.

2.2 Cell Line

1. Phoenix-GP cells (CRL-3215, ATCC, USA): the cells are cultured in Dulbecco's modified Eagle's Medium (DMEM) with 10 % fetal bovine serum (FBS) and 1 % penicillin–streptomycin (10,000 U).

2.3 Plasmid DNAs

1. Retroviral vector plasmids (not commercially available) are murine stem cell virus (MSCV)-based bicistronic vectors named MSCV-F/P-IRES-EGFP and MSCV-IRES-EGFP (mock vector) (*see* **Note 2**) [5].

2. Plasmids for major proteins encoded within the retroviral genome: Gag (M57) and ecotropic Env plasmids [13].

2.4 Cell Culture Media

1. Culture for Phoenix-GP cells: DMEM with 10 % FBS and 1 % penicillin–streptomycin (10,000 U).

2. Medium for harvesting viral supernatant: pH 7.9 high glucose DMEM with 10 % FBS and 20 mM HEPES buffer. Adjust medium to pH 7.9 then add HEPES to 20 mM.

3. IMDM culture medium: IMDM (Iscove's Modified Dulbecco's Medium) with 10 % FBS and 1 % penicillin–streptomycin (10,000 U).

4. Transduction media: Add recombinant mouse (rm) IL-3 (6 ng/mL), rm stem cell factor (10 ng/mL), and IL-6 (10 ng/mL) in IMDM.

5. RPMI-1640 with 10 % FBS.

2.5 Buffers

1. Phosphate-buffered saline (PBS).
2. Hank's Balanced Salt Solution (HBSS).
3. 1 M Hepes Buffer solution.
4. Cell dissociation buffer, enzyme-free PBS.
5. 10× NH_4Cl red blood cell (RBC) lysis buffer (BD PharmLyse Lysing buffer, San Jose, CA, USA.). Dilute to 1× with distilled water prior to use.

2.6 Cytokines

Prepare stock solution at 10–50 µg/mL and store at –80 °C.

1. rm IL-3.
2. rm stem cell factor (SCF).
3. rm IL-6.

2.7 Antibodies

1. Allophycocyanin (APC)-conjugated anti-CD11b (clone M1/70; BD Biosciences, San Jose, CA, USA.).
2. R-phycoerythrin (PE)-conjugated anti-CCR3 (clone 83101; R&D, Minneapolis, MN, USA.).
3. PE-conjugated anti-Siglec-F (clone E50-2440; BD Biosciences).
4. APC-conjugated anti-c-kit (clone 2B8; BD Biosciences).
5. PE-conjugated anti-FcεRIα (clone MAR-1; eBiosciences, San Diego, CA, USA.).
6. PE-Cy7-conjugated anti-CD45 (clone 30 F-11; BD Biosciences).

2.8 Staining Solutions

1. Turk solution: 1 mL glacial acetic acid and 1 mL 1 % aqueous gentian violet in 100 mL distilled water.
2. Discombe's solution: 0.05 % aqueous eosin Y and 5 % acetone in distilled water [14].

2.9 Other Reagents and Equipment

1. 5-fluorouracil (5-FU) (APP Pharmaceuticals, LLC, Schaumburg, IL, USA): 50 mg/mL solution. Just before use for i.p. injection, 5-FU (50 mg/mL) is diluted with HBSS to 10 mg/mL.
2. HISTOPAQUE 1083 to obtain low-density bone marrow (LDBM) cells by density gradient fractionation.
3. Calcium phosphate transfection kit with 2 M $CaCl_2$ and 2× Hepes Buffered Saline (HBS).
4. Polybrene: Prepare a stock solution at 5 mg/mL with sterile water and store at –20 °C; use at 5 µg/mL.
5. Chloroquine: prepare 25 mM stock solution.
6. 7-Aminoactinomycin D (7-AAD), store at 1 mg/mL in DMSO. Use 7-AAD to exclude dead cells.
7. Liberase CL and DNAse.

8. Scales to measure the weight of donor mice.

9. Earthenware mortar and pestle: autoclaved before use.

10. Disposable sterile injection needles (27 G, 1/2 in.), syringes (1 mL) and 29G insulin 1 mL syringes.

11. Falcon Conical 50 mL Tubes.

12. Cell strainer, 40 μm blue: fits into a 50 mL BD Falcon Conical Tube.

13. Syringe filter, 0.45 μm: Diameter 25 mm, Sterile.

14. 6-well Multiwell Plate. Non tissue culture-treated polystyrene, flat-bottom plate.

15. 24-well Multiwell Plate. Non tissue culture-treated polystyrene, flat-bottom plate.

16. 100×20 mm tissue culture dish, tissue culture-treated polystyrene.

3 Methods

3.1 Retroviral Supernatants [13, 15]

1. Culture Phoenix-GP cells on 100-mm tissue culture dish to 70 % confluence.

2. To prepare plasmids (for one dish), add the retroviral plasmids (8 μg F/P or control), 10 μg Gag (M57) plasmid, 3 μg env plasmid, and 36 μL of 2 M CaCl (calcium phosphate transfection kit) in 300 μL sterile H_2O (calcium phosphate transfection kit).

3. Transfection mixture (for one dish): Add 300 μL 2× Hepes buffer in a 50-mL Falcon tube and slowly add plasmids drop-wise while bubbling air through 2× Hepes buffer with sterile Pasteur pipettes (see also manufacturer instructions). Incubate at room temperature, 30 min.

4. Remove the spent medium and add 10 mL fresh medium containing 25 μM chloroquine.

5. Add transfection mixture (total 600 μL) and incubate for 12 h (>6 h) at 37 °C in a CO_2 incubator.

6. Remove the spent medium; add 10 mL fresh medium without chloroquine and incubate for 12 h.

7. Remove the spent medium; add 8.5 mL complete medium to harvest the viral supernatant and incubate for 12 h.

8. Collect the viral supernatant using 10-mL sterile syringes, pass it through a 0.45-μm sterile filter; divide into 4-mL aliquots in polypropylene round-bottom tubes and store at −80 °C. Add 8.5 mL fresh medium to harvest the viral supernatant.

9. Collect the viral supernatant every 12 h up to 48 h after culture initiation.

3.2 Retroviral Transduction into Hematopoietic Progenitor Cells (See Fig. 1)

One or three different control groups may be required, depending on the experiment (*see* Table 1) [8].

1. Prepare donor CD2-IL-5Tg BALB/c mice and age-matched wild-type mice. The numbers of donor and recipient mice should be equivalent, if possible.

2. Administer 5-FU (150 mg/kg body weight) by intraperitoneal injection 6 days prior to BM harvest.

3. After 6 days, sacrifice the donors and harvest the femora, tibiae, and iliac crests; submerge them completely in HBSS in a 50-mL Falcon tube. Transfer to an autoclaved mortar and grind with a pestle.

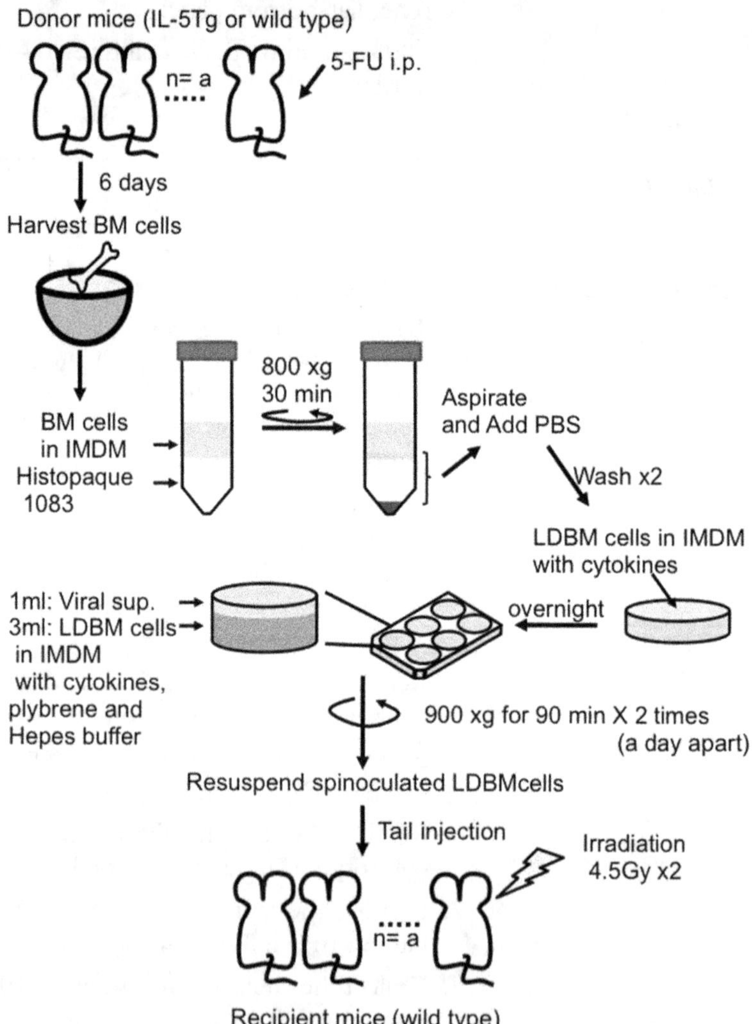

Fig. 1 This figure describes an outline of retroviral transduction and subsequent transplantation for the development of murine chronic eosinophilic leukemia and its controls. *Tg* transgenic, *5-FU* 5-fluorouracil, *BM* bone marrow, *LDBM* low density bone marrow. *Rotation arrows* indicate centrifugation

Table 1
Combinations of viral vector, donor, and recipient

Viral vector	Donor	Recipient	Phenotype[a]
F/P	Wild type	Wild type	MPN
F/P	IL-5 Tg	Wild type	CEL
Mock	Wild type	Wild type	Wild type
Mock	IL-5 Tg	Wild type	IL-5 Tg

[a]Developed phenotypes
F/P, MSCV-F/P-IRES-EGFP; Mock, MSCV-IRES-EGFP; *Tg* transgenic; *MPN* myeloproliferative neoplasm; *CEL* chronic eosinophilic leukemia

4. Pass the ground material through 40 μm cell strainers fitted in 50-mL BD Falcon Tubes. The bone marrow cells are isolated in the Falcon tube.

5. Centrifuge the collected BM cells at $400 \times g$ for 5 min and resuspend in IMDM (about 10 mL/5 mice).

6. Add 15.0 mL HISTOPAQUE 1083 to new 50-mL Falcon tubes, then carefully and slowly layer 10–15 mL resuspended BM cells onto the HISTOPAQUE 1083 surface and centrifuge at $800 \times g$ for 30 min at room temperature. The acceleration and brake on the centrifuge should be turned off.

7. After centrifugation, use a plastic pipette to carefully aspirate the opaque interface containing the mononuclear cells to just above pellet; transfer to a new 50-mL Falcon tube, add PBS to 50 mL and centrifuge at $400 \times g$ for 5 min.

8. Remove the supernatant, resuspend cells in PBS and centrifuge at $400 \times g$ for 5 min.

9. Resuspend them with transduction media (8–10 mice/10 mL, about 2×10^6 cells/mL), seed on 100-mm non-tissue culture plates and then incubate overnight at 37 °C in a CO_2 incubator.

10. Place the media containing cells in 50-mL Falcon tubes and thoroughly wash the plates with 5 mL PBS.

11. Use a microscope to check the plate for remaining cells and repeat pipetting until all but the most firmly adhered cells have been removed.

12. Centrifuge the collected cells at $400 \times g$ for 5 min.

13. Resuspend in IMDM and adjust to about $0.5–1 \times 10^6$ cells/mL.

14. Thaw each viral supernatant at 37 °C in a thermostatic bath.

15. Plate 3 mL resuspended cells in each well of a 6-well plate.

16. Add 1 mL viral supernatant to each well. Viral supernatants derived from 12 h and 24 h cultures should be effective.

17. Add 40 µL 1 M Hepes buffer (10 mM final concentration), 4 µL polybrene (5 µg/mL final concentration) and cytokines: mrIL-3 (6 ng/mL), rm stem cell factor (10 ng/mL), and IL-6 (10 ng/mL) to each well.

18. Centrifuge the 6-well plates at $1,800 \times g$ for 90 min (first spinoculation process), then incubate at 37 °C for 3 h in a CO_2 incubator.

19. Collect the supernatants, add 1 mL transduction medium, centrifuge at $400 \times g$ for 5 min, and resuspend in half the volume of the collected supernatant.

20. Add 2 mL resuspended cells with transduction medium back into each well for 3 mL total and incubate overnight at 37 °C in a CO_2 incubator.

21. Thaw a new viral supernatant at 37 °C in a thermostatic bath.

22. Add 1 mL viral supernatants with 40 µL 1 M Hepes buffer (10 mM final concentration), 4 µL polybrene (5 µg/mL final concentration) and cytokines mrIL-3 (6 ng/mL), rm stem cell factor (10 ng/mL), and IL-6 (10 ng/mL) in each well

23. Centrifuge the 6-well plates at $1,800 \times g$ for 90 min (second spinoculation process).

24. Transfer the plates to a CO_2 incubator and incubate at 37 °C for 3 h.

25. Collect the spinoculated cells with supernatants in a tube and store on ice.

26. Wash the plates with PBS and collect the supernatant; add cell dissociation buffer, repeat pipetting, and check the plate under a microscope to ensure removal of all remaining cells.

27. Centrifuge the collected cells with media and buffers at $400 \times g$ for 5 min and resuspend in PBS (0.2 mL/recipient mouse).

28. Count the cells and adjust to approximately 1×10^6 cells/0.2 mL/mouse.

29. Keep them on ice until transplantation.

30. Place aliquots of transduced cells ($\geq 0.1 \times 10^6$ cells) in non-tissue culture treated 24-well plates and incubate 2 days before analyzing the transduction efficiency of EGFP-expressing bone marrow cells (*see* **Note 3**).

3.3 Bone Marrow Transplantation

1. Prepare wild-type recipient mice.

2. Irradiate the recipient mice at 4.5 Gy with a ^{137}Cs irradiator in the morning on the day of the second spinoculation. Repeat after 3 h.

3. Inject the retrovirus-transduced low-density bone marrow cells into the tail vein with a sterile 29 G 1 mL insulin syringes.

3.4 Confirmation of Disease Development

Recipients typically develop disease 3–4 weeks after transplantation. The mice should be used 4 weeks after transplantation, as most will die by 5 weeks (*see* **Note 4**).

3.5 Cell Counts

1. Draw peripheral blood by retro-orbital bleeding from recipient mice using hematocrit tubes in EDTA Microtainer tubes.

2. Count total leukocytes manually after tenfold dilution with Turk solution and perform differential counts using smears stained with Diff-Quick.

3. For eosinophil count, dilute whole blood tenfold with Discombe's solution and count cells containing stained granules (*see* **Note 5**).

3.6 Confirmation of EGFP⁺ Cells and Eosinophils by Flow Cytometry

1. No antibodies should be required to detect EGFP⁺ cells. To detect eosinophils, stain peripheral blood with the following monoclonal antibodies: APC-conjugated anti-CD11b and PE-conjugated anti-CCR3 or PE-conjugated anti-Siglec-F.

2. Prepare 100 μL peripheral blood for each tube, add antibodies and 2 μL mouse serum; vortex and maintain in the dark at room temperature for 15 min.

3. To lyse red blood cells (RBC), add 2 mL NH_4Cl RBC lysis buffer and incubate in the dark for 15 min at room temperature.

4. Collect the cells and resuspend in PBS containing 1 μg/mL 7-Aminoactinomycin D (7-AAD).

5. Use a flow cytometer (e.g., FACSCalibur) with more than four colors for analyses (*see* **Note 6**).

3.7 Analysis of Mast Cell Infiltration in Tissues (See Note 7)

1. Prepare single cell suspensions of bone marrow, spleen, and intestine [9, 16, 17].

   (a). Bone marrow: the isolation of bone marrow contents are the same as mentioned above (*see* **steps 3–5** in Subheading 3.2 in method of retroviral transduction into hematopoietic progenitor cells). Then add 3–10 mL NH_4Cl red blood cells (RBC) lysis buffer, incubate in the dark for 10 min at room temperature, collect the cells and resuspend in PBS.

   (b). Spleen: grind individual spleen between ground-glass-portion of glass slides and pass the ground material through 40 μm cell strainers fitted in 50-mL BD Falcon Tubes. The cells including red blood cells are isolated in the Falcon tube. To lyse RBC, resuspend 3–10 mL of NH_4Cl RBC lysis buffer and incubate in the dark for 10 min at room temperature, collect them and resuspend in PBS.

   (c). Intestine: obtain intestinal cell suspensions from the ileum. After thoroughly washing in PBS, mince the tissue, treat with liberase CL (0.12 mg/mL) and DNAse (0.25 mg/mL) and then squeezed through 40 μm cell strainers in a sterile dish or 6 wells plate. Resuspend in RPMI-1640 with 10 % fetal bovine serum (FBS). Then, spin the cells down and resuspend them in PBS.

2. To detect mast cells, stain single cell suspensions with the following monoclonal antibodies: APC-conjugated anti-c-kit and PE-conjugated anti-FcεRI, in addition, for intestinal cells, PE-Cy7-anti-CD45 to exclude epithelial cells.

3. Prepare 100 μL resuspended cells for each tube, add antibodies and 2 μL mouse serum; vortex and maintain in the dark at room temperature for 15 min.

4. Collect the cells and resuspend in PBS containing 1 μg/mL 7-Aminoactinomycin D (7-AAD).

5. Use a flow cytometer (e.g., FACS Canto) with more than five colors for analyses.

4 Notes

1. Mice transgenic for IL-5 (on a CBA background) were originally obtained from (Sanderson C, Institute for Child Health Research, Perth, Australia), backcrossed into the BALB/c background and analyzed after ten backcrosses before breeding (Rothenberg ME, Cincinnati Children's Hospital).

2. The retroviral plasmids were kindly provided by Drs Gary Gilliland and Jan Cools, Harvard Medical School, Boston, MA at that time.

3. After 2 days culture, collect the cells and supernatant by repeated pipetting, centrifuge, and resuspend in PBS containing 1 μg/mL 7-AAD. Use a flow cytometer for analysis. The transduction efficiency should be average 10 %.

4. Confirmation of tissue eosinophil infiltration is also useful to determine disease development; however, to avoid sacrificing the animals, it is sufficient to assess peripheral blood for leukocytosis with eosinophilia. Upon opening the abdominal cavity, marked splenomegaly should be detectable in CEL mice. For tissue histology, eosinophils should be detectable even in hematoxylin–eosin staining. To identify eosinophils more clearly, immunohistochemistry using anti major basic protein are recommended.

5. F/P-CEL (chronic eosinophilic leukemia) mice usually exhibit leukocytosis with eosinophilia (approximately 150×10^9 leukocytes/L containing 35×10^9 eosinophils).

6. EGFP⁺ cells should be detected using the excitation wavelength at 488 nm. Eosinophils should be appear as $CCR3^+/CD11b^{+/low}$ and $Siglec\text{-}F^+/CD11b^{+/low}$ populations.

7. This F/P-CEL is also characterized by systemic mastocytosis. Therefore, increased number of mast cells in bone marrow, spleen, and intestine has been observed in this model after successful development of disease.

Acknowledgments

A Part of this project was supported by Research on Intractable Diseases, Health and Labour Sciences research grants from the Ministry of Health, Labour and Welfare of Japan and by a Grant-in-Aid for Scientific Research C from the Ministry of Education, Culture, Sports, Science and Technology of Japan.

References

1. Bain B, Pierre R, Imbert M, Vardiman JW, Brunning RD, Flandrin G (2001) Chronic eosinophilic leukaemia and the hypereosinophilic syndrome. IARC Press, Lyon, France

2. Cools J, DeAngelo DJ, Gotlib J, Stover EH, Legare RD, Cortes J, Kutok J, Clark J, Galinsky I, Griffin JD, Cross NC, Tefferi A, Malone J, Alam R, Schrier SL, Schmid J, Rose M, Vandenberghe P, Verhoef G, Boogaerts M, Wlodarska I, Kantarjian H, Marynen P, Coutre SE, Stone R, Gilliland DG (2003) A tyrosine kinase created by fusion of the PDGFRA and FIP1L1 genes as a therapeutic target of imatinib in idiopathic hypereosinophilic syndrome. N Engl J Med 348:1201–1214

3. Griffin JH, Leung J, Bruner RJ, Caligiuri MA, Briesewitz R (2003) Discovery of a fusion kinase in EOL-1 cells and idiopathic hypereosinophilic syndrome. Proc Natl Acad Sci U S A 100:7830–7835. doi:10.1073/pnas.0932698100, 0932698100 [pii]

4. Gotlib J (2012) World Health Organization-defined eosinophilic disorders: 2012 update on diagnosis, risk stratification, and management. Am J Hematol 87:903–914. doi:10.1002/ajh.23293

5. Cools J, Stover EH, Boulton CL, Gotlib J, Legare RD, Amaral SM, Curley DP, Duclos N, Rowan R, Kutok JL, Lee BH, Williams IR, Coutre SE, Stone RM, DeAngelo DJ, Marynen P, Manley PW, Meyer T, Fabbro D, Neuberg D, Weisberg E, Griffin JD, Gilliland DG (2003) PKC412 overcomes resistance to imatinib in a murine model of FIP1L1-PDGFRalpha-induced myeloproliferative disease. Cancer Cell 3:459–469

6. Roche-Lestienne C, Lepers S, Soenen-Cornu V, Kahn JE, Lai JL, Hachulla E, Drupt F, Demarty AL, Roumier AS, Gardembas M, Dib M, Philippe N, Cambier N, Barete S, Libersa C, Bletry O, Hatron PY, Quesnel B, Rose C, Maloum K, Blanchet O, Fenaux P, Prin L, Preudhomme C (2005) Molecular characterization of the idiopathic hypereosinophilic syndrome (HES) in 35 French patients with normal conventional cytogenetics. Leukemia 19:792–798

7. Klion AD, Law MA, Noel P, Kim YJ, Haverty TP, Nutman TB (2004) Safety and efficacy of the monoclonal anti-interleukin-5 antibody SCH55700 in the treatment of patients with hypereosinophilic syndrome. Blood 103:2939–2941

8. Yamada Y, Rothenberg ME, Lee AW, Akei HS, Brandt EB, Williams DA, Cancelas JA (2006) The FIP1L1-PDGFRA fusion gene cooperates with IL-5 to induce murine hypereosinophilic syndrome (HES)/chronic eosinophilic leukemia (CEL)-like disease. Blood 107:4071–4079

9. Yamada Y, Sanchez-Aguilera A, Brandt EB, McBride M, Al-Moamen NJ, Finkelman FD, Williams DA, Cancelas JA, Rothenberg ME (2008) FIP1L1/PDGFRalpha synergizes with SCF to induce systemic mastocytosis in a murine model of chronic eosinophilic leukemia/hypereosinophilic syndrome. Blood 112:2500–2507

10. Fukushima K, Matsumura I, Ezoe S, Tokunaga M, Yasumi M, Satoh Y, Shibayama H, Tanaka H, Iwama A, Kanakura Y (2009) FIP1L1-PDGFRalpha imposes eosinophil lineage commitment on hematopoietic stem/progenitor cells. J Biol Chem 284:7719–7732. doi:10.1074/jbc.M807489200, M807489200 [pii]

11. Li B, Zhang G, Li C, He D, Li X, Zhang C, Tang F, Deng X, Lu J, Tang Y, Li R, Chen Z, Duan C (2012) Identification of JAK2 as a mediator of FIP1L1-PDGFRA-induced eosinophil growth and function in CEL. PLoS ONE 7: e34912. doi 10.1371/journal.pone.0034912. PONE-D-11-17321 [pii]

12. Mishra A, Hogan SP, Brandt EB, Rothenberg ME (2002) IL-5 promotes eosinophil trafficking to the esophagus. J Immunol 168:2464–2469

13. Williams DA, Tao W, Yang F, Kim C, Gu Y, Mansfield P, Levine JE, Petryniak B, Derrow CW, Harris C, Jia B, Zheng Y, Ambruso DR, Lowe JB, Atkinson SJ, Dinauer MC, Boxer L (2000) Dominant negative mutation of the hematopoietic-specific Rho GTPase, Rac2, is associated with a human phagocyte immunodeficiency. Blood 96:1646–1654

14. Discombe G (1946) Criteria of eosinophilia. Lancet 1:195

15. Yang S, Delgado R, King SR, Woffendin C, Barker CS, Yang ZY, Xu L, Nolan GP, Nabel GJ (1999) Generation of retroviral vector for clinical studies using transient transfection. Hum Gene Ther 10:123–132. doi:10.1089/10430349950019255

16. Cancelas JA, Lee AW, Prabhakar R, Stringer KF, Zheng Y, Williams DA (2005) Rac GTPases differentially integrate signals regulating hematopoietic stem cell localization. Nat Med 11:886–891, doi: nm1274 [pii]. 10.1038/nm1274

17. Minns LA, Menard LC, Foureau DM, Darche S, Ronet C, Mielcarz DW, Buzoni-Gatel D, Kasper LH (2006) TLR9 is required for the gut-associated lymphoid tissue response following oral infection of Toxoplasma gondii. J Immunol 176:7589–7597, doi: 176/12/7589 [pii]

A

B

C

D

Garry M. Walsh (ed.), *Eosinophils: Methods and Protocols*, Methods in Molecular Biology, vol. 1178,
DOI 10.1007/978-1-4939-1016-8, © Springer Science+Business Media New York 2014

GPSR Compliance
The European Union's (EU) General Product Safety Regulation (GPSR) is a set
of rules that requires consumer products to be safe and our obligations to
ensure this.

If you have any concerns about our products, you can contact us on

ProductSafety@springernature.com

In case Publisher is established outside the EU, the EU authorized
representative is:

Springer Nature Customer Service Center GmbH
Europaplatz 3
69115 Heidelberg, Germany